Wound Management and Dressings

Wound Management
and Dressings

Stephen Thomas

Director, Surgical Materials Testing Laboratory
Mid Glamorgan Health Authority

London
THE PHARMACEUTICAL PRESS
1990

The opinions expressed are those of the author. While every effort has been made to ensure the accuracy of the information given, no responsibility can be accepted for inaccuracies, omissions, or errors. For more detailed information the manufacturers' literature should be consulted. Names followed by the symbol™ are or have been used as proprietary names in the United Kingdom. These names may in general be applied only to products supplied by the owners of those marks.

Copies of this book may be obtained through any good bookseller or, in any case of difficulty, direct from the publisher or the publisher's agent:

The Pharmaceutical Press
(publications division of the Royal Pharmaceutical Society of Great Britain)
1 Lambeth High Street, London SE1 7JN, England

Australia
The Australian Pharmaceutical Publishing Co. Ltd.,
40 Burwood Road, Hawthorn, Victoria 3122;

and

Pharmaceutical Society of Australia
Pharmacy House, PO Box 21, Curtin, ACT 2605

Japan
Maruzen Co. Ltd.
3-10 Nihonbashi 2-chome, Chuo-ku, Tokyo 103

New Zealand
The Pharmaceutical Society of New Zealand
124 Dixon Street, PO Box 11-640, Wellington

U.S.A.
Rittenhouse Book Distributors Inc.
511 Feheley Drive, King of Prussia, Pennsylvania 19406

Dedication

This book is dedicated with love to Cathy and Richard whose time it took me to write it, and Beth 'the wind beneath my wings'.

Contents

Preface

This book traces the development of modern wound management materials, describes their composition and physical characteristics, and reviews the published clinical data describing their use. Its primary aims are to introduce the reader to the importance of the role that dressings play in the management of different types of wounds; and provide pharmaceutical, nursing, and medical staff with a unique source of reference for those products which are available in the United Kingdom. The role of wound cleansing agents is also reviewed and some guidance is provided on the selection and use of dressings which may be of value to those health care professionals who wish to develop local wound management policies.

In the early 1970s there began a major revolution in the management of wounds of all types. Until that time, dressings were mainly limited to simple woven fabrics, used alone or in combination with fibrous absorbents such as cotton and viscose. The primary function of these materials was to absorb exudate and keep the wound as dry as possible – a condition that was widely regarded as essential for rapid and trouble-free healing. Following the work of Winter, however, it was recognised that wounds that were kept moist healed faster and more successfully than those which were managed using conventional products. This observation led to the production of the semipermeable films which, in turn, were followed by whole new families of dressings, many of which bore no resemblance to

the products that had been used previously. Detailed descriptions of these new dressings are included in the chapters on simple wound contact materials (including paraffin gauze products), films, foams, alginates, polysaccharide beads, hydrogels, and hydrocolloids.

The stages of wound healing and the way in which the healing process is influenced by the properties of the various dressings are described and discussed. Later chapters describe the importance of bandages and bandaging and the development and use of orthopaedic casting materials. The last chapter contains product information sheets for many of the dressings in current use, describing their construction, method of use, indications, and contra-indications.

The final part of the book contains a classification of dressings in which products are grouped together according to their general indications for use together with a series of detailed indexes to proprietary names, generic names, and manufacturers. A list of the names and addresses of all suppliers is also included, making this section of considerable value to any individual who is involved with the purchasing of dressings.

Wound management and dressings are topics of increasing interest, and many developments are expected in the new few years. The author would welcome any information on these subjects together with any other comments or constructive criticisms.

Dr S Thomas
Director, Surgical Materials Testing Laboratory
Bridgend General Hospital
Quarella Road, Bridgend
Mid Glamorgan CF31 1JP

May 1990

Acknowledgements

The author would like to acknowledge the help and co-operation given by many of the companies involved in the surgical dressings industry during the preparation of this book. Particular thanks are due to Steriseal Ltd and ConvaTec Ltd for providing financial assistance towards the reproduction costs of the colour plates, Courtaulds Ltd for producing the SEMs of the wound contact layers shown in chapter 2, and Johnson and Johnson Ltd for the SEM of bacteria bound onto activated charcoal cloth in chapter 10. It is a pleasure to acknowledge *The Source Book of Medical Illustration*, P.Cull (ed.), London, Parthenon Publishing, 1989, for the use of Figure 1-1.

In addition, I would wish to give special thanks to the following individuals.

Dr Mick Boroff, Johnson and Johnson Orthopaedics Ltd, for providing much of the background material on the development of the synthetic casting materials, Mr Keith Morley (Smith and Nephew Medical Ltd) for advice and technical information on the plaster of Paris bandages and Mr Stuart Jackson for information on the manufacture and properties of activated charcoal cloth.

My thanks also to Mr Eddie Watkins for the help and encouragement he gave me when I first started to take an interest in dressings and wound management; without him this book would probably never even have been started. To my wife, Beth, who helped me turn a collection of disjointed thoughts and facts into a manuscript and without whose tolerance it would definitely never have been finished!

I would also like to thank Mrs Eileen Harries for her invaluable assistance in correcting the proofs, and Mid Glamorgan Health Authority for permission to include the Surgical Dressings Information Cards in chapter 15 and for the use of the computer facilities of the SMTL in the latter stages of the preparation of this book.

Chapter 1

Wounds and Wound Healing

CLASSIFICATION OF WOUNDS

A wound may be defined as a defect or break in the skin that results from physical, mechanical or thermal damage, or that develops as a result of the presence of an underlying medical or physiological disorder. Examples of the more common classes of wound are given below.

Mechanical injuries

Mechanical injuries include the following types of wound.

- Abrasions (grazes) are superficial wounds, generally caused by friction as a result of glancing or tangential contact between the skin and a second harder or rougher surface. By definition, abrasions are usually confined to the outer layers of the skin.

- Lacerations (tears) are more severe than abrasions and involve both the skin and the underlying tissues.

- Penetrating wounds may be caused by knives, bullets or other missiles, or may result from accidental injuries caused by any sharp or pointed object. Although the external appearance of a penetrating wound may suggest that the injury is relatively minor, internal damage can be considerable (depending upon the site and depth of penetration, and/or the velocity of the bullet or missile).[1]

- Bites caused by animals or humans may become infected by a range of pathogenic organisms including spirochetes, staphylococci, streptococci and various Gram-positive bacilli. If untreated these infections may have very serious sequelae, involving fascia, tendon and bone.[2]

- Surgical wounds represent a specific type of mechanical injury, and are discussed in greater detail below.

Burns and chemical injuries

There are several different types of burn: thermal, chemical, electrical, and those caused by radiation – thermal injuries being the most common. The severity of a thermal injury is governed by the temperature of the heat source, the thermal inertia (a function of the thermal conductivity, density and specific heat of the object), and the time of contact or exposure.[3] For example, a temperature of 70°C will cause epidermal necrosis in one second but a temperature of 45°C will require an exposure time in excess of six hours to induce tissue damage.[4] Burns and scalds (thermal injuries caused by moist heat) may be classified into three types depending upon the degree of tissue damage (Fig. 1-1). They are most commonly described as follows.

- Superficial (first degree) burns involve only the epidermis and superficial layers of the dermis and usually result from exposure to prolonged low intensity heat.

- Deep dermal (second degree) burns, in which most of the surface epithelium is destroyed, together with much of the dermal layer beneath. Only some isolated epidermal elements in the deeper layers remain viable, such as those within hair follicles and sweat glands.

- Full thickness (third degree) burns, in which all the elements of the skin are destroyed.

A significant burn may have three identifiable zones: the innermost part of the injury, which has suffered irreversible damage, is called the zone of coagulation; the outermost zone, which has undergone minor reversible damage, is called the zone of uraemia; and between these two lies the area known as the zone of stasis. The eventual fate of the cells in the latter region will be largely determined by the nature of the treatment given.

Chronic ulcerative wounds

Ulcers can be divided into different types depending upon their underlying cause.

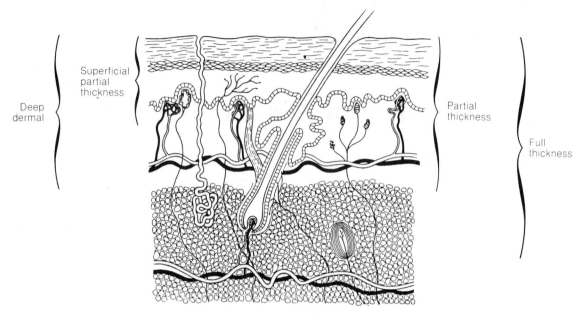

Figure 1-1   Diagrammatic representation of the skin showing the classification of burns.

- Decubitus ulcers (frequently called bedsores, pressure areas, or pressure sores) are usually caused by the sustained application of surface pressure over a bony prominence which inhibits capillary blood flow to the skin and underlying tissue.[5] If the pressure is not relieved it will ultimately result in cell death followed by tissue necrosis and breakdown.

- Leg ulcers, which may be venous, ischaemic or traumatic in origin.

- Ulcers associated with certain systemic infections.

- Ulcers resulting from radiotherapy.

- Ulcers resulting from malignant disease.

MECHANISMS OF WOUND HEALING

Irrespective of the nature or type of wound, the same basic biochemical and cellular processes are required to bring about healing. These are extremely complex, and are only described in sufficient detail to explain how they may be influenced by the application of surgical dressings or the use of different wound management techniques. For additional information, readers are advised to consult more specialised texts.

The following four types of wound healing are generally recognised:

- primary closure, healing by first intention;

- open granulation, healing by secondary intention;

- delayed or secondary closure, sometimes called healing by third intention;

- grafting or flap formation.

Primary closure

Most clean surgical wounds and recent traumatic injuries are managed by primary closure. In this technique the surgeon approximates the edges of the wound and individually sutures the different layers of tissue together. The resulting wound contains minimal quantities of granulation tissue; once it has healed, only a thin scar remains, which may be virtually undetectable when fully mature. Primary closure is generally not appropriate in the treatment of long-standing injuries, or wounds that are infected or contaminated with earth or other foreign material. The following brief outline of the healing process refers to sutured wounds and minor injuries, such as cuts, which are allowed to heal naturally.

Healing begins with the acute inflammatory phase, which commences within a few minutes of the injury and lasts for about three days. As platelets – liberated from damaged blood vessels – flow into the wound, they come into contact with mature collagen, become activated, and aggregate together. During this process, granules within the cells liberate lysosomal enzymes, adenosine triphosphate (ATP), serotonin, growth factors, and other agents that potentiate further platelet aggregation. At the same time, thromboplastin is liberated from injured cells in the vicinity of the wound, activating the clotting mechanism; this results, ultimately, in the cleavage of fibrinogen to form fibrin monomers, which polymerise to produce a fibrin network. Together these two mechanisms produce a plug or clot in the wound, which brings about haemostasis and gives strength and support to the injured tissue. In time this clot dries out to form the familiar scab.

Vasodilatory agents such as histamine and serotonin, which are liberated as a consequence of the original injury, increase the permeability of the local capillary bed, allowing serum and white cells to be released into the area surrounding the wound. The resulting accumulation of fluid in the tissue produces the characteristic swelling and sensations of throbbing and warmth that are experienced by the patient.

Within hours, polymorphonucleocytes (neutrophils) begin to appear in the wound, followed later by macrophages. Both neutrophils and macrophages play an important role in the removal of debris and the ingestion of bacteria. This is the beginning of the 'destructive' phase of healing, in which unwanted fibrin and dead cells are broken down by enzymatic activity. Neutrophils are primarily concerned with bacterial ingestion, and aid macrophages in wound debridement by the release of proteolytic, fibrinolytic and collagenolytic enzymes. In a series of studies in guinea pigs, Simpson and Ross[6] induced a selective neutropenia by administration of an antineutrophilic serum. They showed that, provided the animals were not exposed to significant numbers of pathogenic organisms, wound healing progressed normally, suggesting that neutrophils do not play an essential role in tissue repair. If, however, large numbers of organisms were introduced into the wounds, the animals died of septicaemia and bacteraemia.

The role of the macrophage is more complex. Like the neutrophil, it produces proteinases and other enzymes that break down clots and debris, forming fluid-filled cavities into which fibroblasts and endothelial buds can move. In addition, it produces factors that stimulate the formation of new vascular tissue,[7] and is also believed to play an important part in the initiation and control of fibroblasts – which are, in turn, responsible for the synthesis of collagen. Although the macrophage can function under both aerobic and anaerobic conditions over a range of pH and pO_2,[8] the cell is much less effective in destroying bacteria under hypoxic conditions (see chapter 2).

After about 24 hours, the epithelial cells on the surface of the wound begin to turn down over the edge of the underlying dermis and grow across the defect under the dried scab. Depending upon the size and nature of the wound, this process may be complete within about 2–3 days. At about this time, some evidence of organisation may be detected within the body of the wound itself as fibroblasts begin to lay down strands of collagen, a major constituent of skin, and one which helps to give it strength and form. The production of collagen peaks around the 5th–7th day, although this 'proliferative' phase of healing generally lasts about three weeks in total. It is followed by the final 'maturation' or 'remodelling' phase, which can take up to a year to complete. During this phase, the nature of the final scar is determined and the cellular granulation tissue is changed to a relatively acellular mass. Many of the fibroblasts and capillaries formed during the early stages of healing disappear, and the collagen fibres within the wound are reorganised and replaced. Collagen levels in a wound peak some 2–3 weeks after injury but the tensile strength of the scar tissue continues to increase for up to twelve months or more. This increase in strength corresponds to changes that occur in the structure of the collagen molecule: the material that is formed in the early stages of healing is replaced by a second more stable form as the scar matures. When first laid down, the collagen fibrils are distributed randomly within the wound area but as healing progresses they become orientated in the direction of maximum stress, resulting in an increase in overall wound strength. The closer alignment of the fibres also permits the formation of cross-links which lend further stability to the new tissue.

Open granulation

In wounds that have sustained a significant degree of tissue loss as a result of surgery or trauma, it may sometimes be undesirable or impossible to bring the edges of the wound together. In these situations the surgeon may favour leaving the wound open to heal by secondary intention. A similar decision may be taken if there is considered to be a serious risk of infection, or if there is a likelihood of subsequent wound dehiscence. It has also been found that healing by secondary intention can sometimes give better results than primary closure[9] or split-skin grafting (where the cosmetic results of the latter method can be marred by contraction, wrinkling and pigmentation).[10,11]

Although the basic mechanisms of healing of granulating wounds are similar to those that occur in wounds that heal by primary closure, there are significant differences, particularly in the relative duration of the various stages of the healing process. Like a sutured wound, a defect that is left to heal by secondary intention first undergoes an inflammatory response. During this time the exposed tissue or defect may become covered or filled with a layer of blood or serous fluid, which is released during or soon after the initial injury.

As a result of increased capillary and venous permeability, erythrocytes, leucocytes and platelets are liberated into the wound. Neutrophils predominate during the first 2−3 days but as these decrease in number they are followed by macrophages, which reach their maximum level on day 5−6. As in a sutured wound, macrophages are responsible for the bulk of phagocytic activity but they also produce a host of complex proteins and extracellular products (including a chemotactic factor, which is thought to attract fibroblasts to the wound area). Fibroblasts appear in the base of the developing wound as early as day 4 or 5 and are responsible for the production of intracellular precursors of collagen, which are eventually made into collagen fibrils extracellularly. This process of collagen production is thought to be at least partially under macrophage control.

Around the 2nd−3rd day, endothelial cells appear in the developing inflammatory tissue as capillary buds. Knighton et al.[12] have suggested that the low oxygen tension in the centre of the wound in some way attracts macrophages, the only cells that are able to withstand the severe hypoxia in this situation. The macrophages clear away portions of the fibrous clot and liberate growth factors which stimulate the production of a capillary network. These capillaries retain their permeable nature and thus provide a constant source of cells and fluid for the developing tissue. When the process of repair is complete the demand for oxygen is substantially reduced and much of this new vasculature is lost.

During healing, the wound becomes progressively filled with granulation tissue, which is composed of collagen and proteoglycans (a complex mixture of proteins and polysaccharides together with salts and other colloidal materials; it produces a gel-like matrix which is contained within the fibrous collagen network). The production of granulation tissue continues until the base of the original cavity is almost level with the surrounding skin. At this stage, the epithelium around the wound margin becomes active and begins to grow over the surface of the wound, thus restoring the integrity of the epidermis. Occasionally the production of granulation tissue continues after the wound cavity has been filled, leading to the formation of 'hypergranulation tissue' or 'proud flesh'. This is sometimes associated with the use of occlusive dressings, and can be removed by the application of a caustic agent such as a silver nitrate pencil. A less traumatic method is the short-term local application of a suitable corticosteroid cream or ointment, although this should only be done under medical supervision. Alternatively, a change to a more permeable dressing may be all that is required.

A further, and equally important, part of the healing process is contraction, a mechanism by which the margins of the wound are drawn towards the centre. This produces a small area of scar tissue, which may be only one-tenth of the size of the original wound. Contraction may take place in all healing wounds, but it is particularly important in large wounds that are left to heal by granulation and epithelialisation. Although in many anatomical sites the process of contraction results in a wound with an acceptable cosmetic appearance, contraction of a wound on the face may result in distortion of the features due to the 'purse string' effect. Contraction takes place at a rate of approximately 0.6−0.7 mm/day and is not related to wound size, although it is known that rectangular wounds contract more rapidly than round ones. It has been shown that the contractile forces can be sufficiently powerful to cause severe loss of function,[13] and in wounds on the dorsum of the hand they have even been known to cause dislocation of the knuckles.[14]

Wound contraction generally begins about the

end of the first week and may continue until the wound is completely closed. It is brought about by the action of a specialist cell called a myofibroblast which is formed from a normal fibroblast as a result of major structural and functional changes. Myofibroblasts show many of the properties of both fibroblasts and smooth muscle cells and will respond to agents that cause contraction or relaxation of smooth muscle tissue. The cells are joined together over the entire wound surface; when they contract they gradually pull in the edges of the wound. Some early evidence suggests that there may be a connection between the initiation of myofibroblast activity and the state of hydration (or dehydration) of the surface of the wound.[15] The process of contraction takes place most quickly if a wound is clean and free of infection and is slowed down or prevented altogether by the presence of eschar or adherent dressings.[16]

The healing of traumatic injuries in which large areas of skin are lost, depends upon the extent of the damage. Superficial and shallow partial thickness burns, for example, will heal as the surviving epidermal cells begin to grow and spread across the surface of the wound. In deep dermal burns, these epidermal cells may develop from small numbers of surviving cells present in the lower parts of hair follicles and sweat glands. These will grow up onto the surface of the wound and appear as isolated islands which gradually increase in size and merge. If a burn has been severe, the survival of these isolated areas of epidermis may be prejudiced by dehydration or an inappropriate method of treatment (see chapter 2). In full thickness burns all epidermal elements are lost; without the application of a skin graft, resurfacing of the wound can only take place by migration of epithelial cells from the wound margins, and healing is therefore very slow.

Delayed primary closure

Less commonly used than the other methods of healing, delayed primary closure is generally carried out when, in the opinion of the surgeon, primary closure may be unsuccessful (due to the presence of infection, a poor blood supply to the area, or the need for the application of excessive tension during closure). In these circumstances, the wound is left open for about three to four days before closure is effected. In these situations, sutures may be inserted at the time of the operation but left loose.

Grafting and flap formation

A skin graft is a portion of skin (composed of dermis and epidermis) that is removed from one anatomical site and placed onto a wound elsewhere on the body. If successful, grafting ensures that the wound will heal rapidly, thus reducing the chances of infection and the time spent in hospital. The major disadvantage of this technique is that the patient finishes up with two wounds instead of one, and it is often reported that the pain associated with the donor site is worse than that occasioned by the original injury. Most commonly used are partial thickness or split thickness grafts which are usually 300–375 µm thick. These are removed from a suitable donor site, such as the thigh or buttock, using a special knife which can be preset to ensure that the harvested material is of the required thickness. As elements of epidermal tissue remain in the base of sebaceous glands and hair follicles, the donor site heals rapidly, usually within 10–14 days.

For more specialist applications, such as facial reconstruction, full thickness grafts can be taken – these may contain fat, hair and sebaceous glands. They have the advantages that they are cosmetically more acceptable and less likely to form severe contractures than split thickness grafts. Full thickness grafts are also used when a neurovascular bundle or cortical bone must be covered with tissue. They have the disadvantage that, in many cases, the donor site will itself require the application of a second, partial thickness graft, if the wound is too large to be closed by suture.

The success of a graft depends upon a number of factors, the most important of which is the presence of a good vascular bed to supply the metabolic needs of the transplanted tissue. Stress on the graft itself, infection, and the formation of seromas and haematomas are major causes of graft failure.

Skin flaps differ from grafts in that the relocated tissue is frequently not completely separated from the body. In this technique a portion of skin and subcutaneous tissue is raised on three sides and rotated or transposed to cover an adjacent area of skin loss. In this way the entire flap continues to receive a supply of blood from its original vasculature until it becomes established elsewhere. The maximum size of the flap depends upon the anatomical site from which it is raised, and the nature and distribution of the major blood vessels. In a variation of this technique, a flap of tissue is relocated complete with its attached blood supply: this is known as a free flap transfer. A more detailed summary of the techniques of grafting and flap formation is given elsewhere.[17]

PROBLEMS OF WOUND HEALING

Although the majority of wounds heal uneventfully, problems do occur sometimes. In most instances these are associated with delayed healing, frequently caused by infection resulting from the presence of foreign bodies, sinuses, etc.

A simple method for determining the volume of a wound using an alginate dental impression material has been described;[18] this enables users to assess and compare different forms of treatment, and monitor the healing process. Using this technique, the wound is filled with the impression material, which is allowed to set. The resulting plug is removed, and weighed, and the volume of the wound calculated by dividing the recorded weight by the density of the alginate. This procedure was found to be particularly useful for pressure sores and other irregular lesions which were difficult to measure by alternative means.

The healing rates of hundreds of healthy surgical wounds have been calculated by Marks et al.,[19,20] from which they have derived simple equations which may be used to predict the likely time for a wound of a given size to heal. For example, in abdominal wounds, the predicted time to heal (in days) is given by:

$$(WD \times 1.23) + 3.6$$

where WD is the wound width or depth (in mm), whichever is the greater. Similar equations are available for pilonidal wounds and wounds produced after surgery for hidradenitis suppurativa. Using these equations as a base line it is possible to monitor the progess of a wound and ensure that the rate of healing does not vary significantly from the norm; for example, due to the presence of a subclinical infection.

The isolation of micro-organisms from a wound is not of itself an indication of the presence of an infection, as wounds of all types can rapidly acquire bacteria from any one of a number of sources. Such contamination may result from contact with infected or contaminated objects, the ingress of dirt or dust (either at the time of injury

or later), or from the patient's own skin or gastro-intestinal tract. For example, it has been found that, unless effective measures are taken to prevent contamination, virtually all burns become colonised by bacteria within 12 to 24 hours.[21] The consequences of bacterial contamination of a wound will depend upon a number of factors: these include the number of organisms, their pathogenicity (potential to cause disease), and the ability of the patient's own defence system to combat any possible infection. The latter, in turn, may depend upon the patient's age, general health and nutritional status, and other factors such as the administration of immunosuppressive drugs, which may inhibit the production of leucocytes.

Many wounds will yield a variety of organisms upon microbiological investigation but may never show the classical symptoms of infection − redness and swelling with heat and pain − which were described by Celsus nearly two thousand years ago. Indeed the presence of a whole host of different organisms is virtually inevitable in dirty or sloughy wounds such as leg ulcers or sacral pressure areas (particularly in patients who are doubly incontinent). However a similar pattern of infection in a major burn could, if untreated, rapidly develop into a life-threatening septicaemia. Signs that a previously healthy wound may be developing an unacceptably high bioburden include a change in colour or odour, or an increase in exudate production. If adequate measures are not taken to control the infection, it may lead eventually to the formation of cellulitis and ultimately bacteraemia and septicaemia.

Lawrence, in a series of publications on the effects of bacteria on burns[22] and wound healing,[23,24] described the techniques available for detecting and quantifying the number of bacteria present in a wound, and outlined changes in the types of organism that have been isolated from infected wounds over a thirty-year period. The most common pathogen to be isolated from wounds of all types is *Staphylococcus aureus*. This organism, which is found in the nose of 20−30% of normal persons, may be isolated from approximately one-third of all infected wounds. Other organisms that can cause serious wound infections include *Pseudomonas aeruginosa*, *Streptococcus pyogenes*, and some *Proteus*, *Clostridium* and coliform species. Gilliland *et al.* showed that the presence preoperatively of *Pseudomonas* spp. and *Staph. aureus* significantly reduced skin graft healing; they also demonstrated that, of 16 ulcers which were slow to heal or which recurred after discharge, 15 (94%) contained *Staph. aureus.*[25]

The types of organism present in a given wound may not remain constant but vary as the condition of the wound itself changes.[21] Burns covered with a wet slough frequently contain an abundance of Gram-negative bacilli – including *Ps. aeruginosa, Proteus mirabilis, Klebsiella* spp., and *Escherichia coli* – together with *Streptococcus faecalis, Staph. aureus* and *Strep. pyogenes.* As the slough separates, however, the number of Gram-negative organisms decreases and the Gram-positive bacteria predominate. Of all these organisms, Lowbury and Cason[21] have identified *Strep. pyogenes* and *Ps. aeruginosa* as being amongst the most serious pathogens in a burn. *Strep. pyogenes* will cause the total failure of a skin graft if present at the time of operation and *Ps. aeruginosa* has been found to be an important cause of systemic infections in patients with severe burns, although other organisms may also cause serious problems from time to time.

The number of organisms that might be considered to constitute an infection in a wound was discussed by Lawrence,[24] who considered that the level of 10^5/gram suggested by Pruitt[26] formed a useful guide – provided it was recognised that the bacteriological picture of a wound could change from day to day.

The management of an infected wound usually consists of a combined systemic and local approach, including the use of antibiotics where appropriate and the application of a suitable dressing (which may itself possess inherent antibacterial activity). The use of topical antibiotics is not generally encouraged, as it may cause sensitivity reactions or lead to the emergence of antibiotic-resistant strains of bacteria. More detailed accounts of the causes, diagnosis and treatment of infected wounds may be found elsewhere.[27,28]

Another long-term problem associated with wound healing is the formation of hypertrophic or keloid scars (Plate 1). These unsightly areas result from excess collagen production but the reason for their formation is not fully understood; they are most likely to occur in negroes and in young people around puberty. Hypertrophic scars are limited to the site of the original injury but keloid scars may continue to grow and spread into the surrounding tissue for a number of years.

In the past the treatment of hypertrophic and other raised scar tissue consisted of the long-term application of pressure by means of specially made garments. In 1981, it was discovered that the effects of pressure therapy could be enhanced by the application of a sheet of silicone gel (Spenco). It was reported that the gel appeared to relax or soften the scar tissue, allowing the pressure garments and inserts to hasten their levelling effect on the hypertrophied area.[29] It was also suggested that, for some applications, the gel could be used on its own without the application of pressure. In a second study, published by Quinn et al.,[30] the authors reported that a second silicone gel sheet (Silastic™ Q7-9119 – Dow Corning) produced marked improvement in hypertrophic scars when held in place by surgical tape, a crêpe bandage, silicone adhesive, or a pressure garment. The mechanism of action is currently unknown but the authors suggest that it may be linked to the release of a low molecular weight silicone fluid and hydration of the stratum corneum.

A number of other local and systemic factors are well recognised causes of delayed or impaired wound healing. Foreign bodies introduced deep into a wound at the time of injury can, if not removed, cause a chronic inflammatory response and delay healing or lead to the formation of a granuloma or abscess. Long-standing wounds that heal by epithelialisation, such as burns and leg ulcers, may develop Marjolin's ulcer, an uncommon slow-growing squamous cell carcinoma. Other major factors that have an important effect upon the rate of healing include the age and nutritional status of the patient; underlying metabolic disorders such as diabetes or anaemia; the administration of drugs that suppress the inflammatory process; radiotherapy; arterial disease which may be aggravated by smoking; and the presence of slough and necrotic tissue.

In view of the extreme complexity of the healing process it is perhaps not surprising that the rate, and sometimes the quality, of healing can be adversely affected by the inappropriate application of dressings or wound-cleansing solutions. In view of the nature of some of the materials that are applied to wounds, it is probably more surprising that healing ever takes place at all! It is interesting to consider that whilst surgical techniques have evolved and developed over the centuries, wound management and a recognition of the importance of the correct use of surgical dressings have – with few exceptions – made relatively slow progress. It was not until the early 1960s that the benefits of moist wound healing were first recognised. Until that time the general approach to wound management, and the range of materials which were applied to granulating wounds, probably differed little from those used by Florence Nightingale at the time of the Crimean War; more recently, however, many new wound management products have been developed. As a result there is now a greater understanding of the performance characteristics that are required of a surgical dressing: these are discussed in the following chapter.

REFERENCES

1. Owen-Smith M., Wounds caused by the weapons of war, in *Wound Care,* Westaby S. (ed.), London, Heinemann Medical, 1985, 110–120.
2. Feller N. and Lurie A., The early care of wounds caused by human and animal bites, *Fam. Physn,* 1977, **7**, 29–30.
3. Bull J.P. and Lawrence J.C., Thermal conditions to produce skin burns, *Fire Mat.,* 1979, **3**, 100–105.
4. Nature and types of wounds, in *Wound Treatment and Care in General Practice,* Goode A.W. (ed.), London, Update Publications, 1984, 4–6.
5. Barton A. and Barton M., *The Management and Prevention of Pressure Sores,* London, Faber and Faber, 1981.
6. Simpson D.M. and Ross R., The neutrophilic leukocyte in wound repair; a study with antineutrophilic serum, *J. clin. Invest.,* 1972, **51**, 2009–2023.
7. Thakral K.K. *et al.,* Stimulation of wound blood vessel growth by wound macrophages, *J. surg. Res.,* 1979, **26**, 430–436.
8. Silver I.A., The physiology of wound healing, in Ref.28, 11–32.
9. Silverberg B. *et al.,* Hidradenitis suppurativa: patient satisfaction with wound healing by secondary intention, *Plast. reconstr. Surg.,* 1987, **79**, 555–559.
10. Darnett R. and Stranc M., A method of producing improved scars following excisions of small lesions of the back, *Ann. plast. Surg.,* 1979, **3**, 391–394.
11. Morgan W.P. *et al.,* A comparison of skin grafting and healing by granulation following axillary dissection for hidradenitis suppurativa, *Ann. R. Coll. Surg.,* 1983, **65**, 235–236.
2. Knighton D.R. *et al.,* Regulation of wound healing angiogenesis – effect of oxygen gradients and inspired oxygen concentration, *Surgery,* 1981, **90**, 262–270.
13. Upton J. *et al.,* Major intravenous extravasation injuries, *Am. J. Surg.,* 1979, **137**, 497–506.
14. Rudolph R., Contraction and the control of contraction, *Wld J. Surg.,* 1980, **4**, 279–281.
15. Thomas S. *et al.,* A new approach to the treatment of extravation injury in neonates, *Pharm. J.,* 1987, **239**, 584–585.
16. Foresman P.A. *et al.,* Influence of membrane dressings on wound contraction, *J. Burn Care Rehab.,* 1986, **7**, 398–403.
17. Davies D.M., Plastic and reconstructive surgery, *Br. med. J.,* 1985, **290**, 765–768.
18. Resch C.S. *et al.,* Pressure sore volume measurement, a technique to document and record wound healing, *J. Am. geriat. Soc.,* 1988, **36**, 444–446.
19. Marks J. *et al.,* Prediction of healing time as an aid to the management of open granulating wounds, *Wld J. Surg.,* 1983, **7**, 641–645.
20. Marks J. *et al.,* Pilonidal sinus excision – healing by open granulation, *Br. J. Surg.,* 1985, **72**, 637–640.
21. Lowbury E.J.L. and Cason J.S., Aspects of infection control and skin grafting in burned patients, in Ref.1, 171–189.
22. Lawrence J.C., The bacteriology of burns, *J. hosp. Infect.,* 1985, **6**(suppl. B), 3–17.
23. Lawrence J.C., Bacteriology and wound healing, in *Cadexomer Iodine,* Fox J.A. and Fischer H. (eds), Symposium, Munich, 22 January 1983, Stuttgart, Schattauer Verlag, 1983, 19–31.
24. Lawrence J.C., The effect of bacteria and their products on the healing of skin wounds, in *A Biological Approach to the Wound Healing Process,* Rue Y. (ed.), Proceedings of a Symposium, Royal College of Physicians, London, 5 June 1987, Andover, Medifax, 1987, 9–21.
25. Gilliland E.L. *et al.,* Bacterial colonisation of leg ulcers and its effect on the success rate of skin grafting, *Ann. R. Coll. Surg.,* 1988, **70**, 105–108.
26. Pruitt B.A., The diagnosis and treatment of infection in the burned patient, *Burns,* 1984, **11**, 79–81.
27. Westaby S. and White S., Wound infection, in Ref.1, 70–83.
28. *Wound Healing and Wound Infection,* Hunt T.K., (ed.), New York, Appleton-Century-Crofts, 1980.
29. Perkins K. *et al.,* Silicone gel; a new treatment for burn scars and contractures, *Burns,* 1982, **9**, 201–204.
30. Quinn K.J. *et al.,* Non pressure treatment of hypertrophic scars, *ibid.,* 1985, **12**, 102–108.

Chapter 2

Functions of a Wound Dressing

The ideal dressing should provide an environment at the surface of the wound in which healing may take place at the maximum rate consistent with the production of a healed wound with an acceptable cosmetic appearance.

A surgical dressing is generally applied to a wound to stem bleeding, absorb exudate, ease pain, and provide protection for the newly formed tissue. Historically, a variety of substances have been used for this purpose. A number of texts have been published on the development of dressings and wound management products throughout the ages,[1-3] and they describe the use of cobwebs, dung, leaves, animal fat, honey, and other exotic agents. Undoubtedly, many of these materials would have been heavily contaminated with micro-organisms, making them a potential source of infection.

When Lister demonstrated the importance of cleanliness and good aseptic practice in medicine and surgery in the late 19th century, the quality of the materials used in wound management also began to improve. In 1880 Joseph Gamgee developed the now famous composite dressing pad that still bears his name, and which he sometimes used medicated with iodine or phenol. In the early part of this century, gauzes impregnated with paraffin were introduced as non-adherent dressings for the treatment of burns and similar types of wound; medicated versions of these 'tulle gras' dressings were subsequently manufactured, some of which are still in use at the present time.

However, the most significant advance in the development of wound management materials came in the early 1960s, when George Winter published the results of his studies on the effects of occlusive dressings on the healing rates of experimental wounds in the domestic pig. His observations stimulated a great deal of research into new types of dressing and, as a result, whole families of new products have been developed – including films, gels, foams, and various polysaccharide materials – which have completely revolutionised the treatment of wounds of all types. This chapter examines some of the more important aspects of the performance of these materials in relation to the requirements

of the 'ideal dressing' as defined below.

It is currently believed that for healing to take place at the optimum rate, a dressing should ensure that the wound remains:

- moist with exudate but not macerated;
- free of clinical infection and excessive slough;
- free of toxic chemicals, particles or fibres released by the dressing;
- at the optimum temperature for healing to take place;
- undisturbed by frequent or unnecessary dressing changes;
- at an optimum pH value.

The relative importance of some of these requirements is discussed below.

CONTROL OF MOISTURE CONTENT

Up to and including the late 1950s it was generally accepted that, in order to prevent bacterial infection, a wound should be kept as dry as possible. The dressing materials that were used throughout the first half of this century were therefore designed with the express intention of absorbing and removing all traces of exudate. This philosophy was challenged by Winter[4] and Hinman *et al.,*[5] who demonstrated, both in animals and humans, that wounds that were kept moist healed more rapidly than those that were left exposed to the air or covered with traditional dressings. Other workers have confirmed these findings: in a review of the properties of occlusive dressings, Eaglstein[6] concluded that these materials increase the rate of epidermal resurfacing by some 40%.

In the dry conditions that exist under textile-based products, the wound has been shown to dehydrate, producing a scab (or eschar) which

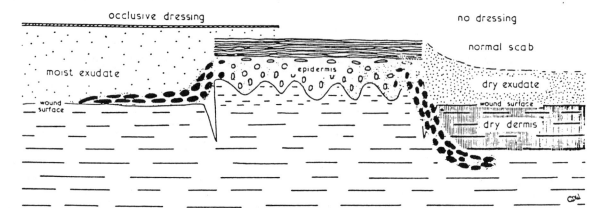

Figure 2-1 Effect of occlusion on epithelial migration (after Winter[11]).

consists of dried serous exudate and a layer of devitalized dermis. This scab, which may also incorporate some of the fibres from the dressing, forms a natural barrier to migrating epidermal cells, forcing them to move deeper beneath the drying eschar, prolonging the healing time, and causing an unnecessary loss of healthy tissue (Fig. 2-1). It is believed that epidermal cell movement is slower under these conditions because the cells are physically impeded by the collagen fibres at the interface of the scab and the underlying dermis. Wounds covered with an occlusive dressing do not form a scab, so epidermal cells are able to move rapidly over the surface of the dermis, through the exudate which collects at the wound/dressing interface.

The application of a totally occlusive or semipermeable dressing to a wound can also be important in preventing secondary damage as a result of dehydration. The capacity of a deep partial thickness wound to undergo spontaneous healing depends upon the survival of epidermal cells in hair follicles and sweat glands in the base of the wound; if these are allowed to become dehydrated and devitalised, the wound will not heal readily and may have to be grafted. Work on burns reviewed by Lawrence[7] has shown that the application of an occlusive dressing will salvage not only dermal tissue but also certain epithelial elements in the zone of stasis surrounding the original injury. The use of traditional dry dressings in these situations can result in progressive dehydration of the threatened zone followed by devitalisation and necrosis, with the result that this zone becomes indistinguishable from the original lesion. The prevention of

dehydration by the application of a suitable occlusive or semipermeable dressing may limit or prevent these secondary effects.

Some wounds, such as deep second degree burns and full thickness burns, produce quantities of plasma which combines with necrotic cells to form a coagulum that dries to form a hard eschar. It has been the experience of the author that the application of a suitable moisture-retaining dressing will prevent the formation of this eschar, or effect its rapid removal if already present. Early work on the use of a starch-based hydrogel (Scherisorb™) in the treatment of extravasation injuries in neonates[8] suggests that the provision of a moist wound environment in this situation may have similar beneficial effects, limiting tissue damage and reducing scar formation.

Occlusive dressings or other materials that have the effect of hydrating dry tissue can also play an important role in the treatment of decubitus ulcers. In such wounds, tissue which has become non-viable as a result of the sustained application of high levels of pressure, rapidly becomes necrotic and takes on a black leathery appearance. In this condition the ability of the skin to regulate the passage of moisture vapour is lost, and as a result, further dehydration of the underlying tissues occurs, causing additional damage and impeding the removal of the dead tissue by the normal autolytic processes. The application of an impermeable dressing in this situation will prevent further moisture vapour loss, bring about rapid rehydration of the black necrotic layer, and facilitate auto-debridement.

Not all wounds require the conservation of moisture, however. Leg ulcers and donor sites frequently produce large volumes of exudate, and some burns have been shown to produce up to 5200 $g/m^2/day$;[9] in these situations the primary function of a dressing may be simple absorption, to prevent maceration and infection.

In their simplest form, absorbent wound dressings consist of a mass of cotton or viscose fibre enclosed in a retaining sleeve. The first product to be produced commercially was Gamgee tissue, developed over a century ago. Although still used for certain orthopaedic purposes, for wound management it has been largely replaced by other more sophisticated products with coverstocks made of non-woven fabric; some of these dressings contain layers of cellulose tissue to distribute blood or exudate more efficiently throughout the body of the pad. Other products are filled with cellulose wood pulp, a fine powdery material which is also used in nappies and incontinence aids. These pads are often highly absorbent but they should never be cut (to fit around drains, for example) because the cellulose filler would be lost into the wound. Absorbent pads are used as secondary dressings in the management of heavily exuding wounds.

Other materials that may be applied to exuding wounds include a number of dressings that have little or no intrinsic absorbent capacity. Some of these materials, such as the semipermeable films and certain thin foam sheets, are permeable to moisture vapour; when one is placed on a wound, the aqueous component of the exudate is lost through the back of the dressing in the form of vapour, whilst the cellular material remains trapped at the surface of the wound. Thus, provided the rate of fluid transfer through the dressing is similar to the rate of exudate production, the wound will be maintained in a relatively constant state of hydration.

A similar effect can be achieved by the use of more sophisticated products, such as the alginate and hydrocolloid dressings which are described in more detail in later chapters. These dressings actually change their physical form as they take up exudate; in so doing they produce an aqueous gel on the surface of the wound which is believed to create an environment that is conducive to healing.

GASEOUS PERMEABILITY

For many years, it was believed that the presence of atmospheric oxygen was essential for rapid wound healing. For this reason it was considered that gaseous permeability was a prerequisite for a surgical dressing and, as such, was one of the required performance parameters of an ideal dressing identified by Winter in 1975.[10] This followed earlier work in which he showed that the mitotic rate of regenerating epidermal cells in a wound that was covered with a gas-permeable membrane could be increased by a factor of 5–10 times by exposing them to an oxygen-enriched atmosphere. This effect could be demonstrated when the partial pressure of oxygen (pO_2) was increased to 100 kPa and beyond.[11] Similar effects were reported by Silver,[12] who demonstrated that, in wounds that were moist but relatively free of exudate, epidermal repair beneath the so-called 'permeable' dressings took place more quickly in the presence of oxygen than under hypoxic conditions. In heavily exuding or grossly contaminated wounds, however, the pO_2 beneath even the semipermeable films was extremely low. Within an hour of applying the dressing, the oxygen that was originally present at the surface of the wound had disappeared; it was suggested that this, together with any additional oxygen which diffused through the film, was metabolised by inflammatory cells or bacteria in the exudate before it could reach the tissue beneath. Further evidence for this theory may be drawn from the work of Varghese,[13] who found that wound fluid under oxygen-permeable films contained more neutrophils than fluid collected from beneath hydrocolloid dressings (which, in their partially hydrated state, are less permeable than the films).

From these findings, it would be reasonable to assume that the use of a dressing with a high oxygen permeability would contribute positively to wound healing. However, angiogenesis (the formation and growth of new blood vessels) is also fundamental to the healing process. Using a rabbit ear chamber technique, Knighton et al.[14] were able to demonstrate that a hypoxic tissue gradient was essential for angiogenesis, and postulated that capillary formation in hypoxic regions is stimulated by the presence of a secondary angiogenic factor produced by hypoxic macrophages. Further support for this theory has come from work that has shown that reduced pO_2 promotes the growth of fibroblasts and the production of angiogenic factors from tissue macrophages in vitro. Studies with oxygen-impermeable dressings have also shown that angiogenesis is increased, both in pig wounds and in the chorioallantoic membrane of a fertile hen's egg, when atmospheric oxygen is excluded.[15] All of these observations confirm that limited hypoxia actually stimulates the formation of new blood vessels and granulation tissue, and thus speeds up the healing process.

In an informative review of the role of oxygen in wound healing, Silver[16] divides the healing process into epidermal and connective tissue repair, as the two processes differ markedly in their response to oxygen. He concludes that, although angiogenesis and the formation of granulation tissue is increased by moderately elevated pO_2, further increases in oxygen tension may reduce fibroblast activity and thus delay healing. The maximum rate of fibroblast growth and replication takes place in areas of oxygen tension of 30–40 mmHg, and it is likely that the greatest activity will be in front of the advancing capillary network in the centre of the wound.[17] In contrast, the growth of epidermal cells appears to be enhanced by increasing pO_2 with no evidence of oxygen poisoning at the highest concentrations used.

It might be assumed that, because oxygen is rapidly metabolised by white cells in wound exudate, the gaseous permeability of a dressing is also important in the prevention or control of infection. However, the results of studies carried out using hydrocolloid dressings appear not to support this theory: it was demonstrated that epithelialisation occurred faster under the 'impermeable' hydrocolloid material than beneath a semipermeable film dressing,[6] with no adverse effects upon the bacteriological picture or wound infection rates.[18] More recent work on the physical characteristics of hydrocolloid dressings has shown, however, that these materials (when hydrated) are far more permeable than was previously recognised; the conclusions that were drawn from the study described above may therefore have to be reviewed (see chapter 8).

In the past, other workers have shown that the local application of oxygen can play an important role in the prevention and control of wound infection, and the healing process in general.[19,20] More recently, Hinz et al.[21] applied an oxygen-liberating, isotonic solution of the tetrachlorodecaoxygen anion complex (Oxoferin™ – OXO Chemie, Heidelberg, FRG) to 271 long-standing or problem wounds. Tetrachlorodecaoxygen is a water-soluble material containing oxygen in a chlorite matrix, which liberates oxygen in the presence of haem moieties. It appeared to have three therapeutic effects in this study: wound cleansing was intensified, the formation of new granulation and epithelial tissue was accelerated, and the rate of wound closure was increased; use of the material on large surface wounds was found also to produce a good terrain for grafting.

It is possible that these beneficial effects are related to the activity of macrophages. Although it is known that these cells can phagocytose bacteria under both aerobic and anaerobic conditions, they are much less effective in destroying bacteria in the absence of oxygen. Under hypoxic conditions, macrophages have been seen to engulf bacteria, carry them in their cytoplasm, and later eject them undamaged; the same cells provided with an adequate supply of oxygen were able to lyse phagocytosed bacteria and cause them to disappear.[22]

One of the mechanisms by which macrophages exert their antibacterial effect is the generation of the superoxide anion (O_2^-) and hydrogen peroxide from molecular oxygen. Laboratory studies involving leucocytes in an anoxic environment showed that their ability to kill *Staphylococcus aureus* was markedly impaired, presumably as a result of their inability to produce these highly active molecular species.[23] In a rare human genetic disorder, chronic granulomatous disease, leucocytes are similarly unable to produce these oxygen-rich moeties (due to a defect in the leucocyte oxidase system), with the result that affected patients are highly susceptible to infections by many pathogenic bacteria, including *Staph. aureus, Escherichia coli,* and *Pseudomonas* and *Salmonella* spp.

From all these observations, it is obvious that the role of gaseous oxygen in wound healing is extremely complex and finely balanced, and this may have important implications when selecting a dressing for use in any given situation. A healthy non-infected wound in the early stages of healing may benefit from the application of a relatively impermeable product, which creates a hypoxic environment favouring angiogenesis and the formation of granulation tissue. This treatment may be continued until the defect is filled in to the level of the surrounding skin; once this stage is reached, a change to an oxygen-permeable product may have some merit, as it will facilitate epithelial growth and discourage the production of excess granulation tissue (which sometimes forms beneath less permeable dressings). In infected – or sloughy and necrotic – wounds, the oxygen supplied by the blood may be insufficient for the macrophages to exert effective phagocytic and bactericidal activity; in these situations, the use of a more permeable dressing or the local application of oxygen may provide the stimulus required for healing to recommence.

In clinical practice, however, it may sometimes be difficult to demonstrate the advantages of so-called 'oxygen-permeable' dressings. The adhesive films, such as Opsite™, are frequently described as 'oxygen-permeable' but, in this context, 'permeable' is a relative term; it is highly likely that, in many instances, insufficient oxygen will pass across the membrane to meet the needs of the tissue beneath (see chapter 4).

The permeability of dressings to carbon dioxide is also important, as surface wounds may develop a respiratory alkalosis (pH 8) as a result of the loss of carbon dioxide into the air. The application of a simple occlusive dressing will help to prevent or reduce this loss, and thus help to maintain the wound in a slightly more acid environment. Under occlusive dressings, the total oxygen requirement of the wound must be supplied by the local circulatory system, as in normal tissue. However, there is some evidence to suggest that this process also may be influenced or enhanced by the application of certain dressings and wound management solutions, which alter the pH of the local wound environment.

pH EFFECTS

In the blood, the release of oxygen from oxyhaemoglobin takes place most rapidly in an acid environment. During exercise, carbon dioxide and lactic acid build up in muscles, lowering the pH and resulting in the maximum release of oxygen to meet tissue needs. Conversely, an alkaline environment will tend to stabilise oxyhaemoglobin and thus reduce the available oxygen. In a detailed study of the effects of pH on oxygen dissociation, Leveen[24] described how a shift of only 0.9 units resulted in a five-fold increase in the oxygen released. In further clinical studies, the same workers showed that a decrease in the pH of a wound brought about by the application of polyacrylic acid resulted in a significant increase in pO_2, from 32 to 61 mmHg (as measured by direct oximetry). Many of the

alkaline wounds they examined also contained histotoxic levels of ammonia, liberated from urea by the enzyme urease (produced by some bacteria). Acidification of such wounds would minimise the toxicity of ammonia (which varies with pH).

The practical effects of applying agents to reduce wound pH were investigated by Wilson et al.,[25] who compared a buffered emulsified ointment (pH 6.0) with a commercial presentation containing malic, benzoic and salicylic acids (pH 2.8). Compared with pretreatment values, the group treated with the commercial material showed a reduction in pH for up to four hours, but the buffered product remained active for over 24 hours. When both materials were applied to leg ulcers in a controlled trial, it was found that the healing rates achieved with the buffered material were significantly better than those achieved with the unbuffered ointment despite the initial difference in the pH of the two products. The authors concluded that these findings added some support to the theory that prolonged chemical acidification of the ulcer surface does increase the healing rate, possibly as a result of increased oxygen availability.

In a comparative study of the local environment in chronic wounds treated with modern wound dressings, Varghese and his co-workers[13] found that the pH of wounds covered with a hydrocolloid dressing was consistently lower (pH 6.1) than that of comparable wounds dressed with a semipermeable film (pH 7.1). Laboratory studies suggested that this effect was due, at least in part, to the inherent acidity of the dissolved hydrocolloid base.

From the evidence currently available, it would appear that dressings that directly or indirectly reduce the pH of wound fluid may help to prevent infection, and will be likely to produce conditions that are more conducive to rapid healing than other materials which produce a more alkaline local environment.

FREEDOM FROM TOXIC AND PARTICULATE MATERIAL

As early as 1913 it was recognised that cellulosic particles entering a wound could cause a foreign body reaction with the formation of a granuloma.[26] As many of the dressing materials in common use are manufactured from cotton or viscose, the problems of fibre and particle loss are still very real. The loss of fine fibrous particles from gauze swabs is easily demonstrated by gently agitating an intact swab in a suitable quantity of filtered water or saline, and passing it through a dark coloured membrane filter. Under a low power lens, this fibrous material is easily visible against the dark background. If examined under an electron microscope, the structure of the fibres and debris can be seen more clearly (Fig. 2-2).

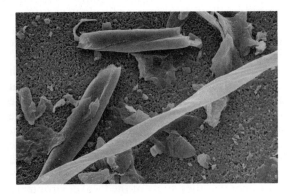

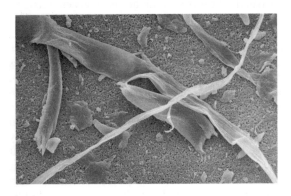

Figure 2-2 Particulate material lost from surgical gauze (× 360).

The problems of fibre loss from gauze materials placed directly onto the surface of a granulating wound have been described in the past. Fibres from the dressing may become incorporated into the drying eschar or, more importantly, may become embedded in the granulation tissue itself, where they may disrupt the normal healing pattern and adversely affect the quality of the healed wound.[27] Similar problems have been reported when wood fibres from disposable paper gowns were introduced into surgical wounds.[28-33]

The fibres were found to cause keloids, wound dehiscence, incisional hernias, and intestinal obstructions (due to the development of peritoneal adhesions). The presence of polyurethane foam particles in animal wounds was also found to provoke bizarre hypertrophy of the epidermis, and an intensive inflammatory cell reaction in the connective tissues.[10]

The presence of foreign bodies may also predispose a wound to infection. In an experimental study using human volunteers, Elek[34] showed that more than 1 000 000 staphylococci had to be injected into the dermis to cause an infection. In the presence of a piece of silk stitch, however, only about 100 viable organisms were required to cause a comparable infection.

It is equally important that the dressing should not contribute any form of contamination (either chemical or microbiological) to the wound. In the past, dressings supplied in sealed packages have been found to be contaminated with blood, oil, pieces of wire, insects, and even a piece of chain − none of which are likely to contribute positively to rapid or uneventful wound healing!

As the dressings on the market increase in complexity and sophistication, so does the potential for contamination by residual quantities of chemicals used in the manufacturing process. Comprehensive testing programs are essential to ensure that these new products will be unlikely to cause any adverse effects in patients.

LOW ADHERENCE

With the exception of the semipermeable films, the hydrogels, and the hydroactive materials, most dressings exhibit some tendency to adhere to the surface of a drying wound. This adherence may be due simply to the intrinsic viscosity and 'stickiness' of serum itself, but more often it is caused by the penetration into the body of the dressing of blood or exudate, which subsequently dries and hardens to form a scab that incorporates the fibres or threads of the dressing like reinforcing bars in concrete, turning a soft supple fabric into a board-like structure. When the dressing is removed, the bond between the eschar and the underlying tissue will fail first, resulting in considerable damage to the newly formed epithelium.

If a fabric with an open structure is placed upon a wound, it is also possible for granulation tissue to grow through the dressing, so that the material effectively becomes part of the healing wound. If this occurs, removal of the dressing will again result in damage and thus delay healing. Dressings manufacturers have made many attempts to overcome this problem by applying so-called 'non-adherent' facing layers to their dressings. Although these layers may be very different structurally, they are all designed to prevent the problem of adherence by reducing the size of the pores or apertures which are brought into contact with the tissue. However, if these pores are reduced below a certain critical size, there may be a danger that exudate from wounds such as leg ulcers, which is too viscous to to pass into the dressing, may accumulate on the surface of the surrounding skin. If this occurs it sometimes leads to an area of inflammation which corresponds exactly to the size of the dressing. This condition has been named 'Melolin leg' although it may occur with any perforated plastic film product (Plate 2).

The various types of facing layers used on low adherence dressings include perforated plastic films (e.g. Melolin™ and Telfa™), heat-calendered non-woven fabrics made from hydrophobic fibres (e.g. Hansapor Steril Plus™), and an apertured cloth coated with a layer of plastic that has been vacuum-ruptured (e.g. Perfron™ and Release II™). Histological studies of wounds dressed with perforated film dressings have shown that, although the bulk of the wound area is protected by the dressing, regular patches of secondary damage are visible on the dermis corresponding to the holes in the plastic film: these are caused by dehydration as a result of moisture vapour loss through the holes. Other dressings with specially modified wound contact surfaces have been produced from foams; these include Synthaderm™, Lyofoam™ and Allevyn™, all of which are claimed to be of low adherence. The effectiveness of the non-adherent layers on all these dressings depends mainly upon the size and uniformity of the pores. (Examples of different wound contact layers are shown in Figs 2-3 to 2-7.)

A laboratory method has been used to provide

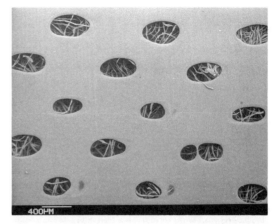

Figure 2-3 Wound contact layer of Melolin™, a perforated polyester film ($\times 20$).

some indication of the degree of adherence that could be anticipated if a particular dressing were to be applied to a drying wound.[35] A cold-cure silicone rubber material is applied to the dressing under test, inside a suitable former. The liquid rubber penetrates the body of the pad and hardens, and the force required to remove the dressing from the silicone rubber block provides a measure of the porosity of the facing layer. The higher the peel force, the greater the porosity and the potential for adherence.

The adherent properties of four different dressings were described by Malone,[36] following a study of 40 patients who had had an ingrowing great toe-nail removed. Their wounds were treated with either a paraffin gauze dressing, a knitted viscose dressing, a hydrocolloid dressing, or a silicone polymer foam. Of the 10 wounds dressed with the knitted viscose, 8 bled upon removal of the dressing, and 7 of the patients treated with this material complained of pain. No bleeding resulted from the removal of the paraffin gauze, but 5 patients complained of pain. One patient complained of pain upon removal of the hydro-colloid but no pain was reported with the use of the silicone foam. The association between pain and wound management has been discussed in more detail elsewhere.[37]

Some 'non-adherent' dressings are available that have no intrinsic absorbency, but which are intended to be used in conjunction with secondary absorbent pads. These include the tulle gras dressings which are described in more detail in chapter 3.

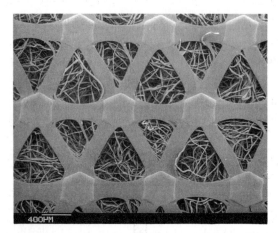

Figure 2-4 Wound contact layer of Melolite™, an apertured polyethylene net (×20).

IMPERMEABILITY TO MICRO-ORGANISMS

The ability of a dressing to act as an effective barrier to pathogenic organisms is of primary importance for two reasons. Airborne bacteria entering the wound may delay healing by producing an infection, which in extreme cases may develop into a life-threatening septicaemia. Equally important is the possibility that contaminated blood or exudate from a wound may pass through a dressing and reach the external surface. If this occurs small particles or fibres contaminated with exudate may become detached and released into the environment, leading to cross-infection and possibly the spread of antibiotic-resistant strains of bacteria. Even more serious is the risk to nursing and other hospital staff should the patient be suffering from a serious blood-borne viral infection.

It is known that, in the dry state, an absorbent pad made from cellulose fibres forms a reasonable bacterial barrier, as the fibres act as a simple depth filter; airborne organisms are invariably associated with dust or other particulate material, which is held back by the cotton or viscose fibres. This property is well recognised, as cotton wool plugs have long been used in microbiological laboratories to preserve the sterility of growth medium in flasks or test tubes. If the fibres of the dressing become wet, however, these barrier properties are lost. 'Strike-through', the passage of blood or serous exudate from a wound to the outer surface of a dressing, provides a liquid pathway along which bacteria may travel in both directions. If this occurs, the dressing should be changed immediately. In a simple study *in vitro*, Colebrook and Hood[38] showed that motile pathogenic organisms such as *Pseudomonas* and *Proteus* spp. could pass through a moist dressing within a few hours. Although non-motile bacteria could also pass through the dressing, they took somewhat longer, up to 48 hours in some cases. The authors suggested that strike-through could be prevented very simply by the inclusion of a plastic film beneath the outer layers of the dressing.

The barrier properties of a number of simple surgical absorbents were investigated in the laboratory by Piskozub,[39] who concluded that a dressing composed of layers of gauze would give more reliable protection than cotton wool or bleached wood pulp.

In order to enhance the absorbent capacity of their products, some manufacturers incorporate fluid-retardent layers into the pads to delay or prevent strike-through. These may take the form of spreader layers made from cellulose tissue, which cause absorbed liquid to be transported laterally within the body of the pad; alternatively, impermeable or hydrophobic layers can be placed towards the back of the pad to prevent strike-through altogether. A laboratory method to compare the performance of absorbent wound dressings has been described by the author.[35]

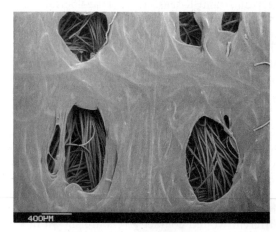

Figure 2-5 Wound contact layer of Release™ II, a vacuum ruptured polyethylene sheet (×20).

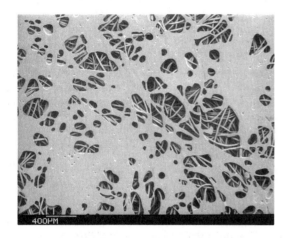

Figure 2-6 Wound contact layer of Hansapor Steril Plus™, consisting of heat calendered polyolefin fibres (×20).

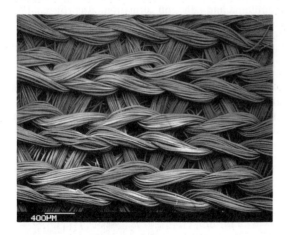

Figure 2-7 Wound contact layer of ETE™, consisting of knitted viscose (×20).

THERMAL PROPERTIES

The importance of wound temperature in the healing process was described by Myers,[40] following a study involving 420 patients. It was found that, after wound cleansing, it took 40 minutes for the wound to regain its original temperature and three hours for mitotic and leucocytic activity to return to normal. Temperature also influences the rate of oxyhaemoglobin dissociation, and a decrease in wound or skin temperature from 37°C

to 23°C can have a very significant effect upon oxygen availability.

The thermal properties of different types of dressing were reported by Lock,[41] following a study in pigs. He showed that, compared with exposed wounds which reached a temperature of 21°C, wounds dressed with conventional materials of gauze and cotton wool attained 25–27°C, those covered with a polyurethane film dressing reached 30–32°C, and those dressed with a polyurethane foam (Synthaderm™) reached 33–35°C. The effects of different types of dressings upon the temperature of intact skin were recorded by Turner,[42] who showed that hydrogel dressings produced a drop in the temperature of the skin as a result of evaporation of moisture vapour. Other dressings, such as gauze and the hydrocolloids, acted more like thermal insulators, tending to maintain the wound at a constant temperature. Similar findings were reported by Cherry and Ryan[15] who found that the application of a hydrocolloid dressing increased the temperature of a leg ulcer from 32.7°C to 35.2°C.

Unexplained and contradictory evidence for the thermal effects of one hydrogel dressing on wounds has been reported previously by Rosin,[43] who found that the application of Geliperm™ produced an increase in wound temperature for the first three days of treatment, compared with traditional materials.

The thermal properties of dressings may have important clinical implications. The application of a hydrogel sheet to a recent minor burn should produce a cooling effect, reducing pain and inflammation. However, application to a wound on an already cold, ischaemic limb would be less appropriate, as phagocytic and mitotic activity are particularly sensitive to temperatures below 28°C, and any additional cooling effects could be undesirable; in this situation, a dressing with good thermal properties may be required if optimum healing rates are to be maintained.

REFERENCES

1. Elliot I.M.Z., *A Short History of Surgical Dressings,* London, Pharmaceutical Press, 1964.
2. Bishop W.J., *A History of Surgical Dressings,* Chesterfield, Robinsons and Sons, 1959.

3. Forrest R.D., Early history of wound treatment, *J. R. Soc. Med.*, 1982, **75**, 198–205.

4. Winter G.D., Formation of the scab and the rate of epithelization of superficial wounds in the skin of the young domestic pig, *Nature*, 1962, **193**, 293–294.

5. Hinman C.C. *et al.*, Effect of air exposure and occlusion on experimental human skin wounds, *Nature*, 1963, **200**, 377–379.

6. Eaglstein W.H., The effect of occlusive dressings on collagen synthesis and re-epithelialization in superficial wounds, in *An Environment for Healing: The Role of Occlusion*, Ryan T.J. (ed.), International Congress and Symposium Series No. 88, London, Royal Society of Medicine, 1985, 31–38.

7. Lawrence J.C., Laboratory studies of dressings, in *Wound Healing Symposium*, Lawrence J.C. (ed.), Proceedings of a Symposium, Birmingham, 1982, Oxford, Medicine Publishing Foundation, 1983, 115–128.

8. Thomas S. *et al.*, A new approach to the treatment of extravasation injury in neonates, *Pharm. J.*, 1987, **239**, 584–585.

9. Lamke L.O. *et al.*, The evaporative water loss from burns and water vapour permeability of grafts and artificial membranes used in the treatment of burns, *Burns*, 1977, **3**, 159–165.

10. Winter G.D., Epidermal wound healing, in *Surgical Dressings in the Hospital Environment*, Turner T.D. and Brain K.R. (eds), Proceedings of a Conference, Cardiff, March 1975, Cardiff, Surgical Dressings Research Unit, Welsh School of Pharmacy, 47–81.

11. Winter G.D., Epidermal regeneration studied in the domestic pig, in *Epidermal Wound Healing*, Maibach H.I. and Rovee D.T. (eds), Chicago, Year Book Medical Publishers, 1972, 71–112.

12. Silver I.A., Oxygen tension and epithelialization, in Ref. 11, 291–305.

13. Varghese M.C. *et al.*, Local environment of chronic wounds under synthetic dressings, *Arch. Derm.*, 1986, **122**, 52–57.

14. Knighton D. *et al.*, Regulation of wound healing angiogenesis: effect of oxygen gradient and inspired oxygen concentration, *Surgery*, 1981, **90**, 262–270.

15. Cherry G.W. and Ryan T.J., Enhanced wound angiogenesis with a new hydrocolloid dressing, in Ref. 6, 61–68.

16. Silver I.A., Oxygen and tissue repair, in Ref. 6, 15–19.

17. Kanzler M.H. *et al.*, Basic mechanisms in the healing of cutaneous wounds. *J. derm. Surg. Oncol.*, 1986, **12**, 1156–1164.

18. Williams D.L. *et al.*, Effects of a new hydrocolloid dressing on healing of full thickness wounds in normal volunteers, in Ref. 6, 77–83.

19. Fischer B.H., Topical hyperbaric oxygen treatment of pressure sores and skin ulcers, *Lancet*, 1969, **2**, 405–409.

20. Perrins D.J., Influence of hyperbaric oxygen on survival of split skin grafts, *ibid.*, 1967, **2**, 868–871.

21. Hinz J. *et al.*, Rationale for and results from a randomised, double blind trial of tetrachlorodecaoxygen anion complex in wound healing, *ibid.*, 1986, **1**, 825–828.

22. Silver I.A., The physiology of wound healing, in *Wound Healing and Wound Infection*, Hunt T.K. (ed.), New York, Appleton-Century-Crofts, 1980, 11–32.

23. Hohn D.C. *et al.*, Effect of oxygen tension on the microbiocidal function of leukocytes in wounds and in vitro, *Surg. Forum*, 1976, **27**, 18–20.

24. Leveen H.H., Chemical acidification of wounds, an adjuvant to healing and the unfavorable action of alkalinity and ammonia, *Ann. Surg.*, 1973, **178**, 745–753.

25. Wilson I.A.I. *et al.*, The pH of varicose ulcer surfaces and its relationship to healing, *Vasa (Bern)*, 1979, **8**, 339–342.

26. Adams J.E., Peritoneal adhesions – an experimental study, *Lancet*, 1913, **1**, 663–668.

27. Wood R.A.B., Disintegration of cellulose dressings in open granulating wounds, *Br. med. J.*, 1976, **1**, 1444–1445.

28. Sturdy J.H. *et al*, Surgical sponges: a cause of granuloma and adhesion formation, *Ann. Surg.*, 1967, **165**, 128–134.

29. Saxen L. and Myllarniemi H., Foreign material and postoperative adhesions, *New Engl. J. Med.*, 1968, **279**, 200–202.

30. Weibel M.A. and Majno G., Peritoneal adhesions and their relation to abdominal surgery, *Am. J. Surg.*, 1973, **126**, 345–353.

31. Tinker M.A. *et al.*, Granulomatous peritonitis due to cellulose fibers from disposable surgical fabrics: laboratory investigation and clinical implications, *Ann. Surg.* 1974, **180**, 831–835.

32. Tinker M.A. *et al.*, Cellulose granulomas and their relationship to intestinal obstruction, *Am. J. Surg.*, 1977, **133**, 134–139.

33. Dragan M.J., Wood fibres from disposable surgical gowns and drapes, *J. Am. med. Ass.*, 1979, **241**, 2297–2298.

34. Elek S.D., Experimental staphylococcal infections in the skin of man. *Ann. N.Y. Acad. Sci.*, 1956, **65**, 85–90.

35. Thomas S. *et al.*, Wound dressing materials – testing and control, *Pharm. J.*, 1982, **228**, 576–578.

36. Malone W.D., Wound dressing adherence; a clinical comparative study, *Arch. emerg. Med.*, 1987, **4**, 101–105.

37. Thomas S., Pain and wound management, *Nurs. Times, Community Outlook Suppl.*, 1989, **85**, 11–15.

38. Colebrook L. and Hood A.M., Infection through soaked dressings, *Lancet*, 1948, **2**, 682–683.

39. Piskozub Z.T., The efficacy of wound dressing materials as a barrier to secondary bacterial contamination, *Br. J. plast. Surg.*, 1968, **213**, 387–401.

40. Myers J.A., Modern plastic surgical dressings, *Hlth Soc. Serv. J.*, 1982 (18 March), 336–337.

41. Lock P.M., The effect of temperature on mitotic activity at the edge of experimental wounds, in *Symposia on Wound Healing; Plastic, Surgical and Dermatologic Aspects,* Lundgren A. and Soner A.B. (eds), Molndal, Sweden, 1980, 103–109.

42. Turner T.D., Semiocclusive and occlusive dressings, in Ref. 6, 5–14.

43. Rosin R.D., A study of environmental temperatures under wound dressings, in *Geliperm: A Clear Advance in Wound Healing,* Woods H.F. and Cottier D. (eds), Proceedings of a Conference, Oxford, 1983, Sheffield University Printing Unit, 1984, 147–153.

Chapter 3

Primary Wound Contact Materials

Dressings that are used to absorb exudate (from wounds such as burns, donor sites and leg ulcers) are frequently manufactured from cotton or viscose fibres enclosed in a sleeve of gauze or a suitable non-woven fabric. Such dressings are often highly absorbent, but exhibit a tendency to adhere to the surface of the wound as fluid production diminishes. The use of a suitable wound contact material placed at the wound/dressing interface can help to overcome this problem; as this layer may have little intrinsic absorbent capacity, it must be sufficiently porous to allow the passage of blood or exudate away from the surface of the wound into the secondary dressing, in order to prevent maceration of the underlying tissue.

The first modern dressing to be produced specifically for use as a wound contact layer was 'tulle gras,' developed by Lumière during World War I. It was originally made from an open-weave cloth coated with soft paraffin containing 1.25% Balsam of Peru (as a mild antiseptic) but, following reports of skin reactions in some patients,[1] Balsam of Peru was eventually omitted from the formulation.

In an interesting account of the history of tulle gras, Elliot[2] describes how many hospital pharmacies prepared their own from net curtain, which was washed, dried, cut into pieces, and packed in flat 50-cigarette tins, prior to the application of the paraffin base and eventual sterilisation. Tulle gras became very popular and eventually became the subject of a monograph in the British Pharmaceutical Codex of 1949.

Two forms of the dressing are now officially recognised with monographs in the British Pharmacopoeia. Although both types are made from the same base fabric, which consists of a bleached cotton or cotton and viscose gauze of leno weave, the products differ in the content of white soft paraffin. The traditional material contains not less than 175 grams of paraffin base per square metre of cloth, but the alternative formulation bears a lower loading of paraffin, in the range $90-130$ g/m^2. This makes the dressing less occlusive, and therefore less likely to cause maceration of the underlying skin when applied to heavily exuding wounds. Changes in presentation have also been made and both types of dressing are now available individually wrapped. Examples of the official paraffin gauze dressings include:

- Jelonet™ – Smith & Nephew,
- Paranet™* – Vernon-Carus,
- Paratulle™* – Seton,
- Unitulle™* – Roussel.

* low loading material

In addition to the products identified above, a number of alternative materials are available that do not comply with current British monographic requirements. These are mainly produced outside the UK and include Vaseline™ gauze (Sherwood), Lomatuell™ (Lohmann) and Grassolind™ (Hartmann). Unlike the dressings of the British Pharmacopoeia, they are all made from a simple plain-weave gauze fabric impregnated with soft paraffin.

Branolind™ (Hartmann) consists of an open-weave cotton cloth impregnated with an ointment containing lanolin, paraffin and Peru balsam.

MEDICATED TULLE DRESSINGS

It was recognised very early on that the ointment applied to the dressing fabric could act as a carrier for a range of medicaments. As a result, tulle dressings were produced containing local anaesthetic agents, sulphonamides, antibiotics (including penicillin), vitamins, honey, and other agents that were believed to promote healing and control or prevent infection. However, when it was realised that the topical use of antibiotics for the treatment of trivial conditions could lead to the emergence of resistant strains of micro-organisms, and cause sensitivity reactions in some patients, the use of tulle dressings containing these materials declined. As a general guide, it was recommended that antibiotics that were used systemically should not be applied to the skin,[3] although other products containing agents that were too toxic or unsuitable for systemic administration could be used. One such product is Framycetin Gauze Dressing BP, known as Sofra−Tulle™ (Roussel), which is impregnated with a white soft paraffin basis containing 10% anhydrous lanolin and framycetin sulphate 1%. Framycetin is a broad-spectrum antibiotic which is active against both Gram-positive and Gram-negative bacteria, including common skin pathogens such as *Staphylococcus aureus, Escherichia coli* and *Pseudomonas aeruginosa*. Framycetin, which consists mainly of neomycin B, was first isolated in 1947 and was used primarily in ophthalmology, where it was found to be particularly effective against staphylococcal infections. The tulle preparation was developed some time later; its use in the treatment of wounds was first investigated in the early 1960s,[4−6] when it was claimed to reduce the risk of sepsis and promote healing. Similar beneficial results were reported after its use in the treatment of superficial and deep dermal burns.[7,8] The development of Sofra-Tulle has been described in detail by Wicks and Peterson.[9] Although many of the early reports on the use of framycetin stated that the material did not cause hypersensitivity reactions, Kirton and Munro-Ashman[10] reported that they had encountered 70 cases of contact dermatitis due to neomycin or framycetin over a two-year period, and argued that neither of these materials should be used without definite indications and, even then, not for extended periods (Plate 3).

Fucidin-Intertulle™ (Leo) consists of a cotton gauze fabric impregnated with white soft paraffin and lanolin containing 2% sodium fusidate, an antibiotic which is highly active against *Staph. aureus* (including strains that are resistant to other antibiotics). Sodium fusidate is unusual in that it is able to penetrate intact skin; in the form of a dressing, it has been recommended for the treatment of ulcers, skin grafts and burns infected with susceptible organisms. Unlike Sofra-Tulle, Fucidin-Intertulle does not appear to cause skin sensitisation,[11,12] but it has been suggested that the topical use of sodium fusidate on its own may lead to the development of bacterial resistance[13] − which could be very important in view of its

value in the systemic treatment of serious infections, including osteomyelitis and intracranial abscesses.

Because of the problems of skin sensitivity and bacterial resistance associated with the topical use of antibiotics, some manufacturers have produced dressings containing other well proven antimicrobial agents. Bactigras™ (Smith & Nephew) consists of a gauze fabric impregnated with yellow soft paraffin containing 0.5% chlorhexidine acetate, a potent antimicrobial agent which is active against a wide range of micro-organisms.[14] Chlorhexidine does not appear to induce bacterial resistance in normal use[15] and has a low incidence of skin sensitisation.[16] It is strongly bound to cellulose materials, such as fibres of cotton or viscose, and its antimicrobial activity is reduced in the presence of blood and pus.[17] Despite the apparent advantages of chlorhexidine, the likely clinical effectiveness of Bactigras was questioned in the past, following a series of *in-vitro* tests which suggested that chlorhexidine acetate, present in the basis as a dispersed powder, is not easily extracted by serum or wound exudate and is therefore not readily available to exert an antimicrobial effect.[18,19] Other workers have claimed that, despite these unsatisfactory laboratory test results, the dressing does appear to be effective in preventing the colonisation of experimental burns,[20] although the issue remains the subject of some debate.[21,22] Clinical experience with Bactigras suggests that the dressing may be of some value in the treatment of non-infected minor burns as a prophylactic agent, against the growth of bacteria.[23] Since the dressing became the subject of a monograph in the British Pharmacopoeia (under the name of Chlorhexidine Gauze Dressing), two more products have become available, − Serotulle™ (Seton) and Clorhexitulle™ (Roussel).

Dressings containing other antimicrobial agents are also available. Inadine™ (Johnson & Johnson) consists of a knitted viscose fabric impregnated with polyethylene glycol (PEG) containing 10% povidone-iodine, equivalent to 1% available iodine. The use of a hydrophilic basis facilitates the extraction of povidone-iodine (by serum or exudate), which imparts pronounced (though short-term) antibacterial activity to the dressing.[19] The use of PEG has the additional advantage that, should the dressing adhere to the wound, it may be removed by irrigation with sterile water or normal saline.

Other medicated dressings containing a variety of ingredients are also available, though not all are licensed for use in the UK. They include the following.

● M and M Tulle™ (Malam) contains cod liver oil BP 23% w/w, purified honey BPC 23% w/w, and hexachlorophane BP 0.05% w/w.

● Xeroform™ (Sherwood) contains 3% bismuth tribromophenate in a paraffin basis.

● Xeroflow™ (Sherwood) contains 3% bismuth tribromophenate in a bland oil emulsion.

● Scarlet Red™ Ointment Dressing (Sherwood) contains scarlet red (o-tolylazo-o-tolylazo-2-naphthol), an agent that is said to promote the growth of epithelium, in a blend of lanolin, olive oil and soft paraffin.

● Branolind L™ (Hartmann) contains a local anaesthetic agent 'Stadacain' 2% in a basis of lanolin, yellow paraffin and Peru balsam.

The value of some of these medicated products is unclear. In one American study, epithelial cell proliferation in donor sites was determined by measuring the uptake of tritium-labelled thymidine by regenerating epithelial cell DNA. From their results, the authors concluded that the healing rates of wounds dressed with Xeroform and Scarlet Red Ointment Dressing were statistically superior at 48 hours to those obtained with more conventional treatments (such as Betadine™, fine mesh gauze and air exposure).[24]

In contrast, the authors of a second study (which also included both Xeroform and Scarlet Red Ointment Dressing, and which was designed to determine the clinical effectiveness of a range of impregnated dressings on the healing rate of donor sites) concluded that the rate and quality of healing of all wounds were virtually the same, regardless of the type of dressing used.[25]

Although paraffin gauze dressings are generally considered to be of low adherence, it is not uncommon for patients to experience considerable pain when they are removed. In some instances, this can be severe enough to require the use of narcotic analgesics such as pethidine or morphine.[26] Often removal of the dressings leads to additional trauma to the surface of the wound causing bleeding or removal of new epidermal tissue (Plate 4).

ALTERNATIVE FORMS OF DRESSINGS WITH LOW ADHERENCE

Because the greasy, semi-occlusive nature of tulle dressings sometimes causes problems of skin maceration, alternative wound contact materials have been developed. A textile wound contact layer, which is not impregnated with paraffin or PEG, has been introduced. It consists of a knitted viscose fabric and is offered as an alternative to impregnated dressings for the treatment of exuding wounds (such as leg ulcers). The dressing has a monograph in the British Pharmacopoeia and is known as Knitted Viscose Primary Dressing. Two brands are available, N-A™ Dressing (Johnson & Johnson) and Tricotex™ (Smith & Nephew). Little clinical information has been published on the efficacy of these materials.

A totally new approach to the development of a non-adherent wound contact layer has been adopted by Smith & Nephew. Transite™ consists of two thin layers of polyurethane bonded together to form a transparent plastic film, which is perforated with a series of slits. The two components of the film differ in their chemical structure and their affinity for water: one layer is hydrophilic, the other is hydrophobic. In use, the dressing is placed over an exuding wound and held in place by means of adhesive handles on two opposite sides; a simple absorbent pad is then placed on the back. In the presence of wound exudate, the hydrophilic layer absorbs moisture and swells, causing the slits in the film to open, allowing exudate to pass through into the pad behind. As the wound dries, the film loses moisture, and the slits close once more. In this way, the dressing is able to exert a degree of control over the environment at the surface of the wound. When the pad becomes saturated with exudate it can be changed without disturbing the primary dressing, which may be left in place until the wound is healed.

A number of absorbent dressing pads are available that have one surface modified to prevent the dressing adhering to a drying wound. Examples of some of these materials are shown in Figs 2-3 to 2-7. The most familiar products of this type are Melolin™ (Smith & Nephew) and Telfa™ (Kendall), the Perforated Film Absorbent Dressings of the British Pharmacopoeia. Both products have a simple fibrous absorbent layer covered with a perforated plastic film, and are intended for use on minor injuries and other low exudate wounds. It is generally accepted that such dressings should not be applied to leg ulcers or other lesions producing quantities of viscous exudate, as the exudate may be unable to pass through the pores in the dressing – leading to maceration of the skin or, occasionally, the production of an inflammatory reaction (sometimes known as Melolin leg!).

Other manufacturers have approached the problem of adherence in a different way. A few have chosen to apply a coating of metallic aluminium to the wound contact surface of their dressings. One such product is Metalline™ (Lohmann), which consists of an absorbent pad faced with a layer of non-woven tissue coated with a thin layer of aluminium (by vacuum deposition). This is said to provide an effective low adherence surface which will not stick to a granulating wound. The dressing is available in a range of sizes and is sometimes used as a bed sheet for patients who have suffered extensive burns. Although not widely used in the UK at present, Metalline is used extensively in Europe. Laboratory studies carried out by the author suggest that, in some production batches at least, there is a possibility that some of the aluminium may be lost from the dressing during normal use and remain in the wound. The clinical significance of this observation is not known.

Other products that have an aluminium wound contact layer include Absderma™ (LIC Hygien, Solna, Sweden) and Alutex™ (Ortmann). Laboratory tests suggest that aluminium loss of the sort described above, does not appear to be a problem with these two dressings.

There is little doubt that there will continue to be a demand for tulles and other low adherence dressings for some time to come. However, the development of new, more sophisticated wound management materials – such as alginates, hydrogels and hydrocolloids (some of which do not require the application of a secondary absorbent layer) – will continue to have a significant impact upon the market share of the low adherence products. It is likely that (in the management of donor sites and ulcers in particular) paraffin gauze dressings, both plain and medicated, will gradually be replaced by these alternative new materials.

REFERENCES

1. Trevethick R.A., Sensitization to tulle gras dressings, (letter), *Br. med. J.,* 1957, **2**, 883–884.

2. Elliot I.M.Z., *A Short History of Surgical Dressings,* London, Pharmaceutical Press, 1964.

3. D'Arcy P.F., Drugs on the skin: a clinical and pharmaceutical problem, *Pharm. J.,* 1972, **209**, 491–492.

4. Lunn J.A., Controlled trial of a wound dressing: Sofra-Tulle, *Practitioner,* 1962, **188**, 527–528.

5. Jackson P.W., Sofra-Tulle in the treatment of minor wounds, *ibid.,* 1962, **189**, 675–678.

6. Currie J.P. and Sinclair D.M., Framycetin in the treatment of cutaneous injuries, *ibid.,* 1963, **190**, 112–113.

7. Ramirez A.T. *et al.,* Topical framycetin in the treatment of burns, *Philippine J. surg. Special.,* 1969, **24**, 1–14.

8. Smith R.A., The treatment of burns: a clinical evaluation of Sofra-Tulle, *Clin. Trials J.,* 1972, **9**, 37–40.

9. Wicks C.J. and Peterson H.I., Medicated wound dressings – a historical review, *Opusc. med.,* 1972, **17**, 90–95.

10. Kirton V. and Munro-Ashman D., Contact dermatitis from neomycin and framycetin, *Lancet,* 1965, **2**, 138–139.

11. Ritchie I.C., Clinical and bacteriological studies of a new antibiotic tulle, *Br. J. clin. Pract.,* 1968, **22**, 15–16.

12. McCormack B.L. *et al.,* Practical evaluation of a new sodium fusidate (Fucidin) wound dressing, *J. Ir. med. Ass.,* 1968, **61**, 137–141.

13. *Martindale; The Extra Pharmacopoeia,* 29th edn, Reynolds J.E.F. (ed.), London, Pharmaceutical Press, 1989, 235.

14. Davies G.E. *et al.,* 1:6–Dichlorophenyldiguanido-hexane ('Hibitane'): laboratory investigation of a new antibacterial agent of high potency, *Br. J. Pharmac. Chemother.,* 1954, **9**, 192–196.

15. Longworth A.R., Chlorhexidine, in *Inhibition and Destruction of the Microbial Cell,* Hugo W.B. (ed.), London, Academic Press, 1971, 95–106.

16. Senior N., Some observations on the formulation and properties of chlorhexidine, *J. Soc. cosmet. Chem.,* 1972, **11**, 1–19.

17. Lowbury E.J.L., Chlorhexidine, *Curr. Ther.,* 1957, **179**, 489–493.

18. Thomas S. and Russell A.D., An *in vitro* evaluation of Bactigras, a tulle dressing containing chlorhexidine, *Microbios Lett.,* 1976, **2**, 169–177.

19. Thomas S. *et al.,* Improvements in medicated tulle dressings, *J. Hosp. Infect.,* 1983, **4**, 391–398.

20. Andrew J.K. *et al.,* An experimental evaluation of a chlorhexidine medicated tulle gras dressing, *ibid.,* 1982, **3**, 149–157.

21. Thomas S., An experimental evaluation of a chlorhexidine medicated tulle gras dressing, (letter), *ibid.,* 399–400.

22. Andrew J.K. *et al., idem.,* 401.

23. Lawrence J.C., Minor burns, *Nurs. Mirror,* 1977, **144,** 58 – 60.

24. Salomon J.C. *et al.,* Effect of dressings on donor site epithelialization, *Surg. Forum,* 1974, **25,** 516 – 517.

25. Gemberling R.M. *et al.,* Dressing comparison in the healing of donor sites, *J. Trauma,* 1976, **16,** 812 – 814.

26. Thomas S., Pain and wound management, *Nurs. Times, Community Outlook Suppl.,* 1989, **85,** 11 – 15.

Chapter 4

Semipermeable Film Dressings

DEVELOPMENT OF FILM DRESSINGS

It is likely that the first transparent film dressings were those manufactured in the 18th century from isinglass, the dried prepared swim bladder of certain species of fish. This, together with other ingredients, was spread (in the form of a solution) onto layers of ribbon, linen, or oiled silk, to form a plaster. The resulting materials were so thin and translucent that the wound was visible underneath. Any fluid that accumulated beneath the dressing could be seen; if this became excessive, it could be drained off through a small hole cut in the fabric. Robert Liston (1846), quoted by Elliot,[1] said that isinglass plaster was not irritating to wounds and – unlike the common adhesive plasters – it did not become loose or give rise to erythema. It was therefore considered to represent a great advance over other dressings in current use (such as compresses, pledgets and bandages), which generally did no real good and often hindered the healing of the wound. In 1880, isinglass plaster was used successfully as a dressing after skin grafting, an indication for which it was thought to be particularly well suited.

Another early film dressing was manufactured from pyroxylin or gun cotton, which was prepared by nitrating cotton fibre with equal parts of nitric and sulphuric acid. After purification and drying, the highly inflammable residue was dissolved in a mixture of ether and rectified spirit to form a clear colourless solution known as collodion. When poured onto the skin, the solvent evaporated, leaving a thin transparent plastic film which contracted on drying. In 1848, collodion was used in America for dressing suture lines, and later formed the subject of a monograph in the first edition of the British Pharmacopoeia (1864). In the 1867 edition, it was joined by a second formulation – containing Canada balsam and castor oil – which was known as Flexible Collodion, and was used as a dressing for burns, ulcers and abrasions of the skin. Squire's

Companion to the British Pharmacopoeia (1874) described both of these materials, together with two non-official preparations: Dr Richardson's Styptic Colloid (containing tannic acid), and Dr Pavisi's Haemostatic Collodion (which contained carbolic acid, tannic acid and benzoic acid). In 1903, it was said that the thin film that formed when a solution of collodion was allowed to dry on a sheet of glass made a valuable dressing for open wounds.

Collodion proved to be a very popular material and the British Pharmaceutical Codex of 1934 contained thirteen monographs for various medicated preparations, some of which contained ether and benzene! The use of collodion in its various forms has declined over the years because of the toxic and inflammable properties of some of the solvents used, although modified formulations are still available for use as wart removers. More modern versions of these solvent-based film dressings have been developed, using different solvent systems and more modern synthetic polymers.

- Opsite™ Spray Dressing (Smith & Nephew) consists of an ethoxyethyl methacrylate-methoxyethyl methacrylate copolymer ('Hydron') dissolved in a mixture of ethyl acetate and acetone.

- Nobecutane™ Spray (Astra), is a solution of acrylic resins dissolved in ethyl acetate.

Once applied to the skin and allowed to dry, the materials mentioned above form tough protective films, which are said to be impervious to bacteria. They have been used in the past for application to minor injuries and suture lines following surgery.

The development of modern polymers has also led to the production of a range of new plastic films, a number of which have been used for medical applications. In 1945, Bloom[2] described the use of 'Cellophane' in the treatment of 55 patients with burns, following his experiences with the material in an Italian prison camp during

World War II. He reported that wounds treated with the film healed rapidly and even infected wounds healed normally, under a thin layer of 'inspissated purulent serum' and that patients found that the application of the material resulted in an immediate relief of pain. In 1948, Bull *et al.*[3] described the development of a dressing in which a semipermeable window, manufactured from a nylon derivative, was supported in an adhesive polyvinyl frame. The nylon film formed an effective bacterial barrier and was sufficiently permeable to prevent maceration of the underlying skin. The results of a clinical trial into the use of this dressing were reported some two years later by Schilling *et al.*[4] Following this early work, the first major study into the effects of occlusive or semi-occlusive dressings on wound healing was carried out in the early 1960s by Winter[5] and Hinman *et al.*[6] Some of the films they used were impermeable to water vapour, and, although developments of these materials were employed successfully as incise drapes to cover the area around an operation site, it was found that their extended use on large wounds frequently led to bacterial proliferation and skin maceration, making them unsuitable for use as dressings.

In 1971 Smith & Nephew introduced Opsite™, a film dressing that effectively overcame the problems of skin maceration. Originally produced as an incise drape, the film was manufactured from a type 1 polyurethane, coated with a vinyl ether adhesive system. In 1974, this was changed to a type 2 polyurethane, and the product was also marketed as a dressing. Opsite is permeable to water vapour and oxygen but impermeable to water and micro-organisms.

Because of the success that Opsite enjoyed in the market-place, a number of film dressings were soon developed and produced by other manufacturers, subject to licences given by Smith & Nephew. As the potential for significant improvement to the basic film was somewhat limited, Smith & Nephew's competitors were forced to identify aspects of the performance of the dressing that they could develop or improve and use as the basis of their marketing strategy. One obvious area for improvement lay in the method of application, as the original presentation of Opsite had one well-recognised disadvantage. Prior to use, the film had to be removed completely from its backing sheet; once free, it had a marked tendency to curl up and stick firmly to itself. If this happened, the dressing had

to be discarded, which was wasteful in terms of both time and material costs.[7] Considerable attention was paid to this problem; as a result, a number of interesting new application systems were developed, which the manufacturers claimed made their dressings much easier to apply. The problems with the early presentation of Opsite were referred to by Haessler[8] in a study of dressings for catheter sites. She compared Opsite with Tegaderm™ (3M) and with gauze. Although the two films were found to be broadly equivalent, and superior to gauze in most respects, Tegaderm was preferred to Opsite because of its ease of application. As a result of these commercial pressures, Smith & Nephew eventually introduced an improved presentation of Opsite.

The other area in which it was thought that improvements could be made was the type of adhesive system applied to the film. The vinyl ether adhesive used by Smith & Nephew is thought by some to be more likely to cause a sensitivity reaction or an allergic response than the acrylic-based adhesives used by most of the other manufacturers. To date, however, the only instances of adverse reactions said to be linked to the use of film dressings – of which the author is aware – have been associated with a product bearing an acrylic adhesive. In most instances, these sensitivity reactions have been shown to be caused by the use of preparations containing iodine or other medicaments, which were applied to the skin before the dressing. The formulation of the adhesive system can have other important effects, which are discussed later in the chapter.

More recently, medicated film dressings have been introduced and other more sophisticated products have been developed, which are able to cope with larger volumes of exudate than the simple adhesive membranes.

At the time of writing, the plain unmedicated film dressings available on the British market are:

- Bioclusive™ – Johnson & Johnson,
- Dermafilm™ – Vygon,
- Dermoclude™ – BritCair,
- Ensure-it™ – Becton Dickinson,
- Opraflex™ – Lohmann,
- Opsite – Smith & Nephew,
- Tegaderm – 3M.

Because of the importance attached to the method

of application, by manufacturers and users alike, the presentation of each product is described briefly below.

Bioclusive

The adhesive film is carried upon a piece of release paper which is divided into three. The dressing is applied in much the same way as a first-aid finger dressing. The central portion of the paper is removed and the dressing placed in position before the two outer pieces of the backing paper are removed.

Dermafilm

The adhesive film is carried upon a single piece of release paper; the ends of the film, which are not coated with adhesive, form handles (which may be removed by tearing along a perforated line once the dressing is in position).

Dermoclude

The adhesive film is sandwiched between a coated paper release layer and a sheet of thicker plastic on the outer surface (to give the film stability). The adhesive film, together with its plastic backing, is removed from the release paper by means of a semi-rigid yellow tab which runs along one end of the sheet. Once the dressing has been placed in position on the wound, the supporting film is removed by means of a second white paper tab.

Ensure-it

The adhesive film is sandwiched between a layer of release paper on the adhesive side and a sheet of thicker plastic on the outer surface. The adhesive film, together with its plastic backing, is removed from the release paper by means of a semi-rigid blue plastic handle which runs along one edge of the sheet. After the dressing has been placed in position on the wound, the plastic backing sheet is removed by means of a white paper tab. The blue handle, which is an integral part of the dressing, may then be removed or left in position as required.

Opraflex

The film is sandwiched between a coated paper release layer and a semi-rigid plastic backing bearing two tabs or handles. Running across the centre of the release paper is a red plastic strip through which a continuous wavy line is cut, penetrating both the red plastic strip and the release paper itself. When the dressing is folded backwards, the two halves of the paper separate along the cut and tend to form 'fingers' that lift away from the adhesive film, because of the rigidity imparted by the plastic strip. In this way, the release paper is easily removed and the dressing is left adhering to the plastic backing sheet. The dressing is positioned over the wound by means of the two tabs; the backing sheet is removed once the dressing is in position.

Opsite

As with Bioclusive, the adhesive film is carried upon a piece of release paper that is divided into three, and the dressing is applied in much the same way. The central portion of the release paper is removed and the dressing is placed in position before the two outer pieces of paper are removed. Green adhesive handles of a thicker plastic material are attached to two opposite edges of the dressing; these facilitate correct application and overcome the problem of wrinkling, which was experienced with the earlier presentation.

Tegaderm

The film is sandwiched between a sheet of release paper on the adhesive side and a thin card on the outer surface. The card is cut through approximately 12 mm from the outer edge, forming a border surrounding a central panel. In use, the central portion of the card is removed and the release paper is peeled away from the adhesive surface, leaving the dressing suspended on a card 'frame' to give it stability. Once positioned over the wound, the dressing is applied and the carrier frame removed.

All the dressings are supplied sterile in paper/plastic peel pouches, in a range of different sizes. Larger sizes of Opsite, Opraflex and Dermafilm are also available for use as incise drapes, although these generally have modified application systems.

PHYSICAL PROPERTIES OF FILM DRESSINGS

The physical properties of the films used in these dressings are important because they have a direct influence on the clinical performance of the products. Six of the dressings described above have been reviewed previously[9] and the major aspects of their performance identified and compared. These include:

- thickness and weight of film,
- extensibility of film,
- moisture vapour permeability,
- gaseous permeability,
- tissue compatibility.

The thickness of the film will influence both the permeability and extensibility of the final dressing. An elastic film that requires a relatively high force to bring about a small extension may, when placed over a joint, restrict movement or cause tissue damage by a shearing effect;[10] a more extensible product will tend to stretch or move with the joint, allowing maximum mobility whilst reducing the possibility of skin damage. Although the majority of the dressings examined[9] were similar in performance in this respect, one product – Dermafilm – gave results for residual tension after stretching that were significantly higher than the rest. This suggests that Dermafilm should not be applied under tension, and should be used with care on sites that are subject to flexing, such as knees and elbows, particularly in elderly patients or those with fragile skin.

Moisture vapour permeability

One of the principal advantages claimed for the film dressings is that they permit the passage of excess exudate away from the surface of the wound in the form of water vapour. In the laboratory,[9] the permeability of six of the dressings described previously was found to range from 436 to 862 g/m^2/24 hours – equivalent to 18–35 g/m^2/hour.

Dressing	MVP g/m^2/24hr
Opsite	862
Bioclusive	605
Tegaderm	846
Ensure-it	436
Opraflex	477
Dermafilm	472

However, as the water vapour loss from uncovered wounds has been reported to vary from 3400 to 5200 g/m^2/24 hours (140–215 g/m^2/hour),[11] such relatively small variations are unlikely to be significant in this situation. Even with the most permeable of the products, it has been reported that large volumes of exudate often accumulate beneath the dressing, and may leak from around the edge unless they are aspirated with a syringe. The problems of excess fluid production from donor sites were addressed by Richmond and Sutherland,[12] who demonstrated that the intravenous administration of ethamsylate (1g) immediately after the induction of anaethesia reduced the accumulation of liquid beneath an Opsite dressing. (Ethamsylate is a haemostatic agent which reduces haemorrhage from small blood vessels by increasing platelet adhesiveness.) In contrast, intact skin transpires water vapour at a rate varying between 10 and 80g/m^2/hour. It has been shown that with a transpiration rate of 60g/m^2/hour through skin, only about 20 g/m^2/hour is lost through an Opsite dressing, and therefore some two-thirds of the total transpired water vapour are sequestered under the film.[13] Accumulations of sweat and secretions beneath a dressing – on the intact skin surrounding a wound – are likely to reduce the performance of the material, leading to failure of the adhesive bond and the formation of wrinkles, through which bacteria may reach the area of the wound.[14] Alternatively, exudate may accumulate under the wrinkled dressing, causing irritant dermatitis.[10] Excess moisture beneath a dressing may also produce tissue maceration and an increase in the bioburden of the skin, thereby increasing the possibility of wound infection. It is in this context that the differences in the moisture vapour permeability of the various dressings are likely to become important.

Smith & Nephew has announced a new version of Opsite designed specifically to overcome these problems. Opsite™ I.V. 3000 is manufactured from a hydrophilic polyurethane coated with an acrylic emulsion adhesive which is applied in regular pattern on the surface of the dressing. The film is much more permeable than that used in the standard Opsite, and thus allows water to evaporate much more rapidly from the patient's skin – reducing the risk of infection. At the present time the dressing is intended specifically for use as a cannula dressing, but it is likely that larger sizes will be introduced for wound management in due course.

Gaseous permeability

In his early work on film dressings, Winter[15] found that the rate of epidermal wound healing in his animal model varied with the oxygen permeability of the film he used. Under polyethylene film, 90% of the wound surface was covered by new epidermis in three days; under polypropylene film, which has 60% of the permeability of polyethylene, only 70% wound cover was achieved in the same time; and under polyester, which has only 1% of the permeability of polyethylene, 52% of the wound surface was covered with new epithelium. From these observations, Winter concluded that, for rapid epithelialisation, a dressing with high oxygen permeability is required. Similar findings were reported by Silver,[16] who recorded the partial pressures of oxygen beneath different types of dressings in the treatment of superficial wounds. Under polyethylene film the oxygen concentration was relatively high (123 mmHg) but under polyester it was very low (21 mmHg). Pure oxygen directed onto the surface of each dressing resulted in an increase in the oxygen concentration beneath, but once again the size of the increase was proportional to the permeability of the film. Like Winter, Silver concluded that the rate of migration of epidermal cells under occlusive dressings is related to the oxygen permeability of the film: the greater the permeability, the faster the rate of epithelial growth.

The presence of bacteria in a wound can also have an important effect upon oxygen concentration. Silver showed that the common skin pathogens, *Proteus, Pseudomonas* and *Staphylococcus* spp. brought about a considerable reduction in oxygen tension, followed by epidermal cell detachment; this effect was detectable long before any signs of clinical infection were evident.

Later work by Silver[17] and others has shown that the concentration of oxygen beneath commercial film dressings on heavily exuding wounds is very low. It is likely that that much of the oxygen that does penetrate through the dressing is rapidly metabolised by bacteria or neutrophils before it can exert any beneficial action on the wound itself.

The results of the laboratory study referred to previously[9] indicate that the permeability of the dressings currently available ranges from 0.5 to 2 L/m^2/24 hours. A sample of polyethylene film tested at the same time had a permeability of 1.8 L/m^2/24 hours.

Dressing	Oxygen permeability
Opsite	1.84
Bioclusive	1.65
Tegaderm	2.00
Ensure-it	0.88
Opraflex	0.78
Dermafilm	0.54
Polyethylene	1.79

In view of the findings of Winter and Silver, the differences in permeability of the various dressings may have important implications for the healing rates of the wounds to which they are applied.

Equally important is the permeability of the film to carbon dioxide. Wounds that are exposed to the air or covered with a very permeable dressing may become progressively more alkaline as the carbon dioxide is lost to the environment; this too can have important implications for wound healing. The importance of the permeability of dressings to both moisture vapour and other gases has been discussed in more detail in chapter 2.

Tissue compatibility

Any material that comes into contact with a wound should not liberate any agent that may be toxic or have any adverse effect upon the healing process. A useful technique for detecting the presence of such agents is cell culture, which provides a rapid sensitive screening method that can be performed in the laboratory. It is sometimes possible to induce cells to grow upon the surface of some film dressings, which suggests that the products concerned are free of any acute toxicity and would be unlikely to cause problems in the clinical situation. When the tissue compatibility of six film dressings was determined in the laboratory,[9] the dressings were found to vary significantly in their ability to support the growth of mouse connective tissue fibroblasts (L 929). On three of the dressings – Ensure-it, Tegaderm and Dermiflex – the cells were able to form a continuous monolayer on the film with no evidence of any inhibition. Growth on Bioclusive was partially inhibited and no growth at all was seen on Opraflex or Opsite. When extracts of the films were tested for inhibitory activity, only Opsite showed evidence of cytotoxicity at the dilutions used.

The clinical significance of these findings is uncertain. In principle, it would seem preferable to select a product that is apparently free from the toxic effects described above; however, the wealth of published data describing the successful use of Opsite in wound management suggests that the cytotoxicity demonstrated in the laboratory (which is believed to be associated with a component of the adhesive system) is likely to be of only limited relevance *in vivo*.

EFFECT OF SEMIPERMEABLE FILM DRESSINGS ON SKIN BACTERIA

By virtue of their semipermeable nature, all the film dressings are claimed to provide a barrier to bacteria; and this property is easily demonstrated in the laboratory. In a study into the effects of a number of different dressing materials on the growth of pathogenic bacteria and the re-epithelialisation of superficial wounds,[18] a series of standard wounds (made on human volunteers) were inoculated with heavy cultures of *Staph. aureus, Ps. aeruginosa, Staph. epidermidis* and *Streptococcus pyogenes*. The wounds were covered with the test dressings and quantitative cultures taken after 6, 24 and 48 hours. The results were expressed relative to 'Saran', an impermeable plastic film which acted as a control. The authors concluded that, in the test system used, there was no significant difference in the healing rates recorded beneath any of the materials examined (including the control). However, the number of micro-organisms recovered from beneath the dressings varied according to species and the time of sampling. With the exception of *Ps. aeruginosa*, the number of organisms isolated from the Opsite-covered wounds tended to be significantly lower than those recorded beneath the other semipermeable films (which were not significantly different from those found under the impermeable control).

The ability of a film dressing to act as a bacterial barrier was investigated in an animal study, in which standard wounds on a pig were dressed with Opsite, Vigilon™ and Duoderm™ (Granuflex™).[14] Both the dressing itself and the skin immediately around the perimeter were challenged with suspensions of bacteria (*Staph.*

aureus and *Ps. aeruginosa*) on one, two or three occasions; on removal of the dressings, the wounds were examined for the presence of the test organisms. Although the hydrocolloid dressing, Duoderm, prevented the ingress of both organisms in all the tests, Opsite and Vigilon failed to prevent contamination of 50% of the wounds challenged with *Staph. aureus* and all the wounds challenged with *Ps. aeruginosa*. This failure was considered to be due to bacteria gaining access from the edge of the dressing (through wrinkles or channels formed beneath the film), rather than by direct penetration through the film itself. It was also noted that the total number of normal skin organisms beneath Opsite was reduced, compared with the other dressings. A laboratory comparison of the antimicrobial properties of Opsite and Tegaderm revealed that, although both dressings appeared to possess some intrinsic antimicrobial properties,[19] Opsite was significantly more active than Tegaderm against a range of different organisms. The *in-vivo* activity of the films was investigated in a further study, in which the antibacterial effects of Opsite, Tegaderm and Ensure-it were compared on the skin of volunteers (the bacterial bioburden of which was artificially raised by occlusion).[20] Once again, it was found that Opsite was the only product that had any significant antimicrobial effect, producing a 2×10^3 reduction in numbers compared with the control. The antimicrobial properties of Opsite are thought to be due to an ingredient present in the adhesive which is also responsible for the effects upon the fibroblasts described previously. The identity of this chemical has not been disclosed by the manufacturer and no formal claims for antimicrobial activity have ever been made for the product.

Omiderm

A film dressing developed in Israel by Omikron Scientific, Rehovot, is now marketed in UK by Perstorp. Omiderm™ consists of a hydrophilic membrane 40 µm thick, which is made from polyurethane onto which have been grafted hydrophilic groups such as acrylamide and hydroxyethylmethacrylate. The film is relatively inelastic when dry, but, once wet, it will rapidly absorb water and become very elastic and conformable. It is very permeable to moisture vapour (in the order of 5000 g/m^2/24 hours), and also permits the passage of water-soluble antimicrobial agents. Unlike the films described previously, Omiderm is not coated with an adhesive layer; when applied to an exuding wound in the dry state, the film will rapidly absorb moisture and adhere to the surface without the need for any secondary retention materials. When applied to clean non-infected wounds, such as donor sites or partial thickness burns, the dressing may be left in position until the wound is healed – at which time the film will dry out and separate spontaneously. If applied to dirty or infected wounds the dressing should be changed every 12 or 24 hours. The physical properties of the film, together with the results of an animal study, were described by Behar et al.,[21] who demonstrated that an ointment containing neomycin, bacitracin and hydrocortisone, which was applied to the outer surface of the film on contaminated experimental burns in rats, produced highly significant reductions in the number of viable organisms present in the wound.

The clinical use of the dressing in the treatment of wounds (particularly donor sites, chronic wounds, ulcers and burns) was described by Golan et al.,[22] and Cristofoli et al.,[23] who concluded that, overall, Omiderm was easy to use, and that it reduced pain and prevented infection. It was considered to be particularly useful in the management of donor sites and superficial dermal burns.

COMPOSITE FILM DRESSINGS

The following two composite film dressings have been developed.

- Tegaderm™ Pouch Dressing – 3M,
- Transigen™ – Smith & Nephew.

Tegaderm Pouch Dressing

The dressing consists of a thin transparent polyurethane film coated with an acrylic adhesive system. The central portion of the film is perforated and a second smaller piece of similar film is sealed to the centre of the outer surface, forming a pouch. When the dressing is applied to an exuding wound, exudate passes through the holes in the inner film into the pouch, from where the aqueous component evaporates and passes through the outer film as water vapour. A limited clinical assessment of Tegaderm Pouch Dressing was carried out by Barnes and Malone–Lee,[24]

who concluded that (for financial reasons) it would be inappropriate to use the new product on low exudate wounds, though the improved fluid control offered by the pouch could be of value on more heavily exuding wounds.

Transigen

This product, which is currently undergoing further development by Smith & Nephew, is a three-component dressing. It consists of a thin non-woven absorbent fleece, contained in a pouch formed between an outer hydrophilic polyurethane film and an adhesive wound contact layer. Numerous slits in the inner layer allow the passage of exudate through to the absorbent fabric, where it is retained until the aqueous component is lost as water vapour through the back of the dressing. The nature of the plastic film forming the outer layer is such that its permeability to moisture vapour increases in the presence of liquid, only to decrease once again as the fluid is lost by evaporation. The dressing is therefore claimed to exert some positive control over the local wound environment.

Both composite film dressings are indicated for use on wounds that produce larger volumes of exudate that could not be contained by the simple adhesive film products described previously.

MEDICATED FILM DRESSINGS

In a lecture in 1870, Lister spoke of a transparent film (possibly collodion) which had been brought to his attention, and which could be produced containing a range of medicaments. Somewhat suprisingly, however, he could see little value in its use and dismissed the idea somewhat arbitrarily. In more recent times, medicated films have been more readily accepted, and incise drapes containing iodine and chlorhexidine have become widely used. This has led to the development of film dressings that contain antimicrobial agents incorporated into the adhesive mass.

The two medicated dressings available at the present time are Tegaderm Plus™ (3M) and Opsite CH™ (Smith & Nephew). Both dressings are primarily intended as catheter dressings. Tegaderm Plus is similar in appearance and method of application to standard Tegaderm but the adhesive contains 2% available iodine in the form of an iodophor. Opsite CH is medicated with chlorhexidine acetate (5% w/w of the adhesive mass) and is available in two forms: a standard presentation is available in two sizes for dressing central or peripheral catheter sites, and a special version (Opsite CH Cannula Dressing) is available for application over cannulae that bear injection ports. In the latter presentation, that portion of the dressing that covers the wings and surrounds the port of the cannula is reinforced with a second thicker adhesive plastic film, to ensure that the dressing does not become displaced once in position, but the remainder of the film is transparent and allows visual inspection of the site without disturbing the dressing. Although no specific claims are made for the chlorhexidine, it is implied that this will impart antimicrobial activity to the dressing and thus help to reduce the likelihood of infection.

CLINICAL USE OF FILM DRESSINGS

Over the years, Opsite and other film dressings have been used successfully in the treatment of burns and donor sites,[25-30] decubitus ulcers,[31] and post-operative wounds,[32-33] and the management of arterial and venous catheter sites.[34-35]

Neal et al.[36] reported that, in a trial involving 51 patients with partial thickness burns, wounds dressed with Opsite healed significantly faster than comparable wounds dressed with a paraffin gauze containing chlorhexidine (Bactigras™). Using a questionnaire and a multi-directional scaling technique, the authors also found that patients on whom Opsite was used experienced less pain and inconvenience than those dressed with tulle gras. In addition, considerable cost savings were achieved by the use of the film dressing.

In 1982, two semipermeable film dressings (Opsite and Tegaderm) were compared with fine mesh gauze in a controlled trial as a dressing for donor sites.[37] In all, 26 scalp sites and 34 other sites were compared. It was found that, overall, scalp sites healed faster than non-scalp sites (4.9 vs 9 days) but scalp sites dressed with Opsite and Tegaderm were ready to reharvest after 5 days, compared with 12 days when dressed with fine mesh gauze. Using film dressings, one patient was able to have a single site harvested four times in four weeks.

An early assessment of the use of a transparent film dressing for central venous catheter care was reported by Jarrard,[38] following a study involving 30 patients for a total of 938 catheter days. He concluded that the film had many advantages over traditional dressings: the wound was easily visible, and the dressing adhered well to the skin, required infrequent changing and induced no significant adverse effects. Similar findings were reported by Palidar et al.,[39] who compared Opsite and gauze for dressing hyperalimentation catheter sites. They reported that the use of Opsite saved both time and money and did not result in an increase in the rate of wound infection.

In a comparative trial into the use of Tegaderm and gauze following breast surgery in 120 patients,[40] staff and patients found that Tegaderm was easier to apply and more comfortable to wear. Visual inspection of the wound was possible at all times and patients could bath or wash with no adverse effects upon the dressing. The appearance of the healed wound was also improved by the use of the film. It was estimated that the cost of the dressing treatment was less than one-third of the cost of using gauze.

A semipermeable film dressing was compared with gauze coated with lanolin for the treatment of skin reactions following radiotherapy.[41] Although the authors only detected a non-significant trend towards a decrease in healing time in wounds dressed with the film, it was considered that there were other benefits to be obtained from its use. The film dressing required less frequent replacement and did not need to be removed prior to therapy. It was was also said to be less bulky, and cause less pain upon removal, than the lanolin-impregnated gauze.

A significant amount of data has also been produced describing both the physical properties of the dressings and the micro-environment that exists beneath them when they are applied to burns and donor sites.[13,19,20,42,43] The studies by Buchan et al.,[42,43] and Alper et al.[44] showed that, although the concentrations of electrolytes and proteins in the fluid that collected beneath Opsite dressings fell into the normal range of blood values, there were significant differences in other measurements. In particular, the number of white blood cells was found to be some 30 times greater in wound exudate than in burn blister fluid, and significantly higher than in blood taken from the same patient. In contrast, glucose levels in wound exudate were lower than those in burn blister fluid and circulating blood. One possible explanation is that glucose is consumed by the elevated numbers of white cells present (which are probably also responsible for the rapid removal of oxygen from the exudate, as described previously). The similarity between the compositions of blood and exudate suggests that beneath the film dressing there exists a relatively free diffusion of ions from the circulatory system to the surface of the wound. In a recent study, dilutions of moist wound healing fluid (collected from beneath Opsite dressings applied to cutaneous ulcers) were added to a synchronised fibroblast cell culture system. It was found that, although the highest concentrations of wound healing fluid had an adverse effect upon the cell system, dilutions prepared with serum appeared to enhance cell growth – possibly owing to the presence of materials such as platelet-derived growth factors.[44] It is possible that these (as yet unidentified) agents are responsible, at least in part, for the beneficial effects associated with the use of film dressings.

INDICATIONS FOR THE USE OF FILM DRESSINGS

The exact position of the film dressings in wound management is not easy to define, and some of the indications for which they were originally recommended are now perhaps better addressed by newer wound management materials. However, there is little doubt that the films are of value for dressing surgical wounds and protecting the site of insertion of in-dwelling catheters. They can also be used with advantage in the treatment of superficial partial thickness burns and early decubitus ulcers, where they serve a protective function. Indeed, a significant proportion of all film dressings purchased are used to aid in the prevention of skin damage due to friction on sites that are liable to break down and form ulcerated areas.

For all these applications, the films offer a number of advantages over traditional dressings. They are highly conformable, convenient to use, and permit constant observation of the wound, whilst providing a warm moist wound-healing environment. Like all dressing materials, however, they do have their limitations: they are not well suited for application to large heavily exuding wounds, and are probably not indicated for the treatment of chronic leg ulcers.

REFERENCES

1. Elliot I.M.Z., *A Short History of Surgical Dressings*, London, Pharmaceutical Press, 1964.
2. Bloom H., Cellophane dressing for second degree burns, *Lancet,* 1945, **2**, 559.
3. Bull J.P. *et al.,* Experiments with occlusive dressings of a new plastic, *ibid.,* 1948, **2**, 213–215.
4. Schilling R.S.F. *et al.,* Clinical trial of occlusive plastic dressings, *ibid.,* 1950, **1**, 293–296.
5. Winter G.D., Formation of the scab and the rate of epithelization of superficial wounds in the skin of the young domestic pig, *Nature,* 1962, **193**, 293–294.
6. Hinman C.D. *et al.,* Effect of air exposure and occlusion on experimental human skin wounds, *ibid.,* 1963, **200**, 377–379.
7. Myers J.A., Ease of use of two semipermeable adhesive membranes compared, *Pharm. J.,* 1984, **233**, 685–686.
8. Haessler R.M., Transparent IV dressing vs. traditional dressings, *J. natn. intraven. Ther. Ass.,* 1983, **6**, 169–171.
9. Thomas S. *et al.,* Comparative review of the properties of 6 semipermeable film dressings, *Pharm. J.,* 1988, **240**, 785–789.
10. Alper J.C., Recent advances in moist wound healing, *Sth. med. J.,* 1986, **79**, 1398–1404.
11. Lamke L.O. *et al.,* The evaporative water loss from burns and water vapour permeability of grafts and artificial membranes used in the treatment of burns, *Burns,* 1977, **3** , 159–165.
12. Richmond J.D. and Sutherland A.B., A new approach to the problems encountered with Opsite as a donor site dressing; systemic ethamsylate, *Br. J. plast. Surg.,* 1986, **39**, 516–518.
13. May R.S., Physiological activity from an occlusive wound dressing, in *Wound Healing Symposium,* Lawrence J.C. (ed.), Proceedings of a Symposium, Birmingham, 1982, Oxford, Medicine Publishing Foundation, 1983, 35–49.
14. Mertz P.M. *et al.,* Occlusive wound dressings to prevent bacterial invasion and wound infection, *J. Am. Acad. Derm.,* 1985, **12**, 662–668.
15. Winter G.D., Epidermal regeneration studied in the domestic pig, in *Epidermal Wound Healing,* Maibach H.I. and Rovee D.T. (eds), Chicago, Year Book Medical Publishers, 1974, 71–112.
16. Silver I.A., Oxygen tension and epithelialization, in Ref. 15, 291–305.
17. Silver I.A., Oxygen and tissue repair, in *An Environment for Healing: The Role of Occlusion,* Ryan T.J. (ed.), International Congress and Symposium Series No.88, London, Royal Society of Medicine, 1985, 15–19.
18. Katz S. *et al.,* Semipermeable occlusive dressings, *Arch. Derm.,* 1986, **122**, 58–62.
19. Holland K.T. *et al.,* A comparison of the *in-vitro* antibacterial and complement activating effect of Opsite

and Tegaderm dressings, *J. Hosp. Infect.*, 1984, **5**, 323–328.

20. Holland K.T. *et al.*, A comparison of the *in-vivo* antibacterial effects of Opsite, Tegaderm and Ensure dressings, *ibid.*, 1985, **6**, 299–303.

21. Behar D. *et al.*, Omiderm, a new synthetic wound covering: physical properties and drug permeability studies, *J. biomed. Mat. Res.*, 1986, **20**, 731–738.

22. Golan J. *et al.*, A new temporary synthetic skin substitute, *Burns*, 1985, **11**, 274–280.

23. Cristofoli C. *et al.*, The use of Omiderm, a new skin substitute, in a burn unit, *ibid.*, 1986, **12**, 587–591.

24. Barnes K.E. and Malone-Lee J., Tegaderm Pouch Dressing, *Nurs. Times,* 1985, **81**, 45–46.

25. James J.H. and Watson A.C.H., The use of Opsite, a vapour permeable dressing, on skin graft donor sites, *Br. J. plast. Surg.*, 1975, **28**, 107–110.

26. Bergman R.B., A new treatment of split-skin graft donor sites, *Arch. Chir. neerl.*, 1977, **29**, 69–72.

27. Lobe T.E. *et al.*, An improved method of wound management for pediatric patients, *J. pediat. Surg.*, 1980, **15**, 886–889.

28. Dinner M.I. *et al.*, Use of semipermeable polyurethane membrane as a dressing for split-skin graft donor sites, *Plast. reconstr. Surg.*, 1979, **64**, 112–114.

29. Barnett A. *et al.*, Comparison of synthetic adhesive moisture vapour permeable and fine mesh gauze dressings for split-thickness skin graft donor sites, *Am. J. Surg.*, 1983, **145**, 379–381.

30. Conkle W., Opsite dressing: new approach to burn care, *J. emerg. Nurs.*, 1981, **7**, 148–152.

31. Braverman A.M. and Nasar M.A., The treatment of superficial decubitus ulcers, *Practitioner,* 1981, **225**, 1842–1843.

32. Drake D., Surgical wound management with adhesive polyurethane membrane, *Ann. R. Coll. Surg.,* 1984, **66**, 74–75.

33. Tinckler L., Surgical wound management with adhesive polyurethane membrane: a preferred method for routine usage, *ibid.,* 1983, **65**, 257–259.

34. Bragg V. and Martin C., Polyurethane film dressing, *J. enterostom. Ther.,* 1983, **10**, 185–186.

35. Peterson P.J. and Freeman P.T., Use of a transparent polyurethane dressing for peripheral intravenous catheter care, *J. nation. intraven. Ther. Ass.,* 1982, **5**, 387–390.

36. Neal D.E. *et al.*, The effects of an adherent polyurethane film and conventional absorbent dressing in patients with small partial thickness burns, *Br. J. clin. Pract.,* 1981, **35**, 254–257.

37. Barnett A. *et al.*, Scalp as a skin graft donor site – repeated rapid re-use with synthetic adhesive moisture vapour permeable dressings, Paper presented to a meeting of the American Burns Association, Boston, MA, May 1982.

38. Jarrard M., Use of a transparent polyurethane dressing (Opsite) for central venous catheter care, Paper presented to the fourth Clinical Congress of the American Society for Parenteral and Enteral Nutrition, Chicago, IL, 30 January–2 February, 1980.

39. Palidar P.J. *et al.*, Use of Opsite as an occlusive dressing for total parenteral nutrition catheters, *J. parent. ent. Nutr.,* 1982, **6**, 150–151.

40. Moshakis V. *et al.*, Tegaderm versus gauze dressing in breast surgery, *Br. J. clin. Pract.,* 1984, **38**, 149–152.

41. Shell J.A. *et al.*, Comparison of moisture vapour permeable (MVP) dressings to conventional dressings for management of radiation skin reactions, *Oncol. Nurs. Forum* 1986, **13**, 11–16.

42. Buchan I.A. *et al.*, Laboratory investigation of the composition and properties of pig skin wound exudate under Opsite, *Burns,* 1981, **8**, 39–46.

43. Buchan I.A. *et al.*, Clinical and laboratory investigation of the composition and properties of human skin wound exudate under semi-permeable dressings, *ibid.,* 1981, **7**, 326–334.

44. Alper J.C. *et al.*, The *in vitro* response of fibroblasts to the fluid that accumulates under a vapor-permeable membrane, *J. invest. Derm.,* 1985, **84**, 513–515.

Chapter 5

Foam Dressings

Probably the first 'cellular' or 'foam' materials to be used in wound management were naturally occuring marine sponges, similar to those found in the Mediterranean region. An interesting account of the history of these materials in medicine is given by Elliot,[1] who describes their use as absorbents, haemostats and simple cleansing aids. Despite their popularity, they were apparently not without their critics, as they were identified as potent sources of wound infection, being difficult both to cleanse and to sterilise. It was also recorded that when used as dressings, they stuck badly to the surface of wounds.

In 1884, Joseph Gamgee exhibited an 'artificial antiseptic absorbent sponge' composed of gauze, cotton and coconut fibre, in the centre of which was placed a capsule of glass or gelatin (Fig. 5-1). Immediately prior to use the capsule was broken and the antiseptic released.[2] It is interesting to note that these materials were prepared for Gamgee by Burroughs Wellcome & Co., an organisation that later gave rise to the Wellcome Foundation (which, through its Calmic Medical Division, still has a very active interest in the use of foam as a surgical dressing). Despite some interest in the development of artificial sponges in the 1950s – primarily for use in surgery – the potential value of dressings made from foam was not recognised until the 1970s, when both Silastic™ Foam and Lyofoam™ were first used in wound management. These two products proved to be the forerunners of a small range of foam materials, which possess a number of the properties of an ideal dressing as identified in chapter 2. Specifically, they provide thermal insulation, do not shed fibres or particles, are easily cut or shaped, and help to maintain a moist environment at the surface of the wound. They are also gas-permeable, non-adherent, light, and comfortable to wear; in some cases they are able to cope with significant volumes of exudate.

The foam dressings available in the UK are as follows.

- Silastic Foam – Calmic,
- Lyofoam – Ultra,
- Allevyn™ – Smith & Nephew,
- Intrasite™ Cavity Wound Dressing – Smith & Nephew.

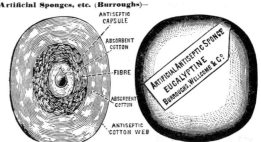

Figure 5-1 Artificial medicated sponge *circa* 1884 (*courtesy of Wellcome*).

In addition to the above, the manufacture of two other foam products – Synthaderm™ and Coraderm™ – previously marketed by Armour, has temporarily been discontinued whilst a new distributor is found.

The properties and uses of these materials are described in more detail below.

SILASTIC FOAM

Silastic Foam dressing is a two-component product that vulcanises at room temperature; it is presented in the form of two liquids, a viscous medical-grade poly(dimethylsiloxane) base and a stannous octanoate catalyst. Because the base is in the form of a suspension, it has a tendency to separate on storage. In order to ensure consistent results, the base should be thoroughly mixed before being removed from the container. The actual dressing, or 'stent', is prepared in situ (in the wound). The two components are measured out (in the ratio of 10 mL of base to 0.6 mL of catalyst), using appropriate sized syringes, immediately prior to use. The two liquids are stirred together in a suitable container for about 15 seconds, and the mixture is then poured directly into the wound cavity. The reaction begins immediately, and the liquid expands to approximately four times its original volume, owing to the release of hydrogen gas. The mixture sets rapidly to form a soft, resilient, open-cell foam that is able to absorb exudate from the surface of the wound. The process takes about three minutes from the initial mixing to the formation of the finished dressing.

Once set, the stent will usually remain in position in a deep wound without the need for bandages or secondary dressings. As healing takes place and the wound becomes more shallow, the stent may be held in position by one or two pieces of surgical tape.

If the foam is allowed to set in contact with intact skin or a smooth or shiny surface, the facing layer of the stent will be smooth, have sealed pores, and be unable to absorb fluid. A similar problem is sometimes encountered in wounds that have a particularly shiny surface. In these circumstances, Calmic have suggested in the past that the wound should be covered with a thin layer of shaving foam before the dressing is prepared. Once formed, the dressing is removed, and both the stent and the surface of the wound are cleansed to remove any soapy residues.

A Silastic Foam stent may often be used for a week, or even longer, provided a simple routine of wound toilet is adopted. The dressing should be removed from the wound twice a day and soaked in a solution of a suitable antiseptic agent, such as chlorhexidine gluconate 0.5% (e.g. a ten-fold dilution of Hibitane™ 5% Concentrate). The stent should be left in the antiseptic solution for a minimum of 10–15 minutes,[3] during which time the patient may wash the wound or take a bath as appropriate. Once the dressing has been adequately disinfected, it must be rinsed very thoroughly under a running tap, with repeated gentle squeezing, to remove all traces of the antiseptic. After a final squeeze to express any remaining water, the dressing can be replaced in the wound. Other antiseptic solutions may also be used: chlorhexidine 0.5% in spirit (where the supply of an aqueous solution can be a problem), or cetrimide 1%. As both of these materials have cytostatic properties, it is important to ensure that all traces are removed from the dressing before reinsertion. Residues of antiseptic in the dressing have been shown to be responsible for irritation of the wound and surrounding skin.[4]

The twice-daily cleansing routine may be varied according to the condition of the wound. Heavily exuding or infected wounds may require more frequent cleansing but, as healing progresses and the amount of exudate becomes less, daily cleansing may be sufficient. As cavity wounds heal and reduce in depth, the use of stents may no longer be appropriate. Although Calmic also produce Silastic Foam in pre-formed flat sheets, at this stage in the healing process, a change to an alternative dressing may be considered more appropriate.

Clinical use of Silastic Foam

Silastic Foam was originally developed by Dow Corning in the 1950s, but it was first used medically in 1962, as a diagnostic aid in the detection of sigmoid cancer. The catalysed base was inserted – as an enema – into the colon, where it expanded and set, taking up the shape and surface characteristics of the gut wall. The resultant cast could provide the surgeon with a useful indication of the presence of a diseased state. This highly novel application of the material became less frequently used with the advent of new instrumentation and improved radiological techniques. The material continued to be used in medicine, however: the soft resilient texture of the cured foam made it well suited to securing skin grafts, particulary in awkward anatomical sites.

The use of Silastic Foam as a primary wound dressing was first reported in 1975, following the treatment of 40 pilonidal sinus excisions in 1972–3. It was found that, compared with traditional treatment regimens, wounds dressed with foam healed faster and patients left hospital much earlier.[5] The successful use of the dressing in this area gave rise to its still-familiar nickname of 'the bung'. This initial publication was followed by a further report[6] of its use in the treatment of 250 patients with a variety of granulating wounds including sacral pressure areas, perineal wounds and abdominal wall breakdown. The results of this study demonstrated that the use of Silastic Foam resulted in increased patient comfort and a reduction in the time required for routine nursing care. A number of similar studies of the use of Silastic Foam in granulating wounds are reported elsewhere,[7,8] and a number of authors have described its use in specific wound types, including donor sites,[9] pressure sores,[10] amputation stump wounds,[11] enterocutaneous[12] and oro-cutaneous fistulae,[13] hidradenitis suppurativa,[14–16] scar control,[17] pinnaplasty,[18,19] epidermoid cancer of the cheek,[20] penile dressings,[21,22] fungating breast wounds,[23] and skin graft fixation.[24]

In addition, two studies have been reported in which the cost of Silastic Foam treatment was compared with that of other dressing materials. A detailed comparison of the cost of treatment of perineal wounds with gauze packs and Silastic Foam was carried out by Culyer et al.,[25] who concluded somewhat non-committally that the 'relative cheapness of foam elastomer was a fairly robust result'. A more positive statement was made by Young and Wheeler,[26] who compared the costs of Silastic Foam and dextranomer beads (Debrisan™) in the treatment of 50 patients with surgical wound breakdown. They concluded that, although the two treatments were apparently equivalent in terms of healing time and patient comfort, the cost of treatment with Debrisan was significantly greater than that with Silastic Foam.

The vast majority of wounds that were treated with foam in the papers cited above were acute or post-surgical; it would appear that this is the area in which the use of Silastic Foam is likely to be of most benefit. The evidence for the product's value in chronic wounds is less convincing; it may well be that for the management of ulcers, for example, the use of alternative materials would be more appropriate.

The major advantages claimed for Silastic Foam are its versatility, a high degree of patient acceptability, and its ease and convenience of use. Many patients are able to manage their own wounds and can therefore be discharged from hospital or allowed to return to work earlier than might otherwise have been the case. Although Silastic Foam is expensive on a unit cost basis, overall treatment costs are not excessively high, as a single dressing may last for a week or more.

Note on the toxicity of Silastic Foam

A recent report in the scientific press has questioned the biological safety of certain chemicals used in plastic manufacture.[27] Although these chemicals are not found in Silastic Foam, one of them is related to a theoretical breakdown product of the catalytic reaction by which the foam is formed. As a result, the US Environmental Protection Agency requested further pre-clinical testing of these chemicals. The manufacturers of Silastic Foam in the USA (Dow Corning) therefore decided, for industrial and commercial reasons, that they would suspend production of the dressing until this information became available.

Silastic Foam was formulated in the United States but the clinical applications were developed in Britain, where it has been used clinically for 16 years and commercially available for eight. During this time, there have been no causally related adverse effects from the use of the material, and the dressing is regarded by leading UK surgical centres as a major advance in the field of wound management. In the light of all the available evidence, neither Dow Corning nor Calmic believed that Silastic Foam posed a significant risk to human health; Calmic therefore continued to market the dressing, whilst conducting further toxicological studies and an in-depth review of all the available scientific data. This work has now been completed and no evidence of any adverse effects resulting from the use of Silastic Foam have been detected. As a result, manufacture of the foam has been recommenced. In view of the versatility and proven cost-effectiveness of Silastic Foam — and the lack of any evidence of toxicity associated with its use —

it would be unfortunate if this unique and valuable dressing were to be withdrawn from the market.

LYOFOAM

Lyofoam evolved from an unsuccessful product called 'Sterafoam' which was manufactured by Bowater Scott. This material had a large open-cell structure, such that exudate and granulation tissue rapidly became incorporated into the cells, causing the dressing to adhere strongly to the wound. It was recognised that some modification to the surface of the dressing was required in order to overcome this problem; as a result of further research and cooperation between Lyo Research International and Dr George Winter of the Institute of Orthopaedics in Stanmore, Lyofoam was eventually developed. Since that time, Lyofoam has undergone several changes of ownership but it is currently owned and marketed by Ultra.

Lyofoam consists of a soft, hydrophobic, open-cell polyurethane foam sheet approximately 8 mm thick. The surface that is to be placed in contact with the wound has been modified, by the application of heat and pressure, to collapse the cells of the foam (Figs 5-2 and 5-3), allowing them to take up liquid by capillary action. The dressing is freely permeable to gases and water vapour but resists the penetration of liquids owing to the hydrophobic nature of the unmodified back. When brought into contact with blood or exudate, fluid is drawn up into the wound contact surface by capillary action and transferred, by this means, laterally across the face of the dressing. The aqueous component of the absorbed fluid evaporates into the larger cells in the back of the dressing and is lost as water vapour to the environment. As this process continues, the small pores in the facing layer of the dressing become progressively more occluded with a mixture of proteinaceous material and cellular debris. This results in the formation of a moist environment, which favours wound healing and auto-debridement by facilitating rehydration and liquefaction of necrotic tissue.

Lyofoam has good thermal insulating properties, and experiments have shown that the surface temperature of wounds dressed with this material is one or two degrees higher than that of comparable wounds dressed with gauze.

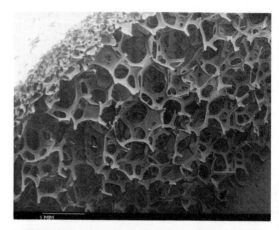

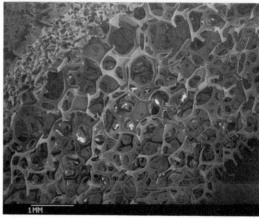

Figure 5-2 Section through Lyofoam Dressing showing collapsed cells of the wound contact layer ($\times$12).

Because Lyofoam is very permeable to moisture vapour, it is of little value in treating dry wounds covered with hard black eschar, unless this is first removed surgically or by some other means. Lyofoam dressings should be held in position with tape or a light bandage; secondary dressings are not usually required. The frequency with which the dressing is changed is governed by the state of the wound. Heavily exuding or very messy wounds may need to be dressed daily or even more frequently, but this may be reduced as healing progresses.

The effects of Lyofoam on the healing of wounds in pigs was determined by Winter,[28] who compared the healing rates of shallow cutaneous wounds dressed with Lyofoam with those of similar wounds dressed with cotton gauze. He

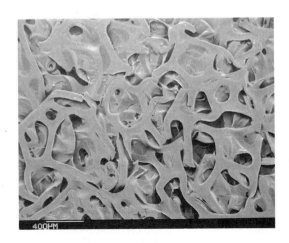

Figure 5-3   Wound contact layer of Lyofoam (×25).

showed that, after four days, wounds covered with the foam were almost completely healed whilst those dressed with gauze were only 56% healed; he concluded from these results that Lyofoam creates good conditions for tissue regeneration.

An early account of the use of Lyofoam dressings in the management of ten skin lesions, including surgical wounds and burns, was given by Baccari et al.,[29] who found Lyofoam to be convenient and easy to use (being absorbent and non-adherent, and promoting rapid wound healing which resulted in minimal scarring).

The use of Lyofoam in the treatment of four patients with leg ulcers has been described by Creevy,[30] who noted that the application of the dressing appeared to reduce pain in the wound. A more detailed evaluation of the use of Lyofoam plus compression in the treatment of 30 patients with leg ulcers was made by Mayerhausen and Kreis.[31] During the course of a six-week study, five patients were healed and 21 others were assessed as making moderate to good progress. Two patients failed to respond favourably to treatment and 4 patients were withdrawn because of pain, intolerance or deterioration. The authors concluded that Lyofoam accompanied by compression produced very promising results in the treatment of leg ulcers.

The largest and most comprehensive trial of Lyofoam dressings yet undertaken was carried out in the community,[32] and involved 200 patients with superficial granulating wounds that were less than 5 mm deep and in the last stage of healing.

Upon entry into the study, patients were randomly allocated into one of two groups: one group had their wounds dressed with Lyofoam, and the second with a perforated plastic film dressing (Melolin™). The cost of all the materials used was recorded, and a figure was also derived for nursing and administrative costs for each individual treatment. Subjective assessments of various aspects of the acceptability of each dressing were recorded by both nurse and patient, on a suitable analogue scale. Analysis of the results of the study revealed the Lyofoam dressing to be significantly less painful in use, and less likely to to adhere to the surface of the wound, than the perforated plastic film dressing.

Financial benefits could also result from the use of the foam, as savings could be demonstrated in both materials and staffing costs. Visits by the community nursing staff to patients treated with Lyofoam were found to be reduced in frequency and duration, compared with those made to patients in the control group. On the basis of these results, the authors suggested that the recent inclusion of Lyofoam in the Drug Tariff should produce significant benefits to patient care.

Larger sizes of Lyofoam are available for dressing burns, and a suitably shaped version is available as a tracheostomy dressing. Pads of polyurethane on thin foam bandages have also been developed for use as first-aid or casualty dressings.

Indications for the use of Lyofoam dressing

Lyofoam is an interesting and versatile material. The smaller sizes may be used as an alternative to perforated film dressings or tulle gras during the final stages of wound healing, whilst the larger sizes may be used in the treatment of ulcers and pressure areas.

SYNTHADERM AND CORADERM

Like Lyofoam, Synthaderm consists of a modified polyurethane foam with two surfaces that are structurally different. The lower hydrophilic surface (which is placed in contact with the wound) consists of a layer of open cells, whilst the upper hydrophobic surface is composed of closed cells. When Synthaderm is placed on the surface of an exuding wound, tissue fluid and exudate are taken up, but prevented from passing right through the dressing by the closed cells of the upper surface. The solid components of the exudate are retained within the foam but the aqueous component is partially lost to the environment by evaporation as moisture vapour. Wounds dressed with Synthaderm are thus maintained in a moist condition, which is said to be conducive to wound healing. It is a feature of the use of Synthaderm that, during the early stages of treatment, there is an apparent increase in exudate production; this may be associated with a slight increase in wound size, as any necrotic material is removed by autolysis. This is normal and should not give rise to concern, provided the dressing is changed frequently (daily or on alternate days). As the wound becomes cleaner, it should be possible to reduce the frequency of dressing changes, so that in the final stages of healing weekly changes are sufficient.

Anecdotal accounts of the use of Synthaderm in the treatment of leg ulcers have been given in the past;[33-35] more recently, a more formal trial has been carried out in 52 patients with pre-tibial lacerations.[36] The authors of the report claim that the results suggest that the wounds treated with Synthaderm healed more rapidly, and with reduced scarring.

The disadvantages of Synthaderm include its poor conformability, and loss of tensile strength when wet. In addition, it has a marked tendency to curl up and wrinkle when it comes into contact with moisture, and so must be bandaged firmly in position to prevent this occurring. The wrinkling is due to the fact that the dressing increases its surface area by almost 20% when wet. This increase in size is accompanied by a seven-fold increase in moisture vapour permeability; thus, to some extent, the permeability of the dressing is related to the moisture content of the wound.[37] Some of these problems are said to be overcome by the development of a second generation product, Coraderm (manufactured under the name Epi-lock™ in the USA). The use of this new material has been described by Wayne,[38] who compared it with a tulle-type dressing in the treatment of three common types of wound – partial thickness burns, deep abrasions, and selected lacerations. He concluded that – in terms of quality and rate of healing, and the patient's perception of pain – Epi-lock appeared to offer significant benefits over the tulle dressing.

Despite the claims that have been made for Synthaderm and Coraderm, and their theoretical advantages, there is little doubt that the dressings have not been widely accepted in practice.

ALLEVYN

Allevyn consists of a hydrophilic polyurethane foam that is backed with a moisture vapour-permeable polyurethane membrane. The surface of the dressing that is placed in contact with the wound is bonded onto an apertured polyurethane net (to render it less adherent in the event of the wound beginning to dry out).

By virtue of its hydrophilic nature, the foam is capable of absorbing large volumes of fluid (in the order of 1400 g/m^2/24hours), even when subjected to pressure. The fluid-handling capacity of the dressing is further enhanced by the presence of the vapour-permeable membrane, which allows a significant proportion of absorbed fluid to be lost (at a controlled rate) by evaporation through the back of the dressing, whilst preserving an effective bacterial barrier. As the wound heals and exudate production diminishes, this backing membrane also helps to prevent excessive dehydration of the wound surface.

Allevyn was originally sold as a burn dressing but its highly resilient nature made it difficult to retain on some anatomical sites. The product has now found a new lease of life as an ulcer dressing, although, as yet, no clinical evidence of its effectiveness has been published.

INTRASITE CAVITY WOUND DRESSING

The highly absorbent properties of the foam used in the manufacture of Allevyn have led to the development of a further product, which is intended to be an alternative to Silastic Foam for the management of cavity wounds (such as deep pressure areas, surgical incisions and excisions, and pilonidal sinus wounds). The dressing consists of chips of the foam encapsulated within a layer of thin, conformable, perforated polymeric film. The dressing is available in a range of shapes and sizes, and more than one dressing can be inserted into a wound at any one time if required. It is claimed that the dressing is easy and quick to change and provides a moist healing environment that prevents slough formation and promotes healing.

REFERENCES

1. Elliot I.M.Z., *A Short History of Surgical Dressings,* London, Pharmaceutical Press, 1964.

2. Gamgee S., A new sponge, *Lancet,* 1884, **1,** 795–796.

3. Thomas E. *et al.,* Silastic foam dressing – an evaluation of the disinfection procedure, *Br. J. pharm. Pract.,* 1983, **5,** 12–13.

4. Evans B.K. *et al.,* The disinfection of silicone foam dressings, *J. clin. Hosp. Pharm.,* 1985, **10,** 289–295.

5. Wood R.A.B. and Hughes L.E., Silicone foam sponge for pilonidal sinus: a new technique for dressing open granulating wounds, *Br. med. J.,* 1975, **3,** 131–133.

6. Wood R.A.B. *et al.,* Foam elastomer dressing in the management of open granulating wounds: experience with 250 patients, *Br. J. Surg.,* 1977, **64,** 554–557.

7. Smith R.C. *et al.,* Treatment of granulating wounds with Silastic foam dressings, *Austral. N. Z. J. Surg.,* 1981, **51,** 354–357.

8. MacFie J. and McMahon M.J., The management of the open perineal wound using a foam elastomer: a prospective clinical trial, *Br. J. Surg.,* 1980, **67,** 85–89.

9. Harding K.G. *et al.,* Silastic foam dressing for skin graft donor sites: a preliminary report, *Br. J. plast. Surg.,* 1980, **33,** 418–421.

10. Macfie J., A liquid alternative to gauze, *Nurs. Mirror,* 1979, **149,** 30–32.

11. Stewart C.P.U., Foam elastomer dressing in the management of a below-knee amputation stump with delayed healing, *Prosthet. Orthot. Int.,* 1985, **9,** 157–159.

12. Streza G.A. *et al.,* Management of enterocutaneous fistulas and problem stomas with silicone casting of the abdominal wall defect, *Am. J. Surg.,* 1977, **134,** 772–776.

13. Regnard C.F.B. and Meehan S.E., The use of a silicone foam dressing in the management of malignant oral-cutaneous fistula, *Br. J. clin. Pract.,* 1982, **36,** 6–8.

14. Morgan W.P. *et al.,* The use of Silastic foam dressing in the treatment of advanced hidradenitis suppurativa, *Br. J. Surg.,* 1980, **67,** 277–280.

15. Cook P.J. and Devlin H.B., Boils, carbuncles and hidradenitis suppurativa, *Surgery,* 1985, **19,** 440–442.

16. Miller L.A., Hidradenitis suppurativa, *Nurs. Times,* 1982, **78,** 524–525.

17. Malick M.H. and Carr J.A., Flexible elastomer molds in burn scar control, *Am. J. occup. Ther.,* 1980, **34,** 603–608.

18. Bandey S.A. *et al.,* Silastic foam dressing in pinnaplasty, *J. Laryng. Otol.,* 1986, **100,** 201–202.

19. Ross J.K. *et al.,* A Silastic foam dressing for the protection of the post-operative ear, *Br. J. plast. Surg.,* 1987, **40,** 213–214.

20. Shukla H.S., Cosmetic and functional advantages of foam elastomer dressing in the management of epidermoid cancer of the cheek, *Br. J. Surg.,* 1982, **69,** 435–436.

21. DeSy W.A. and Oosterlinck W., Silicone foam elastomer: a significant improvement in postoperative penile dressing, *J. Urol.,* 1982, **128,** 39–40.

22. Whitaker R.H. and Dennis M.J.S., Silastic foam dressing in hypospadias surgery, *Ann. R. Coll. Surg.,* 1987, **69,** 59–60.

23. Bale S. and Harding K., Fungating breast wounds, *J. Distr. Nurs.,* 1987, **5,** 4–5.

24. Groves A.R. and Lawrence J.C., Silastic foam dressing: an appraisal, *Ann. R. Coll. Surg.,* 1985, **67,** 116–118.

25. Culyer A.J. *et al.,* Cost effectiveness of foam elastomer and gauze dressings in the management of open perineal wounds, *Soc. Sci. Med.,* 1983, **17,** 1047–1053.

26. Young H.L. and Wheeler M.H., Report of a prospective trial of dextranomer beads (Debrisan) and silicone foam elastomer (Silastic) dressings in surgical wounds, *Br. J. Surg.,* 1982, **69,** 33–34.

27. Ritter E.J. *et al.,* Teratogenicity of di(2-ethyl-hexyl)phthalate, 2-ethylhexanol, 2-ethylhexanoic acid, and valproic acid, and potentiation by caffeine, *Teratology,* 1987, **35,** 41–46.

28. Winter G.D., Epidermal wound healing under a new polyurethane foam dressing (Lyofoam), *Plast. reconstr. Surg.,* 1975, **56,** 531–537.

29. Baccari G. and Boschetti E., Ferite, ustioni e piaghe medicate con spugnoa di poliuretano, Communication to the Sixth National Congress of the Società Italiana di Chirurgia d'Urgenza e Pronto Soccorso, Padua, 9–11 June 1977.

30. Creevy J., Lyofoam – use in the treatment of leg ulcers, in *Advances in Wound Management,* Turner T.D. Schmidt R.J. and Harding K.G. (eds), London, John Wiley, 1985, 39–40.

31. Mayerhausen W. and Kreis M., Ulcus cruris, *Arzt. Prax.,* 1987, **5,** 2033–2035.

32. Hughes L.E. *et al.,* Wound management in the community – comparison of Lyofoam and Melolin, *Care Science and Practice,* 1989, 7, 64–67.

33. Dahle J.S., Conservative treatment of leg ulcers, in *Proceedings of a Symposium on Wound Healing,* Sundell N. (ed.), Espoo, Finland, 1979, 143–151.

34. Lock P.M. and Riddle M.D., The use of Synthaderm in the treatment of ischaemic leg ulcers, in Ref. 33, 135–141.

35. Bayliss D.J., A clinical application for Synthaderm a new plastic dressing material – a new treatment for an old problem, in Ref. 33, 189–200.

36. Martin T. and Kirby N.G., Clinical aspects of Synthaderm, in Ref. 30, 31–38.

37. Thomas S., The role of foam dressings in wound management, in Ref. 30, 23–29.

38. Wayne M.A., Clinical evaluation of Epi-lock – a semiocclusive dressing, *Ann. emerg. Med.*, 1985, **14**, 65–69.

Chapter 6

Alginates in Wound Management

Since their discovery and characterisation in the early 1880s by a British chemist called Stanford,[1] alginic acid and its salts have been put to various commercial uses. They are now used extensively in the food industry as thickening and stabilising agents for products as diverse as ice cream and beer; it is estimated that, worldwide, in excess of 20000 tons of the material are consumed annually. A significant quantity of alginates is also used by the pharmaceutical industry in the production of topical preparations and oral mixtures, and as adjuvants in the manufacture of vaccines.[2] Whilst no evidence of acute toxicity associated with the oral ingestion of alginates has been reported, a daily intake of 25 mg/kg body-weight has been shown to produce speckling of teeth.[3]

A method of manufacturing calcium alginate fibre was first disclosed in a patent in 1898, but production of the material on a commercial scale only became possible after the publication of a further series of patents in the 1930s. The fibre that was produced at that time was used principally in the textile industry as a soluble yarn, which would dissolve in a scouring process, and which could therefore be used as a support during the manufacture of fine lace, or as draw threads in the production of hosiery.[4] The amount of alginate fibre that was used in surgery and wound management represented only some 10% of annual production; when other synthetic yarns began to replace alginates for textile applications in the 1970s, it became uneconomic to continue to produce the relatively small quantities of fibre required for medical applications. For this reason, the use of alginate fibre in surgery has been limited, and its potential value in wound management has never been fully recognised.

HISTORY OF ALGINATES IN WOUND MANAGEMENT

An early assessment of the use of alginates as haemostats and wound dressings was made by Blaine,[5] who also reported their apparent lack of toxicity (following a series of animal studies in which fibres were implanted into animal tissues, and gels made from alginates were used to treat experimentally produced burns). Clinical studies followed, and the successful use of alginate-derived materials in aural surgery and neurosurgery was reported by Passe and Blaine[6] and Oliver and Blaine,[7] respectively. In 1951, a comparative evaluation of absorbable haemostatic agents, including alginates, was described in a further paper by Blaine.[8]

In all of these studies the sodium and calcium salts of alginic acid were found to be absorbed with no evidence of adverse local histological changes, although the rate of absorption varied with the location and vascularity of the surrounding tissue. However, in the presence of antiseptic agents such as cetylpyridinium bromide, the absorption process was generally incomplete, and some histological changes were noted (including encapsulation and giant cell production).[7]

A mixture of sodium alginate and calcium penicillin, in powder form, was used by Blockley[9] as a styptic, whilst Rumble[10] reported that alginate wool was rapidly absorbed when used as a haemostat in the prevention and control of post-extraction haemorrhage.

Other, more general, areas of clinical usage were described in 1948, when the results of a three-month trial into the use of alginate in the casualty department of Croydon Hospital were reported by Bray et al.[11] In this study, alginates — in the form of films, wool, gauzes, and clots (formed in situ by mixing sterile solutions of calcium chloride and sodium alginate) — were applied to a wide range of wounds, including burns, lacerations, trophic ulcers and amputations. In all cases, healing was found to be rapid and uneventful.

The long-term administration of sodium alginate as an adjuvant for repository hypo-sensitisation agents (covering some 15 000 administrations and 330 patients) was described by Jaros and Dewey,[12] who concluded that the material was 'well tolerated with less of a reaction rate than expected using regular allergenic extracts'.

Other, less favourable, observations upon the toxicity of alginates have also been reported in the literature. Frantz,[13] in a poorly designed and badly reported study, disregarded her own findings (which showed that alginic acid fibres implanted into rats were absorbed completely within two days without any significant undesirable effects) and concluded that alginates were toxic on the basis of additional results obtained from studies involving a nitrated sodium alginate, a material that has no clinical application.

Chenoweth[14] tested the toxicity of alginic acid and sodium alginate in cats by both intravenous and intraperitoneal routes, and reported that dose levels of 250 and 500 mg/kg body-weight caused death or major damage to internal organs such as the heart and kidneys. Dose levels of 25 and 100 mg/kg were found to be much less toxic, although precise details were not given. As neither the method of test nor the dose of alginate used bears any relationship to the use of the material as a haemostat or wound dressing, the relevance of these observations is clearly open to question.

Gosset and Martin,[15] in a presentation to the Academy of Surgery in Paris in 1949, considered that the two papers cited previously were primarily intended as a defence of oxycellulose, and presented experimental data that showed that calcium alginate – injected intramuscularly into both rabbits and rats, using volumes of 0.5 and 3 mL – failed to produce any of the effects described by the American authors; they concluded that calcium alginate was an excellent haemostatic agent that was well tolerated by living tissue.

The biodegradability of alginate fibre residues has been the subject of recent debate,[16,17] and, although it is generally assumed that the polysaccharide molecule is broken down to its monomers by enzymatic activity within the body, this has not been confirmed experimentally.

According to the results of a survey carried out by Stansfield (and reported by Blaine[8]), in the late 1940s and early 1950s, alginates were being used in some 70 hospitals over the range of surgical specialities. Overall, they were found to be highly satisfactory in use; where criticisms were recorded, they were directed mainly at the poor absorption properties of the material and its consequent tendency to induce fistula formation.

It was noted that most of these criticisms related to cases in which the product had been used as packing for large cavities or dead spaces, a function for which it was never originally intended.

Following the early work of Blaine and others, a number of commercial medical alginate products were produced, including an absorbable swab called Calgitex™. When the large-scale manufacture of alginate fibre ceased in the early 1970s, this product was discontinued, owing to the high cost of production.

More recently, however, technological advances and improvements in production techniques in the textile industry, together with an increased understanding of the mechanisms of wound healing, have reawakened interest in the potential value of this unusual and versatile material as a wound dressing.

CHEMISTRY OF ALGINATES

Alginates occur naturally as mixed salts of alginic acid. They are found, primarily as the sodium form, in certain species of brown seaweeds (Phaeophyceae), including giant kelp (*Macrocystis pyrifera*), horsetail kelp (*Laminaria digitata*) and sugar kelp (*L. saccharina*). The yield of alginates varies with the species but is typically in the order of 20–25%. The seaweed that is used for the production of dressings is collected from waters off the Outer Hebrides, the west coast of Ireland, and many other coastal areas all over the world.

Certain species of bacteria – including *Azobacter vinelandii* and *Pseudomonas aeruginosa* – also produce alginates, but these are not used commercially at present.

Extraction of the seaweed with dilute alkali results in the formation of sodium alginate, which is soluble in water, forming a viscous colloidal solution. The calcium salt is, however, insoluble. An ion-exchange reaction is therefore used to manufacture the alginate fibre: a viscous solution of sodium alginate is extruded through a fine orifice into a bath containing calcium ions, and fibres of calcium alginate are precipitated. A reverse reaction occurs when calcium alginate fibres are placed in a solution containing an excess of sodium ions: calcium ions on the fibre are replaced by sodium, and the material becomes soluble.

Sodium alginate has the empirical formula

$(C_6H_7O_6Na)$ and a molecular weight in the range $32\,000-200\,000$. The structural formula is complex, consisting of (1-4)-linked glycuronans comprised of residues of ß-D-mannuronic acid and the C-5 epimer α-L-guluronic acid.[18] These are arranged in homogenous blocks (approximately 20 units long) of one type of acid residue, separated by blocks in which both acid residues occur alternately or randomly. As no evidence of branching has been detected, the molecule is thought to be essentially linear. The relative proportion of mannuronic and guluronic acid residues varies from one species to another; this ratio is extremely important, as it has an effect upon the three-dimensional structure of the polymer, which in turn affects the rheological, gel-forming, and ion-exchange properties of the final dressing. Alginates rich in guluronate form strong but brittle gels, whereas those rich in mannuronate are weaker but more flexible.

COMMERCIAL PRESENTATIONS OF ALGINATES

The following products prepared from alginates are currently available:

- Sorbsan™ – Steriseal,
- Sorbsan Plus™ – Steriseal,
- Sorbsan SA™ – Steriseal,
- Kaltostat™ – BritCair,
- Kaltoclude™ – BritCair,
- Tegagel™ – 3M,
- Stop Hemo™ – Windsor,
- Ultraplast™ – Wallace Cameron.

Sorbsan, which is made from pure calcium alginate, is available as a non-woven fibrous mat (in a small range of sizes) for use as a wound dressing, a loose rope some 30 cm long, which is used for packing deeper wounds, and a thin ribbon 40 cm long, which is supplied with a sterile probe for packing sinuses. Recently, two new presentations based on Sorbsan have been introduced. Sorbsan Plus, which is designed for the treatment of heavily exuding wounds, consists of a layer of alginate fleece bonded onto an absorbent viscose pad and a viscose/polyester backing layer. Sorbsan SA is an island dressing consisting of a piece of alginate fleece located in

the centre of a larger sheet of a waterproof polyurethane foam; the edges of the foam are coated with an acrylic adhesive. The dressing is intended for use on lightly exuding wounds, as the foam helps to conserve moisture and prevent the alginate fibre from drying out.

Kaltostat, which is essentially similar to Sorbsan in appearance, is available both as a dressing and as a 2 g ball for wound packing. When it was first introduced, Kaltostat was manufactured from calcium alginate, but the composition of the dressing has since been modified: it now consists of mixed sodium and calcium salts of alginic acid in the ratio of 20:80. This change has been brought about to increase the rate of gel formation. Kaltoclude, a development of Kaltostat, is an island dressing in which the fibrous pad is placed on a piece of a semipermeable polymeric film. Like Sorbsan SA, Kaltoclude is intended for the treatment of dry or lightly exuding wounds.

Tegagel is made from pure calcium alginate but the fibres are formed into an apertured fabric so that the dressing bears a strong resemblance to a non-woven swab. The manufacturers claim that, because Tegagel maintains its structure in the presence of blood or exudate, it is easier to remove from the wound than either Sorbsan or Kaltostat.

Stop Hemo is presented in two forms, individually wrapped but packed together – a small fibrous haemostatic pad for initial application to a bleeding wound, and a simple first-aid dressing consisting of a small piece of alginate fabric applied to a piece of self-adhesive tape to form an island dressing. Unlike the other alginate products, Stop Hemo is designed primarily as a first-aid dressing for domestic use, and has a product licence for this particular indication.

Ultraplast differs from the other dressings in that it contains a much higher proportion of sodium alginate, and is therefore soluble in water (unlike the pure calcium-based materials, which are soluble only in solutions containing sodium ions). Ultraplast is available in two forms – a knitted gauze sheet approximately 15 cm × 10 cm, and a similar fabric impregnated with 0.15% w/w domiphen bromide in a polyoxyethylene base, supplied as a continuous piece about 2 m × 7.5 cm. Both dressings are intended for use in first aid, the dry form as a haemostatic, and the impregnated version as a non-adherent dressing for burns and similar injuries.

When Kaltostat was first introduced onto the market, it contained a small amount of the quaternary ammonium compound Arquad™, which was introduced during the manufacturing process to improve the handling characteristics of the fibre. Arquad was found to impart pronounced cytotoxic or cytostatic properties to the dressing, when tested by a cell culture method.[19,20] Following correspondence in the pharmaceutical press that discussed the clinical relevance of these findings, the manufacturing process of Kaltostat was modified to reduce the residues of Arquad to a sub-toxic level.

It has subsequently been observed that early batches of Stop Hemo have exhibited cytostatic and antimicrobial properties similar to those associated with the original Kaltostat material. These effects are due to the presence of benzalkonium chloride, which (like Arquad in Kaltostat) is included to improve the handling characteristics of the fibre. Benzalkonium chloride is widely used as an antimicrobial agent and preservative in pharmaceutical formulation, and its presence in Stop Hemo is therefore unlikely to cause any undesirable effects, provided that the use of the dressing is limited to its licensed applications. Indeed, in these situations, the antimicrobial properties could be considered a positive advantage.

CLINICAL USE OF ALGINATES

The earliest studies into the use of one of the modern alginate products were reported by Fraser and Gilchrist,[21] and Gilchrist and Martin.[22] These papers described the use of Sorbsan in the management of foot disorders and a variety of skin lesions, following a clinical evaluation in a group of hospitals in the Sunderland area. The results of these studies were very positive and supported the findings of Blaine (some 40 years earlier). In 1985, a further paper on the use of Sorbsan was published,[23] describing the successful use of the material in the management of a range of problem wounds, including leg ulcers and infected traumatic wounds. The use of Sorbsan in the management of leg ulcers in a diabetic patient was reported by Odugbesan and Barnett.[24]

An obvious potential use for alginate fibre is in the treatment of burns and donor sites, where the haemostatic and absorbent properties of the material should be at their most useful. Groves and Lawrence[25] have described a study in which they compared Sorbsan with a standard gauze pad. They found that, in a simple laboratory test, the alginate absorbed nearly three times as much citrated blood as gauze did, when calculated on a weight for weight basis. In a clinical trial the dressings were applied to fresh, split-thickness donor sites for a period of five minutes after excision; the blood loss from sites treated with Sorbsan was almost half that recorded from comparable wounds treated with gauze.

The effect of longer-term application of alginates to donor sites was investigated by Attwood,[26] who found that sites treated with Kaltostat healed more rapidly than those treated with paraffin tulle (7.0 $\pm$ 0.71 days under alginate, compared with 10.75 $\pm$ 1.6 days under tulle gras). It was also reported that the quality of healing resulting from the use of Kaltostat was significantly better than that achieved using traditional materials, and a reduction in discomfort experienced by patients was also noted.

Following a comparative study of the properties of three modern haemostatic agents used in current surgical practice, Blair[27] found Kaltostat to be more effective than either oxidised cellulose or porcine collagen in controlling bleeding from a surgically inflicted wound in rabbit liver. In addition, the material showed no tendency to cause intestinal obstruction when implanted into mesentery. In contrast, rabbits receiving porcine collagen had to be sacrificed. After six weeks, the oxidised cellulose had completely dissolved, but histological examination of the wound sites treated with alginate showed some evidence of calcium deposition and some fibrous reaction. It is possible that the fibrous reaction was due, in part, to the presence of Arquad in the material at that time.

The haemostatic activity of Kaltostat was investigated by Jarvis,[28] who showed it to be associated with the exchange of calcium ions for sodium in the blood, stimulating both platelet activation and whole blood coagulation.

The principal criticism that is levelled at the alginate dressings, and many other new wound management products, is one of price. There is no question that many of the modern materials are significantly more expensive than traditional dressings, when compared on a unit cost basis. However, such simple cost comparisons are artificial, as they take no account of the effectiveness of the materials concerned.

The method of comparison is particularly

important when calculating the total cost of managing chronic wounds. Leg ulcers that are claimed to be of 20–30 years' duration are commonly encountered, and it is obvious that any dressing or treatment that can facilitate healing in such wounds in a reasonable time, regardless of unit cost, must be worthy of serious consideration. In one community study (involving 64 leg ulcers) carried out by the author,[29] the healing rates obtained with Sorbsan and paraffin tulle were compared. Only 4% of the ulcers treated with tulle healed during the course of the study, whilst 31% of the ulcers treated with Sorbsan healed completely. The healing rates achieved with Sorbsan (measured as a decrease in wound area per day) were over four times those recorded using tulle. Overall, 73% of patients on Sorbsan showed evidence of improvement during the trial, compared with 43% of patients in the control group. When the total costs of both treatments were calculated, it was shown that − on the basis of material costs alone − financial benefits could result from the use of the alginate dressing. If nursing costs were included in the calculation, these savings could be considerable.

ALGINATE DRESSINGS: METHOD OF USE

In use, the plain alginate sheets are simply placed on the surface of the wound and covered with a secondary dressing such as an absorbent pad, which may be retained with tape or a suitable bandage. Alternatively, Sorbsan Plus may be applied, which does not require the use of any additional dressing pads. If the lesion is such that it requires packing, alginate ribbon or rope should be gently laid into the wound, but not packed too tightly.

Once in place, the dressing absorbs exudate and tissue fluid to form a hydrophilic gel over the surface of the wound, providing a moist environment for wound healing. The properties of the gel and the rate at which it is formed differ from product to product, according to the source of the alginate and method of fibre production (as described previously).

The frequency with which dressings should be changed depends upon the amount of exudate produced and the general condition of the wound: initially, a daily change may be required, but this may be reduced as the wound begins to heal. The method of removing the dressings varies from product to product. As Sorbsan rapidly dissolves in solutions containing sodium ions, it is easily removed by irrigation with a sterile solution of 0.9% sodium chloride or 1% sodium citrate, without causing the patient any discomfort or damaging the newly formed tissue. Kaltostat and Tegagel should be removed from the wound using a pair of forceps, after first moistening with sterile saline as required. Although any isolated alginate fibres that become incorporated into the granulating tissue will gradually be absorbed, it is important to ensure that crusts consisting of alginate, dried exudate and skin scales are not allowed to build up around the margin of the wound. In most instances, this is a very minor problem, and simple wound toilet with a saline-soaked swab is all the treatment that is required. However, some patients produce large quantities of scale; if these are not removed, they can act as foci for the formation of small pockets of infection, which can lead to the breakdown of the newly formed epithelium.

Alginates depend for their activity upon the formation of a gel by the absorption of wound exudate. This cannot take place if the dressing is applied to a dry, non-exuding wound, and there is therefore little advantage to be gained by the use of the material in this situation.

Occasionally, it has been reported that, when an alginate dressing is applied to a relatively dry wound, the patient may experience a transient burning sensation. This is thought to be due to the pronounced hydrophilic properties of the fibre, which are causing a degree of local tissue dehydration. The symptoms are usually alleviated by moistening the dressing with a small quantity of sterile saline immediately after application.

Alginates are suitable for the management of most exuding wounds, but should be used with care in deep narrow sinuses or fistulae.

In a recent study using experimental wounds in pigs,[30] it was found that the healing rate achieved with calcium alginate was related to the degree of hydration of the fibrous fleece. Wounds that were dressed with calcium alginate fibre alone and allowed to dry out healed more slowly than comparable wounds that were dressed with alginate and covered with a semipermeable film dressing (Opsite™). It was also found that wounds dressed with a great excess of fibre showed some evidence of a foreign body reaction − a response to the presence of intact fibres of unchanged calcium alginate. These results tend to support the statements made previously: that alginate sheets should be applied to exuding wounds, and used with care in deeper cavities. They are also in accord with a personal observation of the author: that clean non-infected wounds dressed with Sorbsan heal faster if dressing changes are reduced to a minimum.

As a general guide, when a dressing is changed, all the fibre directly in contact with the surface of the wound should have formed a gel. If the dressing is moist but with evidence of significant amounts of unchanged fibre present, it may be appropriate to increase the interval between dressing changes. If, however, the dressing appears to have formed a gel but then dried out, the use of a more occlusive outer dressing may be appropriate. In these situations, it is not always necessary to use a film dressing: the application of a perforated plastic film dressing, such as Melolin™ or Telfa™, may be all that is required. Alternatively, it may be more appropriate to use a composite dressing such as Sorbsan SA or Kaltoclude.

The presence of pathogenic organisms in a wound is not necessarily a contra-indication to the use of an alginate dressing but, in this situation, daily changes are advisable. If obvious signs of clinical infection develop, appropriate systemic antibiotic therapy should be initiated and the use of the dressing suspended (at the discretion of the medical officer in charge). In practice, however, it has been found that alginates can often be used in the treatment of infected wounds – with beneficial results – provided antibiotics are given systemically and the dressings changed daily as described above.

Alginates possess many of the attributes of the ideal dressing identified in chapter 2 but, in addition, they have other interesting and potentially valuable properties. As has been described previously, the polysaccharide material combines with the wound exudate to form a hydrophilic gel, which provides a moist (but not macerated) wound interface – a condition that Winter[31] stated was essential, in order to obtain the benefits of accelerated wound healing. A more detailed review of the properties of wound exudate is provided in chapter 4. It is interesting to speculate that the use of an alginate dressing – which effectively ensures that the wound is covered by an inert, aqueous gel, rich in naturally occurring proteins, amino acids and growth

factors – may have a positive effect upon wound healing. A preliminary communication from Schmidt et al.[19] suggests that pure calcium alginate appears to promote the growth of mouse fibroblasts in culture, indicating that, for the first time, a dressing may be actively contributing to the normal healing process.

It is also possible, though as yet unproved, that the dressing may play a part, in some instances, in controlling microbiological contamination of a wound. It is proposed that bacteria may be physically trapped within the gel itself (and thus removed when the dressing is changed), but it is also possible that lysozyme, which is present in elevated levels in wound exudate, may be incorporated into the gel and exert a mild antibacterial effect.

The exact position and role of calcium alginate in the wound management area has still to be completely determined, but experience would suggest that it is of value in the treatment of most types of exuding wound. However, it is not the product of choice for dry wounds, or those that are completely covered with a hard dry layer of necrotic tissue or slough (unless this is first removed surgically or by some other means). Small amounts of soft yellow slough do not necessarily preclude the use of the dressing, as they will generally be removed by autolysis. Alginates have a high degree of patient acceptability, being comfortable when in position and painless to remove.[32] To date, no sensitivity reactions have been reported associated with the use of alginates, and the material has been used successfully on some patients who have reacted badly to other dressings.

REFERENCES

1. Stanford E., On algin: a new substance obtained from some of the commoner species of marine algae, *Chem. News*, 1883, **47**, 254–257.
2. Amies C.R., The use of topically formed calcium alginate as a depot substance in active immunization, *J. path. Bact.*, 1959, **77**, 435–442.
3. Seventeenth Report of the FAO/WHO Expert Committee on Food Additives, *Tech. Rep. Ser. Wld Hlth Org. No. 539,* 1974.
4. Gilchrist T. *et al.*, Sorbsan – the natural dressing, in *Advances in Wound Management,* Turner T.D. Schmidt R.J. and Harding K.G. (eds), London, John Wiley, 1985, 73–81.
5. Blaine G., Experimental observations on absorbable

alginate products in surgery, *Ann. Surg.,* 1947, **125,** 102–114.

6. Passe E.R.G. and Blaine G., Alginates in endaural wound dressing, *Lancet,* 1948, **2,** 651.

7. Oliver L.C. and Blaine G., Haemostasis with absorbable alginates in neurosurgical practice, *Br. J. Surg.,* 1950, **37,** 307–310.

8. Blaine G., A comparative evaluation of absorbable haemostatics, *Postgrad. med. J.,* 1951, **27,** 613–620.

9. Blockley C.H., A penicillin-styptic for dental work, *Br. dent. J.,* 1947, **82,** 213.

10. Rumble J.F.S., Twenty-five cases treated with absorbable alginate wool, *ibid.,* 1949, **86,** 203–205.

11. Bray C. *et al.,* New treatment for burns, wounds and haemorrhage, *Nurs. Mirror,* 1948, **86,** 239–242.

12. Jaros S.H. and Dewey J.L., Uses of an alginate in hyposensitization, *Ann. Allergy,* 1964, **22,** 173–179.

13. Frantz V.K., Experimental studies of alginates as haemostatics, *Ann. Surg.,* 1948, **127,** 1165–1172.

14. Chenoweth M.B., The toxicity of sodium alginate in cats, *ibid.,* 1173–1181.

15. Gosset M.J. and Martin J., Un nouvel hémostatique chirurgical: l'alginate de calcium, Communication to the Academie de Chirurgie, Paris, 1949.

16. Schmidt R.J. and Turner T.D., Calcium alginate dressings, (letter), *Pharm. J.,* 1986, **236,** 578.

17. Cair Ltd, Calcium alginate dressings, (letter), *ibid.*

18. Gacesa P., Alginates, *Carb. Polymers,* 1988, **8,** 1–22.

19. Schmidt R.J. *et al.,* Alginate dressings, (letter), *Pharm. J.,* 1986, **236,** 36–37.

20. Fry J.R., Alginate dressings, (letter), *ibid.,* 37.

21. Fraser R. and Gilchrist T., Sorbsan calcium alginate fibre dressings in footcare, *Biomaterials,* 1983, **4,** 222–224.

22. Gilchrist T. and Martin A.M., Wound treatment with Sorbsan – an alginate fibre dressing, *ibid.,* 317–320.

23. Thomas S., Use of a calcium alginate dressing, *Pharm. J.,* 1985, **235,** 188–190.

24. Odugbesan O. and Barnett A.H., Use of a seaweed-based dressing in management of leg ulcers in diabetics: a case report, *Pract. Diabet.,* 1987, **4,** 46–47.

25. Groves A.R. and Lawrence J.C., Alginate dressing as a donor site haemostat, *Ann. R. Coll. Surg.,* 1986, **68,** 27–28.

26. Attwood A.I., Calcium alginate dressing accelerates graft donor site healing, Paper presented to the Winter Meeting of the British Association of Plastic Surgeons, England, December 1986.

27. Blair S.D. *et al.,* A comparison of topical haemostatic agents in experimental liver resection, Paper presented to the Eleventh International Congress on Thrombosis and Haemostasis, Brussels, 1987.

28. Jarvis P.M. *et al.,* How does calcium alginate achieve haemostasis in surgery, Paper presented at the Eleventh International Congress on Thrombosis and Haemostasis, Brussels 1987.

29. Thomas S. and Tucker C.A., Sorbsan in the management of leg ulcers, *Pharm. J.,* 1989, **243,** 706–709.

30. Barnett S.E. and Varley S.J., The effects of calcium alginate on wound healing, *Ann. R. Coll. Surg.,* 1987, **69,** 153–155.

31. Winter G.D., Formation of scab and the rate of epithelization of superficial wounds in the skin of the young domestic pig, *Nature,* 1962, **193,** 293–294.

32. Thomas S., Pain and wound management, *Nurs. Times, Community Outlook Suppl.,* 1989, **85,** 11–15.

Chapter 7

Hydrogel Dressings

The potential value of hydrophilic polymers as raw materials for the manufacture of implants, contact lenses and artificial arteries was first recognised by Wichterle and Lim,[1] who described a family of gels based upon glycol methacrylates. The properties of these gels could be varied by changing the monomers used in their manufacture, and the degree of cross-linking produced. Wichterle and Lim suggested that hydrogels for biological use should have a significant water content, be inert to normal biological processes, and be permeable to metabolites; most important of all, they should be non-irritant when embedded into living tissue. A comprehensive review of hydrogel materials – including detailed information on their structure, methods of manufacture, and biological applications – is available in three volumes.[2]

In simple terms, hydrogels consist of insoluble polymers with hydrophilic sites, which interact with aqueous solutions, absorbing and retaining significant volumes of water. The polymers themselves may be prepared from synthetic or semisynthetic materials, or a combination of the two.

Two basic types of gel dressing are currently used in wound management. One group of products has a fixed three-dimensional macro structure and is usually presented in the form of a thin flexible sheet. Dressings of this type do not change their physical form as they absorb fluid, although they may swell and increase in volume. The swelling process will continue until the gel becomes fully saturated or until equilibrium is reached.

Products in the second group, the amorphous hydrogels, do not have a fixed three-dimensional macro structure; when these materials absorb fluid, they progressively decrease in viscosity and may flow to take up the shape of the wound or vessel that contains them. Amorphous hydrogels will continue to absorb fluid until the gel loses all its cohesive properties and simply becomes a dispersion of the polymer in water.

The following hydrogel dressings in sheet form are currently available in the UK:

- Geliperm™ – Geistlich,
- Vigilon™ – Seton.

The amorphous hydrogels are:

- Bard™ Absorption Dressing – Seton,
- Scherisorb™ – Smith & Nephew.

GELIPERM

Geliperm, which was first developed in 1977, consists of two chemically different polymers interlaced together. In the final product, a soft and relatively weak agar gel is stabilised by polyacrylamide (which is included to impart sufficient strength to the material to make it suitable for use as a wound dressing). Geliperm is currently available in a number of different forms.

The first, and probably the most commonly used, preparation is the hydrated sheet, which contains about 96% water, 1% agar and 3% polyacrylamide. This material is strong, moist, flexible and totally transparent. If exposed to a dry, warm environment, however, it will gradually lose much of its water to form a thin, clear, semi-rigid transparent film. This is the basis of the second presentation of Geliperm, the dry sheet form, which is chemically similar to the hydrated sheet in terms of the composition of the basic polymer, but contains about 35% glycerol as a humectant.

The third preparation of Geliperm consists of a hydrated gel that has been reduced to an amorphous mass by a mincing process. Geliperm Granulated Gel, as it is called, is presented in a plastic tube with a short nozzle, which may be used to introduce the gel into small wounds and cavities. As a result of the mincing process, the surface area of the gel is larger, which increases the rate at which at which fluid can be absorbed.

Two other presentations of Geliperm are currently under development – a perforated sheet, and a dry powder form. The perforated sheet is intended for application to heavily exuding wounds such as donor sites, and is similar in composition to the standard Geliperm, except for the presence of holes (which allow the passage of exudate through to a secondary dressing or absorbent pad placed on the outer surface). The dry powder form is manufactured from a starch co-polymer and will be available double-wrapped in sterile sachets containing 2 g of powder.

Properties of Geliperm

Geliperm is permeable to water vapour and gases, and will allow penetration by solutes with a molecular weight of up to about one million, although the rate of diffusion of these materials into and out of the gel is in inverse proportion to their molecular weight. This property has led to the suggestion that the dressing be used as a delivery system for antibiotics and antiseptic agents, and tests have shown that the release of water-soluble materials from the gel can be rapid and complete.[3] Work is currently in progress to investigate the possibility of using Geliperm and a second hydrogel material (KY™ Jelly – Johnson & Johnson) as carriers for placental growth factors (PGFs), in the treatment of chronic wounds. Laboratory and animal studies performed to date suggest that these materials are suitable vehicles for this purpose, and preliminary clinical studies also indicate that PGFs incorporated in the gels stimulate granulation and epithelialisation in chronic leg ulcers.[4] The use of hydrogels as molecular carriers has been described in detail elsewhere.[2]

Although, in theory, any presentation of Geliperm could be used as a drug carrier, the dry sheet form is particularly suitable for this purpose. When placed in an aqueous solution, the dry sheet is rapidly rehydrated, taking up about 50–60% of its total fluid capacity in some 30 minutes. Thereafter, the rate of fluid uptake is reduced, and the gel takes more than 24 hours to reach saturation.[5]

In laboratory studies involving 100 different strains of bacteria and fungi, it has been shown that Geliperm forms an effective barrier to bacteria.[6] It was also shown that the gel itself would not support the growth of a range of clinically important micro-organisms – although, in the presence of a growth medium containing suitable nutrients, bacteria could be cultured on the surface of the dressing after prolonged incubation. Under the conditions of the test, however, no penetration or alteration of the structure of the gel by bacteria or fungi could be detected; and the authors concluded that the material should form an effective bacterial barrier under normal conditions of use. It has been suggested that Geliperm may reduce the concentration of bacterial exotoxins and enzymes in a wound, by absorption.

Geliperm has been used as a coupling agent for ultrasound in the treatment of fractures[7] and soft tissue injuries.[8] The gel, which under experimental conditions transmits 95% of the incident power of the beam, provides a sterile environment and physical protection to the skin, and completely prevents the problems of pin-track infections.

Intramuscular, intraperitoneal and subcutaneous implantation studies in rats showed that Geliperm was well tolerated, when compared with other materials used as tissue implants.[9]

VIGILON

Vigilon (known as Spenco™ in the USA) is a hydrated sheet (containing 96% water) consisting of a radiation cross-linked, high molecular weight polyethylene oxide co-polymer. Because the gel has very little intrinsic strength, in the final dressing it is supported on a centered net of low density polyethylene.

Vigilon is available (sterile) in a sealed plastic pouch, which is enclosed in a non-sterile aluminium outer cover. Inside the pack, both sides of the dressing are covered by a perforated sheet of polyethylene film. Immediately before use, one sheet of polyethylene is removed and the gel is placed directly onto the surface of the wound. The second sheet of plastic may be left in position or removed, as required – depending upon the amount of exudate that may be anticipated. On dry wounds, the sheet will help to conserve moisture in the dressing by reducing the loss of water vapour; on more heavily exuding lesions, it is usually appropriate to remove the backing layer, so that excess fluid may evaporate from the dressing at the maximum possible rate. The gel (with the plastic layers removed) is permeable to water vapour and gases, but impermeable to bacteria.

The manufacturers of Vigilon state that the dressing will absorb approximately 2 cm of fore, aft and lateral shear, and 360° of rotary shear, with a pressure of 30 kPa. It is suggested that this makes the dressing a useful covering for areas of tissue that are liable to frictional damage.

In a controlled study in pigs,[10] it was shown that the average healing time for wounds dressed with Vigilon was 2.5 days, compared with 4.5 days for untreated wounds; other wounds, dressed with Bard Absorption Dressing, healed in an average of 3.5 days.

In 1982, Mandy[11] recorded the use of Vigilon after 26 hair transplantations, 10 dermabrasions, and 42 excisional surgeries, and concluded that − although the material was of value for all these applications − it appeared to be most useful in situations where the epidermis was disrupted over a large area. Dermabrasions treated with the hydrogel healed faster than those dressed with conventional materials, and there was a noticeable relief of pain.

CLINICAL APPLICATIONS OF SHEET HYDROGELS

Hydrogel dressings in sheet form can be applied and removed without causing pain and trauma, provided that they are not allowed to dry out. Once in place, they are said to reduce pain, and therefore have a high degree of patient acceptability. As accurate placement and retention of the gel can be a problem, it is sometimes an advantage to use the material in conjunction with a piece of dressing retention sheet (such as Mefix™ or Hypafix™) to form a simple island dressing. Because the ability of the dressings to cope with large volumes of fluid is limited, they are best used on low exudate wounds − such as dermabrasions, minor burns, donor sites and superficial pressure areas. The granular version of Geliperm is a little more versatile, and may be used in the treatment of sinuses and similar cavity wounds. Small pieces of gel sheet are sometimes applied to the eyes of unconscious patients in intensive care units. The gel keeps the eyes closed and also helps to prevent them from becoming excessively dry.

If required, in appropriate cases, the dressings may be refrigerated before use, producing a cooling effect that alleviates pain and irritation.

The disadvantages associated with the use of sheet hydrogels include the difficulty of fixing them, the need for frequent dressing changes, and the tendency of the materials to dry out on lightly exuding wounds and to cause maceration on heavily exuding ones. It has also been shown that experimental wounds infected with *Pseudomonas* spp. can deteriorate very rapidly when treated with sheet hydrogels such as Geliperm and Vigilon.[12,13]

There is little doubt that hydrogel dressings in sheet form have never realised their expected potential in routine wound management. This is probably due, at least in part, to their high unit cost and the other disadvantages outlined above, but it is also probable that, for many applications, they have been replaced or superseded by other newer materials (such as the hydrocolloid dressings).

BARD ABSORPTION DRESSING

Bard Absorption Dressing is made from corn starch that has been chemically modified by the addition of carboxyl and carboxamide groups, which increase the capacity and control the rate of absorption of water. When partially hydrated, the dressing forms a mouldable hydrogel which may be applied to a variety of exuding lesions.

The dressing is presented in a plastic pack containing 60 g of dry flakes (sterilised by gamma irradiation). Prior to use, a quantity of the flakes are aseptically mixed with sterile water or saline in the ratio of 5 g of dressing to approximately 25 mL of liquid; the resulting gel is applied to the wound with a sterile spatula or tongue depressor. The wound area is covered with a sterile low adherence dressing, held in position with tape or a bandage as appropriate. The gel exerts a gentle suction pressure and is capable of absorbing large volumes of exudate under normal conditions of use.

An early report of the use of Bard Absorption Dressing was given by Spence and Bates,[14] who described its use in the treatment of 40 assorted animal wounds in veterinary practice, and decubitus or stasis ulcers in 148 human patients. They found that the dressing absorbed large volumes of fluid, reduced odour, and − in some instances − afforded relief from pain. The gel also helped to maintain wounds in a clean, healthy condition, but the authors stressed that − although the material was effective in removing water-soluble secretions − surgical intervention was required to remove 'hardened secreted tissue' or slough.

In a later review of 40 cases in the USA,[15] Jeter and co-workers described the use of the dressing in the treatment of specific exuding wounds, including pressure areas, a dehisced abdominal wound, and a necrotic lesion following a Pirogoff amputation of the foot. They concluded that the dressing cleansed the wound, encouraged the formation of granulation tissue, reduced wound odour, and produced dramatic wound healing in some instances. Some patients did, however, experience significant discomfort during the first 10–15 minutes after the application of the gel but, based upon their experiences, the authors challenged a claim made earlier by Montgomery,[16] that the dressing could have contributed to an episode of hyperkalaemia in one patient; they suggested instead that this was more likely to be due to an electrolyte shift or a decrease in renal function.

Bard Absorption Dressing has not been actively marketed or widely used in the UK, probably due (at least in part) to its high unit cost, and its method of presentation. Although the contents of the plastic pack are sterile when received, this cannot be guaranteed once the pack is opened. In practical terms, the chances of the contents becoming contaminated and causing a wound infection are highly remote, but the repeated use of portions of a dressing from an opened container is not in accord with good nursing practice. Furthermore, the recent introduction of Scherisorb, a premixed starch-based gel in unit dose sachets, has done little to improve the commercial position of the Bard Absorption Dressing.

SCHERISORB

Scherisorb is a colourless to pale yellow, transparent, aqueous gel, based upon chemically modified corn starch onto which hydrophilic side-chains have been grafted. These side-chains form a T-shape with the basic starch molecules, for which reason the final structure is often referred to as a graft T co-polymer. The dressing, which is presented in aluminium laminate sachets, contains 2% co-polymer, 78% water and 20% propylene glycol (as a preservative and humectant). When the dressing was produced without propylene glycol, it was reported to need changing daily, as it showed a marked tendency to dry out or produce unpleasant odours. After it was reformulated, a further study showed that the gel could be left in position for up to three days with no apparent adverse effects upon wound healing.[17]

Originally introduced as a leg ulcer dressing, Scherisorb gel has been found to be extremely useful in the treatment of many types of wound, particularly those covered with slough or black necrotic tissue; in some areas of the country, the gel has largely replaced solutions such as Eusol or hydrogen peroxide for debriding and cleansing wounds of this type. It is believed that the gel acts by rehydrating dead tissue, so that the normal autolytic processes can take place at the interface between the slough and the healthy tissue beneath.

The use of Scherisorb in the treatment of leg ulcers was investigated in a comparative trial involving 98 patients.[18] The study, which was carried out entirely in the community, compared the healing rates of wounds dressed with the gel with those of similar wounds dressed with Iodosorb™. No significant differences were detected between the two therapies in terms of healing rate, odour formation, or granulation tissue production. The authors concluded that, although an acceptable healing rate was achieved with both materials, Iodosorb was significantly more expensive in use. Furthermore, the presence of iodine in Iodosorb (as an antiseptic) did not appear to enhance the rate of healing.

The aqueous nature of Scherisorb makes it a potentially useful carrier for topical medicaments. It has been the experience of the author that the incorporation of 0.8% metronidazole powder into the gel makes it an extremely effective adjunct to systemic treatment for wounds infected with sensitive micro-organisms. Application of the medicated gel can be particularly effective in reducing the odour associated with extensive or infected pressure areas,[19] or fungating carcinomas.

Scherisorb has also been used with advantage in the management of extravasation injuries in neonates.[20] The gel is liberally applied to the affected area (usually the foot, or the dorsum of the hand) and the entire area is enclosed in a sterile plastic bag, specially shaped to form a boot or glove. The treatment offers a number of significant advantages over more traditional techniques: the gel is painless to apply and remove, and – being transparent – permits the wound to be examined at all times; dehydration and further loss of viable tissue is prevented; and the healed wound has a highly acceptable cosmetic appearance (Plates 5 to 7).

There appears to be little doubt that amorphous hydrogel materials like Scherisorb have much to offer in the management of dry, sloughy, or low exudate wounds, being much more versatile and economical in use than the sheet hydrogel materials described previously.

REFERENCES

1. Wichterle O. and Lim D., Hydrophilic gels for biological use, *Nature,* 1960, **185**, 117–118.
2. *Hydrogels in Medicine and Pharmacy,* (Vols 1–3), Peppas N.A. (ed.), Florida, CRC Press, 1987.
3. Butcher G. and Woods H.F., Geliperm as a molecular carrier, in *Geliperm: A Clear Advance in Wound Healing*, Woods H.F. and Cottier D. (eds), Proceedings of a Conference, Oxford, 1983, 77–87.
4. Burgos H., Incorporation and release of placental growth factors in synthetic medical dressings, *Clin. Mat.,* 1987, **2**, 133–139.
5. Wokalek H. *et al.,* Theoretical aspects and clinical experience on a new hydrogel wound dressing material, in Ref. 3, 3–33.
6. Barzokas C.A. *et al.,* Microbiological studies on Geliperm, in Ref. 3, 39–47.
7. Breuton R.N. *et al.,* The effect of ultrasound on the repair of a rabbit's tibial osteotomy held in rigid external fixation, *Bone Joint Surg.,* 1987, **69**, 494.
8. Breuton R.N. and Campbell B., The use of Geliperm as a sterile coupling agent for therapeutic ultrasound, *Physiotherapy,* 1987, **73**, 653–654.
9. Taylor D.E.M. and Penhallow J., Biotolerance of Geliperm: a six week implantation study in the rat, in Ref.3, 63–75.
10. Geronemus R.G. and Robinson P., The effect of two new dressings on epidermal wound healing, *J. derm. Surg. Oncol.* 1982, **8**, 850–852.
11. Mandy S.H., A new primary wound dressing made of polyethylene oxide gel, *ibid.* 1983, **9**, 153–155.
12. Brennan S.S. *et al.,* Infection and healing under hydrogel occlusive dressings, in Ref. 3, 49–62.
13. Leaper D.J. *et al.,* Experimental infection and hydrogel dressings, *J. Hosp. Infect.,* 1984, **5 (Supp. A)**, 69–73.
14. Spence W.R. and Bates I., New absorption dressing for secreting ulcers, Paper presented to the Annual Session of the Texas Medical Association, Texas, 28 May 1981.
15. Jeter K.F. *et al.,* Comprehensive wound management with a starch-based copolymer dressing, *J. enterostom. Ther.,* 1986, **13**, 217–225.
16. Montgomery B.A., Product ingredients: important ramification, *J. enterostom. Ther.,* 1985, **12**, 203–204.
17. Cherry G. *el al.,* Scherisorb gel investigated, *Care Sci. Pract.,* 1985, (Special Edn), 12–14.
18. Stewart A.J. and Leaper D.J., Treatment of chronic leg ulcers in the community; a comparative trial of Scherisorb and Iodosorb, *Phlebology,* 1987, **2**, 115–121.
19. Gomolin I.H. and Brandt J.L., Topical metronidazole therapy for pressure sores of geriatric patients, *J. Am Geriat. Soc.,* 1984, **31**, 710–712.
20. Thomas S. *et al.,* A new approach to the management of extravasation injury in neonates, *Pharm. J.,* 1987, **239**, 584–585.

Chapter 8

Hydrocolloid Dressings

The term 'hydrocolloid' has been adopted to describe a relatively new family of wound management products manufactured from gel-forming agents combined with other materials, such as elastomers and adhesives. Frequently based upon carboxymethylcellulose (CMC), hydrocolloids may also contain other polysaccharides and proteins. Typically, they are presented in the form of a flexible foam or film sheet, coated with a layer of the hydrocolloid base and covered with a piece of release paper. The base itself may also be available in the form of granules or paste, which can be applied to the wound in conjunction with the sheet to increase the absorbency of the system.

DEVELOPMENT OF HYDROCOLLOID DRESSINGS

Granuflex™ (ConvaTec), the first of the hydrocolloid dressings − and current market leader in the UK − evolved in a series of stages from Orabase™, a viscous paste that was originally developed as a treatment for mouth ulcers and other oral lesions. Orabase has the ability to adhere firmly to moist surfaces, where it slowly absorbs water to form a protective gel over the lesion. It was this property that led to its experimental use in the treatment of skin excoriation caused by the effluent from surgical stomas and gastro-intestinal fistulae.[1]

The treatment proved so successful that a more convenient presentation was developed, in which a semi-solid pliable wafer of material was backed with a thin polyethylene sheet. The new material, called Stomahesive™, contained a mixture of gelatin, pectin and CMC − three of the ingredients of Orabase. The dressing had two principal functions: it provided an effective barrier over the excoriated tissue, and the polyethylene back also served as a good base for the attachment of an ostomy appliance.

The obvious benefits derived from the use of Stomahesive led, in 1973, to a preliminary study into the use of the adhesive base without the plastic backing in the treatment of varicose ulcers. This was followed by a second study, in 1975,[2] in which Varihesive™ (as it was called) was applied to a total of 22 ulcers of mixed aetiology, with and without occlusion. It was observed that the new material appeared to stimulate the formation of granulation tissue, but it was recorded that in a number of instances this became so exuberant that it had to be destroyed by the application of silver nitrate. Overall, however, the material was well tolerated and produced no general adverse reactions, although a change of treatment was sometimes required to bring about epithelialisation. The following year, the successful use of Stomahesive in the management of decubitus ulcers was also described.[3,4]

The first major study of the use of Varihesive was reported by Tracy et al.;[5] it involved 43 patients with indolent ulcers that had proved resistant to local therapy for more than ten weeks. Overall, 84% of the ulcers healed. The authors concluded that Varihesive formed an excellent covering for wounds in which there was minimal suppurative infection, and suggested that it might also be of value in the treatment of abrasions, donor sites and bed sores.

The first controlled trial of the use of Varihesive was reported by Baxter, in 1980,[6] who compared healing rates of leg ulcers dressed with the hydrocolloid with those of similar wounds dressed with paraffin tulle. Unfortunately, the results of this study were inconclusive and of questionable value. However, a much more positive statement about Varihesive was made by Allen,[7] who described the value of the material in chiropody.

The encouraging results obtained with both Stomahesive and Varihesive led eventually to the development of the now-familiar Granuflex, which was introduced in the USA in 1983 (as Duoderm™), after extensive pre-clinical and clinical trials. More recently, three further presentations of Granuflex have been introduced, which are described below.

A number of new hydrocolloid dressings have now been introduced, some of which are very similar to Granuflex in terms of the structure of the adhesive mass. They are:

- Biofilm™ – CliniMed,
- Comfeel™ – Coloplast,
- Dermiflex™ – Johnson & Johnson,
- Intrasite™ – Smith & Nephew,
- Tegasorb™ – 3M.

The properties of these dressings are described below.

GRANUFLEX

Granuflex consists of a thin layer of a semi-open-cell polyurethane foam bonded onto a polyurethane film, which acts as a carrier for the hydrocolloid base. The base is composed of gelatin, pectin, and sodium carboxymethyl-cellulose (NaCMC), dispersed as micro-granules in an adhesive mass of polyisobutylene. The hydrocolloid base is also available in the form of granules and a paste, which may be introduced into small cavities or sinuses, or used in conjunction with the dressing sheet to increase the absorbent capacity of the system when used on heavily exuding wounds.

Two new presentations, Granuflex Transparent™ and Granuflex Extra Thin™, consist of a layer of the hydrocolloid base, applied directly onto a piece of polyurethane film. Granuflex Transparent (which is actually thinner than Granuflex Extra Thin) is recommended for securing intravenous catheters and may also be used as an incise drape. The Extra Thin material is intended to be used as a post-operative dressing, and may also be used to dress abrasions, superficial pressure sores, and other lightly exuding wounds. A third new development, Granuflex E™, also contains gelatin, pectin and NaCMC, but differs from the original material in the composition of the adhesives and polymers used. It is said that the dressing is able to cope with large volumes of exudate better than the plain Granuflex, and it is therefore recommended for heavily exuding wounds.

Most of the literature that has been published

on Granuflex describes the dressing as impermeable to water vapour and oxygen, and the results of several clinical studies have been discussed or interpreted in the light of this assumption. However, laboratory studies carried out by the author[8] have shown that, in the hydrated state, Granuflex is actually more permeable than most of the other hydrocolloids – and is even slightly more permeable than the film dressing, Opsite™ as shown below.

Product	MVP g/m^2/24hr
Biofilm	4,082
Granuflex	956
Intrasite	545
Comfeel	453
Tegasorb	135
Dermiflex	79
Opsite (film dressing)	862

When a Granuflex dressing is applied to dry skin, it adheres initially by 'dry tack' (owing to the presence of polyisobutylene). As the base absorbs exudate or water vapour, the method of adhesion changes, and the dry tack is replaced by a more powerful adhesive force known as 'wet tack'. The area of the dressing in direct contact with the wound will continue to absorb moisture until it eventually liquefies and forms a soft gel. During this process, the adhesive base undergoes phase inversion, so that it ceases to consist of a dispersion of hydrophilic granules in an adhesive mass and becomes a dispersion of the adhesive in an aqueous hydrogel. The resulting semi-solid material has a characteristic odour and a superficial resemblance to pus, which can cause some alarm to medical and nursing staff unfamiliar with the use of the dressing. In contrast, when Granuflex E absorbs fluid, the resulting gel is held in a cross-linked matrix and remains an integral part of the dressing.

The mechanism of fluid absorption by Granuflex is such that liquid is transmitted only slowly across the hydrocolloid sheet. As a result, that part of the base in contact with the wound is always maintained in a moist condition. This ensures that the dressing may be easily removed from the surface of the wound without causing damage to the underlying tissue. This ease of removal is in marked contrast to the epidermal stripping that frequently occurs when gauze or similar dressings are removed. These effects were noted by Alvarez et al.,[9] during the course of a study in which they compared a hydrocolloid dressing (Granuflex), a polyurethane film dressing (Opsite), 'wet to dry' gauze dressings, and air exposure, on superficial wounds in the domestic pig. Collagen synthesis was enhanced under both occlusive dressings, compared with the other two groups; the differences were detectable from the first day after wounding and remained evident throughout the course of the study. Although the rate of epithelialisation beneath both occlusive dressings was greater than that in wounds dressed with gauze or exposed to air, the hydrocolloid produced a significantly greater number of resurfaced wounds in the early days of treatment, and had a lower HT_{50} (time to heal 50% of wounds), than the polyurethane film. Alvarez and his co-workers also recorded a tendency for the film dressing to cause occasional rewounding upon removal on later days in the study.

The effect of Granuflex on the bacteriology of normal skin was investigated by Lawrence and Lilly;[10] they demonstrated that, although skin covered with an impermeable plastic tape (Sleek™) showed a significant increase in the number of bacteria present, the application of Granuflex did not produce a similar increase, despite the equally occlusive nature of the dressing. In a second paper, Lawrence[11] reviewed the physical properties of Granuflex and concluded that it formed an effective dressing for minor wounds, acting as a bacterial barrier and enhancing patient comfort. Patients were able to shower or wash, and volunteers who wore the dressing for up to ten days showed no evidence of sensitivity reactions or any other adverse response.

The ability of the dressing to act as a barrier to bacteria was used to good effect by Wilson et al.,[12] who reported on the use of hydrocolloid dressings to control the spread of methicillin-resistant Staphylococcus aureus from patients with leg ulcers colonised by the organism. The preliminary results of their work suggested that the dressing could be a valuable alternative to isolation for such patients.

A detailed comparison of the local environment of chronic wounds under occlusive dressings was carried out by Varghese et al., [13] who examined the fluid that collected beneath the dressings and found that the oxygen tension (pO_2) was zero or very low. The pH of the wound fluid beneath each dressing was also measured, and was found to be more acidic beneath the hydrocolloid material than under the polyurethane film, due – at least in part – to the chemical nature of the hydrocolloid base. The low pH under the hydrocolloid dressing was thought to have an inhibiting effect on the growth of some bacteria, particularly Pseudomonas species. Other beneficial effects of an acidic environment have been discussed in Chapter 2: they include a reduction in the histotoxicity of ammonia (produced by enzymatic breakdown of urea by certain bacteria), and an increase in the dissociation of oxyhaemoglobin (raising the pO_2 of the wound). Viable neutrophils were found under both dressings, but in greater numbers beneath the polyurethane film.

The low pO_2 produced beneath Granuflex was thought by Cherry and Ryan[14] to be responsible for the increase in the rate of formation of vascular tissue that they observed in the chorioallantoic membrane of the chick embryo, and also in experimental wounds in pigs. The significance of these findings is discussed in greater detail in chapters 1 and 2.

A recent study[15] showed that Granuflex has pronounced fibrinolytic activity, breaking down human fibrin clots by both tissue-plasminogen-activator-dependent and independent mechanisms. It was also demonstrated in vivo that Granuflex accelerated the clearance of labelled fibrin clots in porcine full thickness wounds. As a result, it has been proposed that the dressing may help to restore normal capillary function in humans by causing dissolution of the fibrin cuffs often found around blood vessels in patients with lipodermatosclerosis or venous ulceration. The fibrin layer is believed to prevent the diffusion of oxygen from affected vessels, leading to tissue necrosis and cell death. The fibrinolytic activity of Granuflex is thought to be due to the presence of pectin, and it has been proposed that this property makes Granuflex contribute in an active or positive way to the wound healing process.

BIOFILM

Biofilm consists of a non-woven polyester fabric sheet (which is permeable to water vapour and gases) coated with an adhesive mass that consists of polyisobutylene mixed with hydrophilic particles composed of gelatin, pectin and CMC. When placed on an exuding wound, the dressing will absorb liquid and swell, forming a hydrophilic gel. The fabric backing of the dressing is strongly hydrophobic and will resist penetration by aqueous solutions or bacteria, under normal conditions of use.

In the dry state, Biofilm dressing is virtually impermeable to water vapour, but, as it takes up fluid and forms a gel, the permeability increases until a steady state is reached. The ability of the hydrated dressing to allow a significant propor- tion of the absorbed fluid to pass into the atmosphere by evaporation means that the product is able to cope with larger volumes of exudate than might otherwise be the case. This evaporation has a second important function: it helps to ensure that the outer surface of the dressing remains dry and retains its properties as a bacterial barrier.

If the dressing is covered by a second occlusive product, or if exudate is formed faster than the rate of water vapour loss, strike-through may occur, allowing bacteria to pass through the dressing. This potential problem was highlighted in a paper by Lawrence and Lilly,[16] who described a laboratory test that showed that bacteria were able to pass through the dressing in 24 hours. Their work stimulated a considerable amount of interest and subsequent correspon- dence, regarding both the suitability of the test method and the relevance of their results to the clinical situation.[17-24]

COMFEEL

First introduced in France in 1982, the Comfeel sheet consists of a semipermeable polyurethane film coated with a flexible elastic mass (made from a styrene-isoprene block co-polymer together with polycyclopentadiene dioctyladipate), and con- taining 42% NaCMC as the principal absorbent. The sheet has bevelled edges, which help to prevent the dressing snagging on clothes or bedlinen. Other components of the Comfeel wound care system include a paste (made from NaCMC, guar gum and other ingredients), and a powder composed of absorbents such as xanthan gum and guar gum. More recently, a new presentation has been introduced: it is circular and bears a series of removable, concentric foam rings

on the outer surface. Known as the Comfeel Pressure Relieving Dressing, it is intended for application to regions that are liable to develop pressure sores, or that already have established pressure areas. Once the dressing is in place, one or more of the foam rings are removed so that the area at risk is protected from any further damage.

As in Granuflex E, the adhesive matrix in Comfeel is cross-linked, forming a honeycomb- like structure in which the hydrocolloid particles are held. As a result, the dressing does not produce a viscous liquid gel as it absorbs fluid, but forms a firmer, more cohesive mass that retains its integrity as it swells. The dressing is easily removed from the wound surface without causing secondary trauma. The frequency of dressing changes are similar to those recommended for Granuflex — daily or on alternate days during the early stages of treatment, reducing to weekly changes as healing progresses.

A summary of the history and early use of Comfeel is given by Samuelsen.[25]

DERMIFLEX

Dermiflex consists of a PVC foam sheet bonded onto an impermeable plastic film, and coated with an adhesive mass that consists of polyisobutylene mixed with particles of CMC, karaya gum and silica. When the dressing absorbs fluid it does not form a smooth viscous gel like Granuflex or Biofilm, but a thick, rather granular, paste. Few published data are available on the use of Dermiflex, but the material has been reported, in some instances, to delaminate in use. It is known that Johnson & Johnson, the manufacturers of Dermiflex, are currently reviewing the product, and it is likely that a modified version will be available in due course.

INTRASITE

Intrasite is a recent development, which is similar in composition to Granuflex (being composed of gelatin, pectin and CMC, dispersed in a poly- isobutylene base). It differs primarily in the material used as the backing layer: in place of a thin foam sheet, Smith & Nephew have substituted a semipermeable film, similar to that used in Opsite. At the time of writing, Intrasite is too new for the results of any clinical evaluations to have been published, but the manufacturers have suggested that the semipermeable nature of the plastic backing may enhance the fluid-handling capacity of the dressing.

TEGASORB

Tegasorb consists of polysaccharide powders together with gelatin and pectin, dispersed in a polyisobutylene adhesive matrix, and applied to a polyurethane film membrane similar to that used in Tegaderm™. Unlike the other hydrocolloid products, Tegasorb dressings are oval; it is claimed that this makes them more convenient to apply to sacral pressure areas and other sites that may be hard to dress. The clear Tegaderm film extends beyond the hydrocolloid base, and this design feature is claimed to eliminate the need to tape down the edges of the dressing, and to prevent the transfer of adhesive onto clothes and bed linen.

CLINICAL USE OF HYDROCOLLOID DRESSINGS

The majority of the studies that have been published to date on the clinical use of hydrocolloid dressings relate to Granuflex. An early report of the use of the material in the treatment of 24 patients with burns was made by Hermans and Hermans,[26] who found that the healing rate of such wounds compared favourably with others dressed with silver sulphadiazine or human allografts. The dressing proved to be well accepted by patients and produced good long-term cosmetic results.

Similar findings have been reported after the use of Granuflex in the management of split-thickness donor sites.[27] In one study, the healing time was reduced to 7 days, from the 10−14 days normally required for paraffin tulle. The hydrocolloid produced better cosmetic results, and perceived pain was also reduced. Under Granuflex, the healed donor sites were soft and supple, and considered to be ready for re-harvesting, in marked contrast to the dry sensitive areas that had formed beneath the conventional dressing. The accelerated healing, and consequent reduction in time spent in hospital, more than offset the high initial cost of Granuflex.

Biltz et al.[28] compared Granuflex with saline gauze in the management of donor sites, and found that healing time was reduced from 13 to 7 days, also with a reduction in pain. Directly comparable results were obtained by Madden et al.,[29] working in the USA, who found that donor site healing time was reduced from 12.6 to 7.4 days when hydrocolloids were used in place of fine-mesh gauze.

The occlusive properties of the hydrocolloid dressings have also been found to be of value in the treatment of pressure areas, particularly those that occur on the heels of bedridden patients.[30,31] In these situations, the dressing prevents the loss of water vapour from the affected area, and facilitates rehydration and natural enzymatic removal of the eschar. It has also recently been suggested that this cleansing action is assisted by the fibrinolytic activity of the pectin in the dressing, as described earlier. Hydrocolloid dressings can also be used with advantage on pressure areas elsewhere,[32] provided the lesions are neither too deep nor too extensive.

Probably the major application for the hydrocolloid dressings lies in the treatment of leg ulcers of all descriptions. Ryan et al.[33] carried out a multicentre uncontrolled study of 28 patients with venous stasis ulcers, over a three-month period. During this time, 43% of ulcers healed, and there was a mean decrease in ulcer size of 75%. A small (unspecified) number of patients failed to respond favourably, and showed an increase in ulcer size during the third month of treatment. It was considered that, in these patients, the improved local conditions produced under the dressing remained inadequate to overcome the underlying problems caused by the venous stasis. The major problems associated with the use of the hydrocolloid were said to be the odour, and leakage of liquefied gel from beneath the dressing. In addition, two ulcers produced excessive amounts of granulation tissue, which was dealt with by the application of a foam pad and a pressure bandage.

Similar rates of healing of venous ulcers were reported in a second multicentre study, carried out by Cherry et al., in which 52% of ulcers in 54 patients healed in about eight weeks.[34]

In a larger multicentre study, involving 152 ulcers from ten centres in seven countries,[35] 62% of ulcers healed in an average of 51 ± 5 days when dressed with Granuflex. A reduction of pain was reported by 79% of patients, and no cases of wound infection were recorded.

Less formal studies of the use of hydrocolloid

dressings have also produced encouraging results. The experiences of Patrizi et al.[36] with Comfeel in the treatment of 33 soft tissue trophic ulcers (82% of which healed), led them to conclude that 'the product offered many benefits which made it close to an ideal treatment.' Other user assessments led to requests that the hydrocolloids should be made more widely available on prescription.[37-39]

The results of a number of controlled trials have also been published. Hydrocolloid dressings were compared with conventional materials in a randomised controlled trial in South Africa,[40] involving 36 patients with long-standing ulcers. Over an eight-week period, ulcers treated with the hydrocolloid reduced in size by 67.6%, but those treated by conventional means (povidone-iodine, covered with a foam rubber pad and compression bandaging) showed a mean reduction in size of only 23%. Although no serious problems were reported with the use of the hydrocolloid, some leakage of fluid from beneath the dressing did occur, and some patients developed a degree of skin maceration and minor fungal infections. Based upon the results of this study, the author considered that hydrocolloid dressings were best suited to application to non-infected wounds that do not produce excessive quantities of exudate.

A further controlled study, carried out in Sweden,[41] and involving 34 outpatients with chronic venous ulcers, compared the effects on healing rates of a hydrocolloid dressing (Duoderm) and a zinc oxide paste bandage. Over a period of eight weeks, both groups of ulcers decreased in volume by an average of 40% and reduced in area by about 55%. There was no statistically significant difference between the two treatment groups at any point in the study.

Despite the differences in design of the investigations quoted above, it is interesting to note that the average healing rates of all the ulcers treated with Granuflex in these studies were remarkably similar.

The value of occlusive dressings, and Granuflex in particular, was questioned by Backhouse et al.,[42] who carried out a clinical trial in which they compared a simple textile primary dressing (N-A™ Dressing) with Granuflex, in the treatment of 56 patients with chronic venous ulcers. In all cases, the dressing was covered with a standard compression bandage. There was no difference between the two groups at the end of a twelve-week period. The authors concluded that careful graduated compression bandaging

achieves healing in the majority of venous ulcers, and there is little to be gained by applying occlusive dressings. It is interesting to note, however, that the average area of the ulcers included in this study was less than 3.5 cm^2, and ulcers above 10 cm^2 were specifically excluded.

Other, more positive, reports on hydrocolloids record their use after surgery for excision of perianal hidradenitis suppurativa,[43] after colorectal surgery,[44] and as an alternative to island dressings for immediate post-operative wounds following clean elective surgery.[45] In all these situations, the enhanced wound healing and reduction in pain observed in the wounds dressed with the hydrocolloid were considered to represent significant advances over the more traditional materials.

Additional evidence for the rapid rate of healing and the lack of pain resulting from removal of the hydrocolloids was advanced by Eisenburg,[46] following a trial involving three patients suffering from epidermolysis bullosa. A total of 44 wounds were dressed with an impermeable hydrocolloid, paraffin gauze, or a perforated plastic film dressing. The wounds dressed with hydrocolloid or polyurethane film healed significantly faster than those dressed with paraffin gauze, and pain and discomfort were also reduced.

There is little doubt that there are many benefits to be derived from the correct use of hydrocolloid dressings. The decrease in pain and the considerable reductions in healing time associated with their use call into question the rationale, and even the morality, of the continued use of treatments such as dry gauze and paraffin tulle for donor sites, leg ulcers, and similar applications.

REFERENCES

1. Sircus W., Orabase in the management of abdominal-wall digestion by ileostomy and fistulas, Lancet, 1964, 2, 762.
2. Ashurst P.J., Granulation in chronic leg ulcers: a trial with a new material, Practitioner, 1975, 215, 353–358.
3. Leeson M., Stomahesive: the astounding new cure for decubitus ulcers, Nursing, 1976, 6, 13–15.
4. Ryan D.M., Pressure sores: treatment using Stomahesive, Nurs. Times, 1976, 72, 299–300.
5. Tracy G.D. et al., Varihesive sealed dressing for indolent leg ulcers, Med. J. Austral., 1977, 1, 777–780.
6. Baxter R., Varihesive and the treatment of chronic leg ulcers, Austral. Fam. Physn, 1980, 9, 599–601.

7. Allen S.A., Varihesive: a new tool in geriatric practice, *Chiropodist,* 1981, **36**, 25−27.

8. Thomas S. and Loveless P., Moisture vapour permeability of hydrocolloid dressings, *Pharm. J.,* 1988, **241**, 806.

9. Alvarez O.M. *et al.,* The effect of occlusive dressings on collagen synthesis and re-epithelialization in superficial wounds, *J. surg. Res.,* 1983, **35**, 142−148.

10. Lawrence J.C. and Lilly H.A., Bacteriological properties of a new hydrocolloid dressing on intact skin of normal volunteers, in *An Environment for Healing: The Role of Occlusion,* Ryan T.J. (ed.), International Congress and Symposium Series No. 88, London, Royal Society of Medicine, 1985, 51−57.

11. Lawrence J.C., The physical properties of a new hydrocolloid dressing, in Ref.10, 71−76.

12. Wilson P. *et al.,* Methicillin-resistant *Staphylococcus aureus* and hydrocolloid dressings, *Pharm. J.,* 1988, **241**, 787−788.

13. Varghese M.D. *et al.,* Local environment of chronic wounds under synthetic dressings, *Arch. Derm.,* 1986, **122**, 52−57.

14. Cherry G.W. and Ryan T.J., Enhanced wound angiogenesis with a new hydrocolloid dressing, in Ref.10, 61−68.

15 Lydon M.J. *et al.,* Fibrinolytic activity of hydrocolloid dressings, in *Beyond Occlusion: Wound Care Proceedings,* Ryan T.J. (ed.), International Congress and Symposium Series No. 136, London, Royal Society of Medicine, 1988, 9−17.

16. Lawrence J.C. and Lilly H.A., Are hydrocolloid dressings bacteria proof?, *Pharm. J.,* 1987, **239**, 184.

17. Piercey D.A., Are hydrocolloid dressings bacteria proof?, (letter), *ibid.,* 223.

18. Cherry G.W., *idem., ibid.,* 281.

19. Lawrence J.C., *idem., ibid.,* 310.

20. Thomas S. and Hay N.P., *idem., ibid.,* 388−389.

21. Cherry G.W., *idem., ibid.,* 456.

22. Moores J., *idem., ibid.,* 486.

23. Lawrence J.C. and Lilly H.A., *idem., ibid.,* 486.

24. Johnson A., *idem., ibid.,* 486.

25. Samuelsen P., Clinical aspects of the Comfeel ulcer care system, in *Advances in Wound Management,* Turner T.D., Schmidt R.J. and Harding K.G. (eds), London, John Wiley, 1985, 97−100.

26. Hermans M.H.E. and Hermans R.P., Preliminary report on the use of a new hydrocolloid dressing in the treatment of burns, *Burns,* 1984, **11**, 125−129.

27. Doherty C. *et al.,* Granuflex hydrocolloid as a donor site dressing, *Care Crit. Ill,* 1986, **2**, 193−194.

28. Biltz H. *et al.,* Comparison of hydrocolloid dressing and saline gauze in the treatment of skin graft donor sites, in Ref.10, 125−128.

29. Madden M.R. *et al.,* Optimal healing of donor site wounds with hydrocolloid dressings, in Ref.10, 131−139.

30. Tudhope M., Management of pressure ulcers with a hydrocolloid occlusive dressing: results in twenty-three patients, *J. enterostom. Ther.,* 1984, **11**, 102−105.

31. Johnson A., Towards rapid tissue healing, *Nurs. Times,* 1984, **80**, 39−43.

32. Yarkony G.M. *et al.,* Pressure sore management: efficacy of a moisture reactive occlusive dressing, *Arch. phys. Med. Rehab.,* 1984, **65**, 597−600.

33. Ryan T.J. *et al.,* The use of a new occlusive dressing in the management of venous stasis ulceration, in Ref.10, 99−103.

34. Cherry G.W. *et al.,* Trial of a new dressing in venous leg ulcers, *Practitioner,* 1984, **288**, 1175−1178.

35. Van Rijswijk L. *et al.,* Multicenter clinical evaluation of a hydrocolloid dressing for leg ulcers, *Cutis,* 1985, **35**, 173−176.

36. Patrizi P. *et al.,* The treatment of superficial trophic ulcerations with Comfeel Ulcus, *Clin. Eur.,* 1984, **23**, 19−26.

37. Milward P., Doing the legwork, *Nurs. Times,* 1986, **82**, 35−36.

38. Pottle B., Trial of a dressing for non-healing ulcers, *ibid.,* 1987, **83**, 54−58.

39. Milward P., The use of hydrocolloid dressings for the treatment of leg ulcers in the community: Drug Tariff considerations, *Care Sci. Pract.,* 1987, **5**, 31−34.

40. Groenewald J.H., Comparative effects of HCD and conventional treatment on the healing of venous stasis ulcers, in Ref.10, 105−109.

41. Eriksson G., Comparison of two occlusive bandages in the treatment of venous leg ulcers, *Br. J. Derm.,* 1986, **114**, 227−230.

42. Backhouse C.M. *et al.,* Controlled trial of occlusive dressings in healing chronic venous ulcers, *Br. J. Surg.,* 1987, **74**, 626−627.

43. Michel L., Use of hydrocolloid dressing following wide excision of perianal hidradenitis suppurativa, in Ref.10, 143−148.

44. Hulten L., Wound dressing after colorectal surgery, in Ref.10, 149−151.

45. Young R.A.L. and Weston Davies W.H., Comparison of a hydrocolloid dressing and a conventional island dressing as a primary surgical wound dressing, in Ref.10, 153−156.

46. Eisenberg M., The effect of occlusive dressings on re-epithelialisations of wounds in children with epidermolysis bullosa, *J. pediat. Surg.,* 1986, **21**, 892−894.

Chapter 9

Polysaccharide Pastes, Granules and Beads

HONEY AND SUCROSE

One of the oldest – and almost certainly the most enduring – material to be used in wound management is honey, a complex mixture consisting principally of glucose and fructose. The Edwin Smith papyrus (c. 1600BC) records how the ancient Egyptians packed honey combined with lard or resin into wounds sustained in battle, and more than 1000 years later Hippocrates recommended its use as an ointment or salve. The healing properties of honey as revealed in the Koran and documented in the Hadith have been discussed in the light of modern scientific knowledge,[1] and a review of the medicinal use of honey has also recently been published.[2] Honey still remains a popular remedy for the treatment of wounds such as leg ulcers and pressure sores, and is a component of a commercially available tulle dressing (M and M Tulle™).

Honey has a low pH, about 3.7, which creates an unfavourable environment for bacterial growth. In a study reported in 1970, Cavanagh et al.[3] described a small clinical trial in which they applied honey to 12 patients whose wounds had become infected after a radical operation for carcinoma of the vulva. All infections responded promptly, and the wounds became 'bacteriologically sterile' within three to six days and remained so until completely healed. All the wounds healed within eight weeks, and one within three weeks. In a laboratory study performed at the same time, it was shown that neat honey was able to kill or inhibit the growth of a range of pathogenic bacteria, including streptococci and coagulase-positive staphylococci, although it was unable to prevent the growth of Candida species. In an account of surgery in western Kenya, Branicki[4] recorded that honey was used in the management of large septic wounds. Once again, it was found that the wounds became sterile within 3–6 days and formed healthy granulation tissue.

Honey has a high osmotic pressure and will effectively draw water out of the surrounding tissue, thus aiding wound cleansing and reducing oedema. It is also possible that honey provides nutrients and a source of energy for the dividing cells on the surface of the wound, although this has not been confirmed experimentally.

In recent years, there has been an increasing interest in the use of sugar (sucrose) as a dressing, although most of the evidence supporting its use is anecdotal, or based upon uncontrolled studies. In 1973,[5] it was reported that, over a five-year period, an 80% healing rate was achieved in decubitus ulcers dressed with granulated sugar and tincture of benzoin. In 1980, Thomlinson[6] described how icing sugar was applied to malodorous malignant breast ulcers in four patients, using a teaspoon or salt cellar. The treatment was repeated every twelve hours. In all four cases, the smell from the wound was greatly reduced, no adverse effects were recorded, and patients were able to manage their wounds at home.

A much larger comparative study was performed by Knutson et al.,[7] who treated 605 wounds of various types with granulated sugar and povidone-iodine. The healing rates of these wounds were compared with those of a further 154 patients, who were treated with other unspecified therapies. The study was not well controlled, but, overall, the wounds treated with sugar were said to heal faster than those in the control group.

The scientific basis for the use of granulated sugar was discussed by Chirife et al. in 1982,[8] following a study in which they measured the effects of increasing sugar concentrations upon the growth of Staphylococcus aureus. They demonstrated that a level of 195 g of sugar per 100 g of water produced complete inhibition of growth, with the number of viable organisms declining steadily throughout the incubation period. They concluded that granulated sugar could act as a universal antimicrobial agent for the treatment of infected wounds and other superficial lesions, and suggested that 'on grounds of safety, economy and availability this therapeutic use of sugar may have widespread applicability, even in emergencies and disasters.'

These enthusiastic conclusions were challenged by Forrest,[9] who considered that the osmotic pressure of partially dissolved sugar could have harmful or undesirable effects — in that it would also tend to dehydrate epithelial cells, macrophages and fibroblasts — and thus delay healing. He also questioned the description of sugar as a 'universal antimicrobial agent' on the basis of tests carried out on a single organism, and doubted the possibility of sustaining the required concentration of sugar at the wound surface for any length of time. Bose[10] was also unconvinced of the merits of sugar, and considered that honey had a number of practical advantages.

In 1985, Trouillet et al.[11] described the results of an uncontrolled trial of the use of sugar in 29 patients with acute post-operative mediastinitis. In this study, 11 patients were initially treated with gauze soaked in povidone-iodine, which was replaced two days later by granulated sugar packed tightly into the wound. The wounds were cleansed and repacked twice daily, and fresh sugar was added at intervals of 3–4 hours as required. The remaining patients had their wounds subjected to continuous irrigation with a weak solution of povidone-iodine. All patients in both groups also received systemic antibiotic therapy. Eight of the patients treated with povidone-iodine alone failed to respond favourably, and were therefore changed to the sugar treatment. Debridement and granulation tissue production occurred within 5–9 days in the majority of the 19 wounds that were dressed with sugar — only 3 required surgical debridement. Overall, 17 of the 19 wounds responded well to the treatment but two patients had severe acute haemorrhage from exposed vascular sutures which required immediate surgery. Four patients died of unrelated causes and 13 patients were eventually discharged completely healed.

Similar encouraging results were reported by Quatraro et al.,[12] following the treatment of 15 diabetic patients, 13 of whom had dystrophic or ischaemic ulcers of the the lower limbs. One of the remaining patients had a suppurative process of the feet, the other had a burn upon the hand. All the wounds were packed with sugar and covered with gauze, and more sugar was added every 3–4 hours. Granulation tissue formed within 5–6 days and all wounds were completely healed in 9–12 days.

Normal commercial sugar is not always sterile, and may contain calcium phosphate, sodium aluminium silicate or other permitted agents to prevent caking upon storage.[13] A paste made from additive-free caster and icing sugar, polyethylene glycol 400 and hydrogen peroxide was developed in 1985, and its use reported by Gordon et al.[14] and Middleton and Seal.[15] Two versions were produced, a thin form for instillation into abscesses (as an alternative to ribbon gauze packing), and a thicker form for the treatment of large open wounds. The thin paste, particularly, was found to be effective in situations where traditional Eusol packs had failed, and the authors concluded that both formulations had many advantages over conventional materials.

Topham[16] described the use of simple sugar pastes containing povidone-iodine on the island of Zanzibar, and concluded that they offered a cheap and chemically pure aid to wound healing.

Although the topical use of sugar appears to be relatively free of adverse effects, osmotic nephrosis resulting in acute renal failure was reported in one patient — after the extensive use of granulated sugar in a deep infected pneumonectomy wound in the right chest of a 64-year-old male. The sugar was removed from the cavity; when urine flow resumed on the second day, it was found to contain large amounts of sucrose.[17] However, Archer et al.[18] questioned whether this nephrotoxicity might have been related, at least in part, to the use of gentamicin (which was applied to the wound in the form of an irrigation before the application of sugar).

The value of sugar in wound healing was discussed by Keith and Knodel,[19] who reviewed the published literature and concluded that 'based upon available information the use of sugar as the sole treatment of wounds cannot be recommended ... when used alone, sugar has not been shown to be effective in hastening wound healing in controlled clinical testing.' Clearly, however, in view of the encouraging results recorded by some workers, there is a need for further controlled studies of this cheap and freely available material.

POLYSACCHARIDE BEADS

Commercial dressings made from polysaccharides that have been chemically modified and formed into beads or granules are used in much the same way as sugar, although they differ in their mode of action. At present, there are two such products available in the UK. They are:

- Debrisan™ – Pharmacia,
- Iodosorb™ – Perstorp.

Debrisan

Debrisan, the first of the two materials to be used as a wound dressing, is manufactured from a derivative of dextran (a linear polymer of glucose produced by a micro-organism, *Leuconostoc mesenteroides*). In its unmodified form, dextran is soluble in water; however, when it is treated with epichlorhydrin under controlled conditions, crosslinks are formed between the chains – these impart a three-dimensional structure to the molecule, rendering it insoluble. The resulting polymer has been given the approved name 'dextranomer'.

Debrisan is supplied sterile, in the form of spherical beads (0.1–0.3 mm in diameter) which are composed of dextranomer, poloxamer 187, polyethylene glycol 300, and a small quantity of water.[20] The beads are highly hydrophilic; 1 g will take up about 4 g of liquid. About 60% of the absorbed fluid is held within the beads themselves; the remainder is retained in the spaces between them. Water, and solutes with a molecular weight of less than 1000, can pass freely into the structure of the beads; but materials with molecular weights in the range 1000–5000 can penetrate only to a limited extent; and molecules larger than this cannot enter the beads at all.

When Debrisan is placed upon a wound, exudate is rapidly taken up by capillary action into the small spaces between the beads. The beads then absorb some of the water and low molecular weight material, and swell. As the beads in contact with the wound become saturated, the excess liquid is drawn up by the next, dry, layer, taking with it the high molecular weight material that cannot enter the beads. In this way, exudate is drawn progressively away from the surface of the wound, carrying with it bacteria and cellular debris.[21]

The transport of bacteria away from the wound surface was neatly demonstrated in a laboratory model by Jacobsson and others,[21] following earlier work by Juhlin.[22] They allowed a column of Debrisan in a glass cylinder to take up a suspension of micro-organisms in a mixture of plasma and normal saline, until the beads became saturated. The column was then pressed out of the cylinder and divided into four segments, which were examined by standard microbiological techniques. It was found that – regardless of the type of organism studied – at the end of the experiment, approximately 80% of the bacteria taken up by the dressing were present in the upper segment of the column. This ability of the beads to separate dissolved materials by their molecular weight has been known for many years, and has formed the basis of their use in column chromatography (under the name of Sephadex™).

The affinity of Debrisan for aqueous solutions is such that it will create a suction pressure of up to 200 mmHg, initially. As the beads become saturated, however, the suction pressure will eventually return to zero. At this point, bacteria that have been transported to the outer layer of the dressing may start to spread back through the dressing. For this reason, it is important that Debrisan dressings on moist wounds are changed regularly, preferably before the beads become saturated. For heavily exuding wounds, twice daily changes may be required.

Because it is chemically inert, Debrisan is unlikely to cause any allergic reaction. In a study of 192 patients with stasis dermatitis and leg ulcers, 69% were found to be sensitive to one or more components of commonly used topical preparations, such as the antibiotics neomycin and framycetin. When the ulcers of 86 of these patients were treated with Debrisan, no irritant or allergic reactions were encountered. About 90% of all the patients treated reported a reduction in pain once treatment was initiated.[23]

Clinical use of Debrisan

In use, it is recommended that Debrisan beads are poured into a wound to a depth of about 3 mm, and covered with a simple dressing pad or a semipermeable plastic film. The mobile nature of the beads can make this procedure somewhat difficult in shallow wounds and, therefore, alternative methods of presentation have been devised. The data sheet for Debrisan suggests the production of a paste made with glycerol, but Johnson[24] described an alternative formulation using Debrisan beads and polyethylene glycol 400, which proved very successful in the treatment of a number of infected wounds. A commercial preparation of Debrisan paste was launched in 1985, consisting of dextranomer 6.4 g with polyethylene glycol 600 and water to 10 g. This was followed, in 1986, by the introduction of a Debrisan pad, in which a dextranomer paste is enclosed in a non-woven textile bag; the pad is placed directly into or onto the wound. Debrisan paste or pad dressings should be changed before they become saturated with exudate. Depending upon the condition of the wound, this may vary from twice daily to every other day.

The presentation of Debrisan as a paste has an effect upon the fluid-absorbing mechanism of the beads. In such a formulation, no capillary uptake of fluid can take place – although this is compensated for, at least in part, by the water-absorbing properties of the glycerol or poly-ethylene glycol.[20]

All three presentations of Debrisan are rec-ommended for the treatment of infected wounds, and for cleansing wounds containing pus, debris and soft yellow necrotic tissue. Once the dressing has achieved this objective, and healthy gran-ulation tissue is produced, alternative treatments should be considered.

Published studies suggest that Debrisan beads have a positive effect upon developing granulation tissue, causing increased cellularity, augmented vascularization, and enhanced accumulation of connective tissue ground substance.[25] Examination of Debrisan beads removed from the surface of wounds revealed high levels of fibrinogen degra-dation products, indicating marked fibrinolytic activity. No clottable fibrinogen was detected, suggesting that stable clots cannot be formed on the surface of a wound dressed with Debrisan; such a wound will therefore remain soft and free-draining.[26]

The concentration of prostaglandins in the fluid produced by leg ulcers dressed with Debrisan was investigated by Jacobsson et al.[21] They found that the highest values were observed in beads removed from highly inflamed wounds, and noted that these levels often decreased as the wounds became cleaner and less oedematous. The constant removal of mediators like prostaglandins has been claimed to limit the inflammatory reaction, and hence reduce wound pain. Comparative studies of human donor sites and experimental burns in pigs showed that, histologically, the inflammatory reaction to trauma was less pronounced in wounds dressed with the beads than in comparable wounds dressed with a Vaseline™ gauze material, although no difference in the rate of epithelial-isation was detected.[27] The possible consequences of small numbers of beads becoming trapped in living tissue were investigated by Falk and Tollerz,[28] who implanted approximately 500 mg

of the beads intramuscularly into rabbits and guinea pigs, and 100 mg subcutaneously. Upon subsequent examination, each bead was found to be loosely encapsulated by connective tissue. Apparently unchanged beads were present up to three years after implantation. No granuloma formation was detected, and the lack of inflam-matory signs and the limited proliferation of fibroblasts led the authors to conclude that Debrisan was well tolerated with an insignificant locally irritating effect.

Numerous papers have been published record-ing the use of Debrisan in different types of wound. In a controlled study involving 48 patients with discharging burns, Debrisan was shown to reduce inflammation and bring about healing faster than saline dressings.[29] It has also been reported to be of value in the management of burns on the hand.[30,31] In this situation the beads were sprinkled onto the hand, which was then inserted into a plastic bag. In the early stages, the dressings had to be changed three times a day, but the interval between changes was increased as healing progressed. The treatment was relatively painless and the hand and fingers could be moved freely within the bag. No crusts were formed and the areas remained soft and pliable throughout.

Similar beneficial effects were recorded in a trial in which the beads were compared with Eusol and paraffin in the treatment of infected bowel wounds. Time to wound closure was 8 days for Debrisan, compared with 12 days for the control group, and patients treated with Debrisan had a shorter hospital stay (by a median of 2.2 days). The authors considered that this reduction in the time spent in hospital compensated for the high cost of the Debrisan treatment.[32] The clinical efficacy of Debrisan was compared with that of streptokinase-streptodornase (Varidase™) in a controlled study involving 87 infected wounds.[33] Both treatments proved to be effective, overall, but the dextranomer seemed to act more quickly; it also appeared to stimulate more effective growth of granulation tissue.

The results of a prospective trial comparing Debrisan beads with a silicone foam dressing in the treatment of 50 open surgical wounds were reported by Young and Wheeler,[34] who found that, although the healing rates obtained with the two dressings were comparable, the cost of Debrisan treatment was considerably higher than that of the silicone foam.

Debrisan has also been used in the treatment of

leg ulcers,[35,36] pressure areas,[37–39] infected wounds,[40,41] and other miscellaneous wound types. In a trial involving the treatment of infected sockets following tooth extraction in 82 patients,[42] sockets dressed with Debrisan (held in place with Orabase™) became pain-free in five days, compared with 12 days for the control group, which were treated with a paste made from zinc oxide and clove oil. In this particular study, however, it is not certain whether it was the beads or the Orabase paste that was mainly responsible for the rapid healing reported by the authors.

In a comparative study reported by Goode et al,[43] Debrisan pads were compared with ribbon gauze soaked in saline in the treatment of 67 patients with infected surgical wounds. It was found that the dextranomer-treated wounds were cleaned 32% quicker than the saline control group, and the authors concluded that the use of the pads provided a simple and efficient method of managing moist infected wounds.

Iodosorb

Iodosorb is similar in appearance and mode of action to Debrisan, consisting of microspheres 0.1–0.3 mm in diameter, formed from a three-dimensional network of cadexomer – starch chains cross-linked by ether bridges. The hydrophilic beads contain 0.9% w/w of iodine, which is firmly held within the structure of the microspheres and is not liberated from them in the dry state, despite the high vapour pressure of elemental iodine. Laboratory studies have shown that the release of iodine is governed both by the physico-chemical characteristics of the carrier and by the solubility of iodine in the solvent medium.[44] Solvents such as polyethylene glycol and propylene glycol are not taken up by the beads and no detectable levels of iodine can be found in them, despite the fact that iodine is soluble in both solvents. If water or an aqueous solution is added to the beads, it is taken up rapidly (1 g of Iodosorb is said to be able to absorb up to 7 mL of fluid); the beads swell and iodine is slowly liberated. In a wound, the iodine is carried – by the capillary movement of fluid – away from the damaged tissue, resulting in a concentration gradient with the lowest levels of iodine at the surface of the wound. Lawrence[45] has suggested – as a result of laboratory studies – that, although the mechanisms of fluid transport and the removal of debris and bacteria from the surface of a wound

are generally similar in both Iodosorb and Debrisan, cadexomer iodine has the advantage of considerably reducing the number of viable organisms present.

A new presentation of Iodosorb has been developed in which the beads are formulated in an inert ointment base containing 0.9% w/w iodine. This new preparation, called Iodosorb Ointment™, is intended for the treatment of chronic leg ulcers.

Unlike Debrisan, Iodosorb is biodegradable – being sensitive to enzymatic hydrolysis by an α-amylase that is present in most body fluids. The breakdown products consist of low molecular weight fractions (mainly maltose and glucose).[46]

Clinical use of Iodosorb

Iodosorb is indicated for the management of sloughy and infected wounds. In an early randomised trial of the treatment of 38 decubitus ulcers,[47] it was found that cadexomer iodine was superior to standard treatments in removing pus and debris from the surface of the ulcer; wound healing rates, as measured by a decrease in wound area, were also significantly improved. During the course of the study, a small number of patients complained of transient smarting during the first hour after application of the dressing.

The major indication for the use of Iodosorb, however, is in the management of leg ulcers. In a multicentre trial carried out in Sweden, involving 93 patients over a six-week period,[48] it was found that cadexomer iodine was more effective than the standard treatment in terms of reduction of pain, removal of exudate and debris, stimulation of granulation and reduction of erythema. Overall, the mean area of the ulcers treated with the beads decreased by over 30%, while those in the control group showed a small increase in area. A significant correlation was also observed between the use of the beads and a reduction in infection with Staph. aureus and other pathogenic species.

In a second optional crossover trial,[49] involving 61 selected patients with venous ulcers, Iodosorb was compared with a standard treatment regimen (which included the use of gentian violet and an ointment containing polymyxin and bacitracin). In this study, patients were encouraged to manage their ulcers by themselves, and, although both treatments were found to be effective, ulcers dressed with the beads healed nearly twice as quickly as those in the control group. The authors concluded that daily bandaging and renewal of a non-adherent dressing may have distinct advantages over less demanding regimens. Following the publication of this paper, Shuttleworth and Mayho[50] commented upon the problems of handling the dressing, and described the use of a paste made from Iodosorb (3 g) and polyethylene glycol (0.5 mL), which they found easier to apply and remove. It was also reported that this formulation appeared to cause less stinging than Iodosorb sometimes did.

In a further multicentred randomised crossover trial,[51] 72 patients had their ulcers managed entirely in the community by general practitioners. In the first four weeks of the study, ulcers treated with standard dressings and changed daily decreased in area by 10%, whereas those dressed with Iodosorb decreased by 36% in the same time. This trend toward increased healing continued after the crossover point. It was also recorded that ulcers dressed with cadexomer iodine produced less odour and pain than those in the control group.

A similar study to that described above was carried out by Lindsay et al.,[52] in which the dressings were changed on alternate days. Once again, Iodosorb proved to be superior to the alternative treatments, in terms of wound debridement, odour, improvement in pain relief and reduction of erythema and oedema. Ulcers dressed with traditional materials reduced in size by about 4% in four weeks, but those dressed with Iodosorb reduced in size by over 33%, a figure that is in close agreement with the results of earlier studies.

In one eight-week study,[53] the clinical efficacy of Iodosorb and that of Debrisan were compared in the treatment of 27 patients with venous leg ulcers. Of those patients treated with Iodosorb, 65% healed completely, compared with 50% of those in the Debrisan group. Relative wound reduction also appeared to be greater in the cadexomer iodine group, but this did not reach statistical significance. The authors concluded that, although both products effectively reduced the symptoms caused by venous leg ulcers, the overall clinical response was significantly better in the cadexomer iodine group. It was suggested that this might be due to the enhanced absorbency of the beads and the antibacterial properties of the iodine, although the results of the bacteriological studies did not correlate well with ulcer healing.

INDICATIONS FOR THE USE OF BEAD DRESSINGS

Although both Debrisan and Iodosorb can be, and have been, used as a single treatment throughout the entire healing process of wounds such as leg ulcers and pressure areas, there is probably little doubt that the major indication for their use is in the early part of the healing cycle – for cleaning or debriding sloughy or infected wounds. Once they have achieved this objective, a change to an alternative treatment may be considered desirable.

REFERENCES

1. Abu T.M.M. Ali, The pharmacological characterization and the scientific basis of the hidden miracles of honey, Saudi med. J., 1989, 10, 177–179.
2. Zumla A. and Lulat A., Honey – a remedy rediscovered, J. R. Soc Med., 1989, 82, 384–385.
3. Cavanagh D. et al., Radical operation for carcinoma of the vulva; a new approach to wound healing, J. Obstet. Gynaec. Br. Commonw., 1970, 77, 1037–1040.
4. Branicki F.J., Surgery in Western Kenya, Ann. R. Coll. Surg., 1981, 63, 348–352.
5. Anon., Sugar sweetens the lot of patients with bed sores, J. Am. med. Ass., 1973, 223, 122.
6. Thomlinson R.H., Kitchen remedy for necrotic malignant breast ulcers, (letter), Lancet, 1980, 2, 707.
7. Knutson R.A. et al., Use of sugar and povidone iodine to enhance wound healing: five years experience, Sth. med. J., 1981, 74, 1329–1335.
8. Chirife J. et al., Scientific basis for use of granulated sugar in treatment of infected wounds, Lancet, 1982, 1, 560–561.
9. Forrest R.D., Sugar in the wound, (letter), ibid., 861.
10. Bose B., Honey or sugar in the treatment of infected wounds, (letter), ibid., 963.
11. Trouillet J.L. et al., Use of granulated sugar in treatment of open mediastinitis after cardiac surgery, ibid., 1985, 2, 180–184.
12. Quatraro A et al., Sugar and wound healing, (letter), ibid., 1985, 2, 664.
13. Addison M.K. and Walterspiel J.N., idem., ibid., 665.
14. Gordon H. et al., idem., ibid., 663–664.
15. Middleton K.R. and Seal D., Sugar as an aid to wound healing, Pharm. J., 1985, 235, 757–758.
16. Topham J.D., Sugar paste in treatment of pressure sores, burns and wounds, ibid., 1988, 241, 118–119.
17. Debure A. et al., Acute renal failure after use of granulated sugar in deep infected wound, (letter), Lancet, 1987, 1, 1034–1035.
18. Archer H, et al., Toxicity of topical sugar, ibid., 1485–1486.

19. Keith J.F. and Knodel L.C., Sugar in wound healing, *Drug Intell. clin. Pharm*, 1988, **22**, 409–411.

20. Schmidt R.J., Xerogel dressings: an overview, in *Advances in Wound Management*, Turner T.D., Schmidt R.J. and Harding K.G., (eds), London, John Wiley, 1985, 65–71.

21. Jacobsson S. *et al.*, A new principle for the cleansing of infected wounds, *Scand. J. plast. reconstr. Surg.*, 1976, **10**, 65–72.

22. Juhlin I., Distribution of micro-organisms in a Debrisan column, *Sv. Kir.*, 1974, **31**, 69–71.

23. Fraki J.E. *et al.*, Allergy to various components of topical preparations in stasis dermatitis and leg ulcer, *Contact Dermatitis*, 1979, **5**, 97–100.

24. Johnson A., Cleansing infected wounds, *Nurs. Times*, 1986, **82**, 30–34.

25. Niinikoski J. and Renvall S., Effect of dextranomer on developing granulation tissue in standard skin defects in rats, *Clin. Ther.*, 1980, **3**, 273–279.

26. Aberg M. *et al.*, Fibrinolytic activity in wound secretions, *Scand. J. plast. reconstr. Surg.*, 1976, **10**, 103–105.

27. Jacobsson S. *et al.*, Studies on healing of Debrisan-treated wounds, *ibid.*, 97–101.

28. Falk J. and Tollerz G., Chronic tissue response to implantation of Debrisan: an experimental study, *Clin. Ther.*, 1977, **1**, 185–191.

29. Gang R.K., Debrisan and saline dressing, *Chir. plast.*, 1981, **6**, 65–68.

30. Paavolainen P. and Sundell B., The effect of dextranomer (Debrisan) on hand burns, *Ann. Chir. Gynaec.*, 1976, **65**, 313–317.

31. Arturson G. *et al.*, A new topical agent (Debrisan) for the early treatment of the burned hand, *Burns*, 1978, **4**, 225–232.

32. Goode A.W. *et al.*, The cost effectiveness of dextranomer and eusol in the treatment of infected surgical wounds, *Br. J. clin. Pract.*, 1979, **33**, 325 and 328.

33. Hulkko A. *et al.*, Comparison of dextranomer and streptokinase-streptodornase in the treatment of venous leg ulcers and other infected wounds, *Ann. Chir. Gynaec.* 1981, **70**, 65–70.

34. Young H.L. and Wheeler M.H., Report of a prospective trial of dextranomer beads (Debrisan) and silicone foam elastomer (Silastic) dressings in surgical wounds, *Br. J. Surg.*, 1982, **69**, 33–34.

35. Floden C.H. and Wilkstrom K., Controlled clinical trial with dextranomer (Debrisan) on venous leg ulcers, *Curr. ther. Res.*, 1978, **24**, 753–760.

36. Groenwald J.H., An evaluation of dextranomer as a cleansing agent in the treatment of the post-phlebitic statis ulcer, *Sth Afr. med. J.*, 1980, **57**, 809–815.

37. McClemont E.J.W. *et al.*, Pressure sores: a new method of treatment, *Br. J. clin. Pract.*, 1979, **33**, 21–25.

38. Parish L.C. and Collins E., Decubitus ulcers: a comparative study, *Cutis*, 1979, **23**, 106–110.

39. Nasar M.A. and Morley R., Cost effectiveness in treating deep pressure sores and ulcers, *Practitioner*, 1982, **226**, 307–310.

40. Bewick M. and Anderson J., A new method for treating infected wounds: studies on dextranomer (Debrisan): case reports, *Clin. Trials J.*, 1978, **15**, 120–126.

41. Soul J., A trial of Debrisan in the cleansing of infected surgical wounds, *Br. J. clin. Pract.*, 1978, **32**, 172–173.

42. Mathews R.W., An evaluation of dextranomer granules as a new method of treatment of alveolar osteitis, *Br. dent. J.*, 1982, **152**, 157–159.

43. Goode A.W. *et al.*, A study of dextranomer absorbent pads in the management of infected wounds, *Clin. Trials J.*, 1985, **22**, 431–434.

44. Gustavson B., Cadexomer iodine: introduction, in *Cadexomer Iodine*, Fox J.A. and Fischer H. (eds), Symposium, Munich, 22 January 1983, Stuttgart, Schattauer Verlag, 1983, 35–41.

45. Lawrence J.C., Bacteriology and wound healing, in Ref.44, 19–31.

46. Personal communication from Perstorp AB, on the *in-vitro* enzymatic hydrolysis of Iodophore gel and other modified starch gels by endogenous α amylase.

47. Moberg S. *et al.*, A randomised trial of cadexomer iodine in decubitus ulcers, *J. Am. geriat. Soc.*, 1983, **31**, 462–465.

48. Skog E. *et al.*, A randomized trial comparing cadexomer iodine and standard treatment in the out-patient management of chronic venous ulcers, *Br. J. Derm.*, 1983, **109**, 77–83.

49. Ormiston M.C. *et al.*, Controlled trial of Iodosorb in chronic venous ulcers, *Br. med. J.*, 1985, **291**, 308–310.

50. Shuttleworth G.J. and Mayho G.V., Controlled trial of Iodosorb in chronic venous ulcers, (letter), *ibid.*, 605–606.

51. Harcup J.W. and Saul P.A., A study of the effect of cadexomer iodine in the treatment of venous leg ulcers, *Br. J. clin. Pract.*, 1986, **40**, 360–364.

52. Lindsay G. *et al.*, A study in general practice of the efficacy of cadexomer iodine in venous leg ulcers treated on alternate days, *Acta ther.*, 1986, **12**, 141–148.

53. Kero M. *et al.*, A comparison of cadexomer iodine with dextranomer in the treatment of venous leg ulcers, *Curr. ther. Res.*, 1987, **42**, 761–767.

Chapter 10

Odour-absorbing Dressings

Infected wounds — such as pressure sores, leg ulcers, and fungating carcinomas — sometimes produce an extremely noxious odour which, even in moderate cases, can be distressing for the patient and unpleasant for hospital staff and visitors. In extreme cases, however, such an odour can become a major source of embarrassment or cause serious psychological problems; a badly affected patient may become withdrawn and avoid all kinds of social contact — even with family and close friends.[1]

Possibly the best known malodorous wounds, although fortunately relatively uncommon, are those infected with *Clostridium welchii*, the causative organism of gas gangrene — a condition which has a particularly penetrating and distinctive smell. Other, more commonly encountered organisms that are also implicated in odour production include *Bacteroides* species and other anaerobes, although infections caused by aerobic organisms such as *Proteus, Klebsiella* and *Pseudomonas* spp. can also cause wounds to smell very badly. Obviously, the most effective way of treating a foul-smelling wound is to prevent or eradicate the infection causing the odour. Although this may sometimes be achieved by the administration of antibiotics or the topical application of antiseptics or antimicrobial agents, it is often not possible to obtain an effective concentration of the antibiotic at the site of the infection by this method, and in these situations, some other method of combating the smell is required. One method is by the use of a dressing that acts like a filter and absorbs the odoriferous chemicals liberated from the wound, before they pass into the air. The most effective material available for this purpose is activated charcoal (which is used in the manufacture of air filters, gas masks and other specialised items of military clothing). This was originally used in the form of granules, but for many applications, these have been replaced by a charcoal fabric; it is this material that forms the basis of most of the dressings in current use.

In 1976, Butcher *et al.*[2] described the use of a charcoal cloth that had been developed by the Chemical Defence Establishment, Porton Down. This was incorporated into pads of surgical gauze containing a layer of a water-repellant fabric, and was used in the treatment of fungating breast cancer, gangrene, and immediately after colostomy operations. In all cases it was reported that following the application of the dressing, the odour from the wounds was totally suppressed.

Activated charcoal cloth is manufactured from a suitable cellulose fabric, which is heated to about 350°C in an inert atmosphere. Under these conditions, the cellulose decomposes, leaving a residue of pure carbon. This is then activated by further heating to 800–900°C in the presence of carbon dioxide or steam, when the surface of the carbon breaks down to form large numbers of pores, some 2 nm in width. By the end of this process, the cloth is very fragile; it has been found, however, that pre-treatment of the cellulose with a solution of certain metallic chlorides (prior to carbonisation) will reduce the loss of carbon by lowering the temperature at which activation takes place. The pre-treatment also has the effect of generating smaller pores in the fibre, which causes less damage to the fabric and prevents it falling apart.

The presence of pores increases the effective surface area of the carbon fibres, and hence their adsorptive capacity. The total area may be determined by measuring the amount of nitrogen that is required to cover the surface with a layer one molecule thick.[3] For the activated charcoal cloth that is used in the manufacture of most of the dressings, this technique gives a result of about 1300 m²/g — the specific surface area of the fabric.

The odours that are produced by necrotic wounds are due mainly to the formation of diamines such as cadaverine and putrescine. These molecules are relatively small (up to about 1 nm across) and are able easily to enter the pores on the charcoal fabric. Protein molecules are much larger, in the range 2–50 nm, and are therefore too large to enter the pores; they are nevertheless, adsorbed onto the activated charcoal, possibly by electrical forces.

A number of dressings that contain activated charcoal have been developed. They are:

- Actisorb Plus™ – Johnson & Johnson,
- Carbonet™ – Smith & Nephew,
- Carbosorb™ – Seton,
- Kaltocarb™ – BritCair,
- Lyofoam C™ – Ultra.

ACTISORB PLUS

Actisorb Plus consists of a porous spun-bonded nylon sleeve containing an activated charcoal cloth that incorporates 0.15% silver, chemically bound onto the carbon. The charcoal cloth is produced by carbonising and activating a knitted viscose fabric made from continuous filament yarn. The continuous yarn is said to produce less

dust than the staple yarns used in the manufacture of the other products, and the knitted structure of the cloth is claimed to make the dressing particularly conformable. Actisorb Plus is a primary wound contact material, and is designed to be placed directly into or onto a wound and covered with a secondary dressing (such as a simple absorbent pad).

When first produced, the dressing was manufactured without the silver; called Actisorb™, it was originally developed to absorb wound odour. However, laboratory studies carried out by Frost et al.[4] showed that when the charcoal cloth was shaken with a suspension of bacteria the number of organisms present in suspension was reduced by a factor of up to 10^5 (i.e. five log reductions) as the cells became adsorbed onto the cloth (Fig. 10-1). When a similar test was carried out using a control fabric, less than one log reduction was obtained. In these tests, Gram-negative bacilli were found to be bound more firmly to the charcoal than either Gram-positive cocci or bacterial spores, both of which were subsequently released by washing. As a result of this work, it was proposed that the dressing could play an

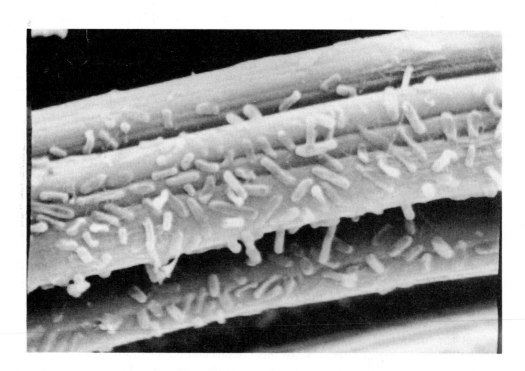

Figure 10-1   *Escherichia coli* bound on to fibres of activated charcoal ($\times 3600$) (*courtesy of Johnson & Johnson*).

important role in reducing the bioburden of wounds such as leg ulcers, thus improving the healing environment.

Although these laboratory studies showed that many of the bacteria were firmly bound onto the charcoal, the organisms remained viable; a method was sought, therefore, of imparting antibacterial properties to the fabric. Eventually, Actisorb Plus was developed, which is identical to Actisorb except for the presence of the silver residues that impart antimicrobial properties to the dressing. When Actisorb Plus was shaken with bacterial suspensions, 5–7 log reductions in viable numbers were obtained, showing that the product performs significantly better than the original material. Similar results were obtained when Actisorb Plus was tested on an animal model[5] – in which experimental wounds on guinea pigs were inoculated with test organisms and sampled by swabbing. After 24 hours, it was reported that control wounds (dressed with a semipermeable film) gave counts of the order of 2×10^8 colony forming units (cfu)/swab, but wounds dressed with Actisorb gave counts around 5×10^4 cfu/swab. An even greater improvement was noted in wounds dressed with Actisorb Plus which gave counts of 5×10^3 cfu /swab.

These observations may have important clinical implications. In a leg ulcer study carried out by Lookingbill et al.,[6] it was found that, whilst the majority of ulcers with less than 10^5 organisms/cm^2 healed, those with more than 10^5 did not. If Actisorb Plus is able to maintain the bioburden of a wound below this critical level, it may make a significant contribution to the healing process. It has also been suggested that, as the dressing is placed directly upon the wound bed, it will also remove bacterial toxins and other other potentially toxic or inhibitory materials present in exudate.

On the negative side, tissue culture work carried out by the author (unpublished data) has shown that, in the presence of activated charcoal cloth, fibroblast cells in culture rapidly become non-viable, because serum proteins and other materials essential for cell growth are removed from the culture medium by the dressing. It is interesting to speculate whether this effect has any relevance to the clinical situation – in view of the beneficial properties attributed to clean moist wound fluid by Alper et al.[7] – and suggests that the use of Actisorb Plus should be reserved for the treatment of malodorous and infected wounds, as the manufacturers recommend.

CARBONET

Carbonet is a multi-component dressing which has both fluid- and odour-absorbing properties. Unlike Actisorb Plus, the dressing can be used on its own, without a secondary dressing. The structure of Carbonet is relatively complex, consisting of six layers bonded together, as follows:

> a wound contact layer consisting of warp-knitted rayon (Tricotex™),
> a layer of cotton/viscose absorbent wadding,
> a fine polyethylene net,
> a layer of woven activated charcoal cloth,
> a second layer of polyethylene net,
> a layer of polyester fleece.

The activated charcoal layer of Carbonet is similar in appearance and specific surface area to that of Actisorb Plus, but it is not in direct contact with the wound, and is therefore less likely to adsorb bacteria and wound toxins. Carbonet is also somewhat less conformable than Actisorb Plus, as a result of its multi-component structure.

CARBOSORB

Carbosorb consists of a rectangle of charcoal cloth sandwiched between two layers of a polyester-nylon non-woven fabric. The charcoal cloth, which has a specific surface area similar to that of Actisorb Plus and Carbonet, is firmly bonded to the back of the dressing by a thick film of adhesive, which acts like a plastic film – preventing the passage of liquid through the dressing. The product literature for Carbosorb suggests that it acts like a semipermeable film dressing, maintaining a moist environment at the surface of the wound. It is questionable, however, whether this is desirable if the wound is dirty, and the exudate copious and infected. At the time of writing, Seton, the distributors of Carbosorb have indicated that the dressing may soon be discontinued.

KALTOCARB

Kaltocarb is a combination product, consisting of a wound contact layer of calcium alginate fibre bonded onto a woven activated charcoal cloth. The dressing is backed with a layer of a non-woven fabric composed of polyester and viscose.

The dressing is said to combine the wound-healing properties of calcium alginate fibre with the odour-adsorbing properties of activated charcoal.

LYOFOAM C

Lyofoam C consists of a piece of Lyofoam polyurethane dressing that is heat sealed to a sheet of plain polyurethane foam around the perimeter. The activated charcoal is enclosed between these two layers in the form of granules, which are bonded onto a piece of non-woven fabric. The specific surface area of the activated charcoal in Lyofoam C is significantly less than that of the charcoal cloth used in the manufacture of the other odour-absorbing dressings. However, in normal use, the charcoal layer present in Lyofoam should not become wet with wound exudate, and thus all the active sites remain available to adsorb the odour-producing chemicals in the gaseous phase. Clinical experience with the dressing appears to support this hypothesis, and the dressing combines odour-absorbing properties with the clinical advantages of the Lyofoam wound-facing layer.[1]

CLINICAL USE OF ACTIVATED CHARCOAL DRESSINGS

Although activated charcoal dressings were originally developed to remove wound odour, and have been found to be particularly effective for this purpose,[1,2] several of them are also said to possess other properties that contribute favourably to the healing process. However, despite the fact that charcoal dressings are widely used, little has been published in the medical press on their clinical use, and most of the data available have been obtained using Actisorb or Actisorb Plus. Laboratory studies that demonstrated the ability of these materials to take up and kill bacteria have been described above, and these are supported by the results of unpublished clinical investigations which suggest that the dressings have other useful properties when used as a treatment for infected leg ulcers. In one multicentre study involving 97 patients, 65 were treated with Actisorb and 32 with conventional dressings. During the course of the trial, the Actisorb group showed a mean reduction in size of 1.23 cm² per week, compared with only 0.20 cm² for the control group. It was

also recorded that the patients treated with Actisorb showed a significant reduction in exudate, and demonstrated a marked improvement in the general condition of their ulcers.[8]

In a more recent study involving 19 patients with venous ulcers, 10 had their wounds dressed with Actisorb Plus and the remainder with alternative treatments (which included Granuflex™ and Scherisorb™ gel).[9] It was reported that, compared with the control group, ulcers dressed with Actisorb Plus achieved a significantly greater reduction in size, and showed a marked reduction in the degree of exudate, pus, odour and necrotic tissue present.

In an uncontrolled study of ten malodorous wounds, it was found that Carbonet reduced the odour in eight cases; a marked improvement was noted in seven wounds after a single dressing change.[10] Schmidt et al.[11] have described a semi-quantitative assay procedure, which they used to compare the sorptive capacities of the charcoal components of some of these dressings (based upon their ability to take up diethylamine from aqueous solution). Although a spurious result was obtained with Actisorb Plus, owing to the presence of silver ions, the test was able to demonstrate differences in the performance of some of the other dressings: Actisorb, for example, appeared to be considerably more active than Lyofoam C. However, as the structure and method of use of the various dressings is also very different, the results of these tests must be interpreted with care.

There is little doubt that activated charcoal dressings do have an important role to play in wound management by absorbing odour, but further controlled studies are required to substantiate some of the additional claims made for the products.

REFERENCES

1. Johnson A., Dressings and rehabilitation: a case report illustrating the benefit of a new 'odour eating' dressing Lyofoam C, Sittingbourne, Ultra Laboratories, 1988.
2. Butcher G. et al., The treatment of malodorous wounds, Nurs. Mirror, 1976, 142, 76.
3. Freeman J.J. and McLeod A.I., Nitrogen BET surface area measurement as a fingerprint method for the estimation of pore volume in active carbons, Fuel, 1983, 62, 1090–1091.
4. Frost M.R. et al., The adsorption of bacteria onto

activated charcoal cloth — an effect of potential importance in the treatment of infected wounds, *Microbios Lett.,* 1980, **13**, 135 – 140.

5. Personal communication, Johnson & Johnson, 1988.

6. Lookingbill D. *et al.,* Bacteriology of chronic leg ulcers, *Arch. Derm.,* 1978, **114**, 1765 – 1768.

7. Alper J.C. *et al.,* The *in vitro* response of fibroblasts to the fluid that accumulates under a vapour-permeable membrane, *J. invest. Derm.,* 1985, **84**, 513 – 515.

8. Mulligan C.M., A controlled, open comparative study to evaluate the safety and performance characteristics of Actisorb activated charcoal cloth dressings when used as part of the treatment regimen for leg ulceration in community medicine, Data on file, Johnson & Johnson, 1985.

9. Simpson J.M., Personal communication, 1988.

10. Data on file, Smith & Nephew, 1988.

11. Schmidt R.J., *et al.,* An assay procedure to compare sorptive capacities of activated carbon dressings; the detection of impregnation with silver, *J. Pharm. Pharmacol.,* 1988, **40**, 662 – 664.

Chapter 11

Wound Cleansing Agents

Wounds such as leg ulcers, burns and pressure areas are frequently covered by a viscid, yellow layer, commonly referred to as slough. Depending upon the type and condition of the wound, the slough may be composed of necrotic tissue, or a mixture of fibrin and pus which contains bacteria, leucocytes and significant quantities of deoxyribonucleoprotein. Inflammatory mediators may also be present, which can cause inflammation of the skin surrounding the wound. The presence of slough and devitalised tissue will predispose a wound to infection, by acting as a bacteriological culture medium and inhibiting the action of leucocytes in controlling invading organisms.

In a study in guinea pigs,[1] it was found that the incidence of infection was increased significantly by the introduction of small quantities of devitalised tissue (skin, fat or muscle) into the wound. It was also shown that skin that had been damaged by dry heat was more likely to promote infection than either scalded skin or skin not subjected to thermal injury. It has been suggested that this effect is due to the production of a 'burn toxin', which is generated by the dehydration of a substance that occurs naturally in the epidermis. The effect of different types of devitalised tissue upon *in-vitro* phagocytosis was examined by the same authors: they demonstrated that, although all reduced the bactericidal capacity of leucocytes, devitalised fat and dry-burned skin had the greatest inhibitory effect upon phagocytosis and bacterial kill. Hohn[2] also demonstrated that, whilst leucocytes (obtained from human blood) incubated with *Staphylococcus aureus* were able to bring about a substantial decrease in bacterial numbers, white cells from mastectomy wounds that were engorged with fat were unable to exert any antibacterial effect.

It follows, therefore, that effective wound cleansing is essential if infection is to be avoided and healing is to take place at the optimum rate. Although surgical debridement is by far the most rapid method, this may not always be appropriate (for a number of reasons), and alternative techniques may sometimes be required. A number of solutions have been used as wound cleansing agents and a few of the more common preparations are described below.

HYPOCHLORITE SOLUTIONS

Hypochlorite solutions have been known for over two hundred years. Eau de Javelle, a solution of potassium hypochlorite, was first used as a bleaching agent in 1782, and a solution of sodium hypochlorite (known as Eau de Labarraque) was used as a disinfectant as early as 1820. Similar solutions were later used to great effect by Semmelweis in preventing the spread of puerperal sepsis.

Chemically, hypochlorite solutions are highly reactive, combining rapidly with amine groups on proteins, to bring about chlorination, oxidation and hydrolysis of nitrogenous material.[3] It is this interaction with protein that gives hypochlorites their antimicrobial activity and leads to their use as disinfectants, lavatory cleaners and water purification agents. Hypochlorite solutions, even at very low concentrations, have a marked inhibitory effect on enzyme systems; because they react with all forms of protein, they are rapidly inactivated by the presence of pus, serum and other organic matter.

Solutions of sodium hypochlorite are very alkaline (pH 11) and are consequently irritant to the skin. This problem was recognised by Dakin, who (in 1915) described the buffered hypochlorite solution that stills bears his name. Both the biological activity and the stability of sodium hypochlorite solutions are pH-dependent.

When stored correctly, a solution of sodium hypochlorite at pH 11 is stable for several months, but at lower pH values the stability is dramatically reduced. Unfortunately, undissociated hypochlorous acid, the chemically active form, reaches a maximum concentration around pH 5.5, at which point the solution is at its most unstable.

Under these conditions, decomposition is very rapid. For this reason, solutions of hypochlorites used in wound management are sometimes buffered to a point somewhere between these two values in order to reduce their irritant effect and achieve a compromise between biological activity and chemical stability.

Dakin's solution (Surgical Chlorinated Soda Solution BPC 1973) contains 0.5% w/v available chlorine and is buffered with boric acid to a pH of 9.5. The solution has to be freshly prepared and is only stable for a period of two to three weeks.

Eusol (Edinburgh University Solution of Lime; Chlorinated Lime and Boric Acid Solution BP) is a solution of calcium hypochlorite containing not less than 0.25% w/v of available chlorine, buffered with boric acid to a pH of 7.5−8.5. Like Dakin's solution, Eusol has to be freshly prepared and is only stable for about two weeks when stored in a full, tightly closed bottle.

Because of the stability problems associated with the two solutions described above, many pharmacies now supply an alternative product, which is a dilution of Milton™.

Milton solution (Richardson-Vicks) is a commercially available solution containing 1% sodium hypochlorite and 16.5% sodium chloride. It is widely used as a 1 in 80 dilution to sterilise babies' feeding utensils; and a 1 in 20 dilution is isotonic with body fluids. For wound management applications, a 1 in 4 dilution is generally used; this contains 0.25% w/v available chlorine and has a pH of 10.5−11.2. Despite the difference in pH of the two solutions, this dilution of Milton is often supplied as a Eusol equivalent. Because of its high pH, the diluted solution is stable for several months in unopened containers.

Chlorasol™ (Seton-Prebbles) is a sterile solution of sodium hypochlorite containing 0.3−0.4% w/v available chlorine, presented in 25 mL sachets. It is an unbuffered solution with a pH of 11−11.5, and is stable for eighteen months.

Chloramine BP is an organic derivative of chlorine with a bactericidal activity similar to that of the inorganic hypochlorites. It is sometimes used as a 2% solution for irrigating wounds, and is said to be relatively non-irritant. Chloramine is stable at an alkaline pH but is much more active under acid conditions.

A comprehensive study of the stability and irritant properties of a number of hypochlorite solutions has been published previously.[4]

Clinical usage of hypochlorites

Solutions such as those described above were originally introduced for the treatment of infected wounds − before antibiotics or antiseptic agents such as cetrimide and chlorhexidine became available. Dakin's solution was used extensively during the first World War as an antiseptic and wound cleansing agent,[5] which had a dramatic effect in reducing wound sepsis. However, in order to be effective, the solution had to be used in large volumes. Dakin suggested that for small lesions, 5−10 mL of the solution should be introduced into the wound every two hours by means of a rubber tube connected to a pipette or syringe. For larger necrotic wounds, up to 2 L of solution could be introduced daily by frequent or continuous irrigation, the treatment continuing for a week or more. During this time, Dakin also observed that the hypochlorite solution had the additional property of assisting in the rapid dissolution of necrosed tissue, and suggested that this was probably due to the ability of the hypochlorites to react with proteins to form soluble products.

The ability of hypochlorite and other antiseptic solutions to dissolve necrotic tissue was investigated in the laboratory by Taylor and Austin,[6] who found that Dakin's solution (in the concentration used clinically) was able to dissolve necrotic tissue, pus, and plasma clots; two other antiseptic solutions, Chloramine and Dichloramine-T, were much less effective in this respect. They also showed that, although the solvent action of Dakin's solution was dependent primarily upon the hypochlorite concentration, the effect was enhanced at an alkaline pH. In a second study, involving standard wounds produced on rabbit ears,[7] the same workers demonstrated that the use of the hypochlorite solution led to the eventual separation of necrotic tissue, hair and coagulated serum, corresponding to a rapid fall in the concentration of chlorine. When in contact with healthy skin, the chlorine concentration fell much more slowly. Chloramine was found to be much less effective than the hypochlorite in removing dead tissue, and the decrease in the concentration of chlorine was also very slight.

Chronic wounds such as decubitus ulcers are frequently covered with a thick layer of necrotic epidermis. This layer is highly permeable to water vapour, and, if exposed to the atmosphere, will rapidly dry out and take on a black leathery appearance. Until this layer is removed, the prospects for healing are poor. As these wounds are sometimes extremely painful, surgical debridement without anaesthesia is often inappropriate; therefore, alternative methods of removing the dead tissue will be required.

In laboratory studies carried out by the author on material removed from a pressure sore, it was found that about 100 mL of a solution containing 0.25% w/v available chlorine was required to solubilise 1 g of soft yellow slough. It follows, therefore, that, in order to achieve any significant cleansing effect in a deep sloughy pressure area, it would be necessary to irrigate the wound with very large volumes of solution (as recommended by Dakin in 1915.) In a further experiment, a sample of necrotic epidermis remained completely unchanged after 24 hours' immersion, confirming that there is little advantage to be gained from applying Eusol to the surface of a pressure area covered with a necrotic skin, unless this layer is first removed surgically or by some other means.

In a much quoted publication on the management and prevention of pressure sores, Barton and Barton[8] suggested that the use of hypochlorites, in common with other antiseptics and antibiotics used topically, can cause the release of endotoxins and other toxic materials from bacteria present in pressure sores – which, in turn, can cause acute oliguric renal failure. Fortunately, additional reports of this effect are hard to find.

With the development of antibiotics and newer and more effective antiseptic solutions, the importance of the hypochlorites has diminished, but they continue to be used in the form of packs and wet dressings for their supposed debriding properties.

Recently, it has been demonstrated that dressings such as the hydrocolloids and hydrogels can enhance wound debridement.[9-12] It is thought that they do this by increasing the hydration of slough or necrotic tissue, which is then removed by autolysis (a process that takes place at the interface between the slough and the healthy tissue beneath). It is highly likely that this simple mechanism is responsible for much of the success claimed for the debriding action of the hypochlorite solutions, rather than any direct chemical action upon the slough itself. If this is the case, it is probable that plain saline soaks would be almost as effective for cleaning the wound, without causing irritation either of the wound itself or of

the surrounding skin. At the present time, the author is unaware of any published data that support the claims made for the value of hypochlorite solutions when used in the form of wet dressings or packs; anecdotal evidence is all that can be found in their favour.

Indeed, in one prospective study, it was shown that pressure sores treated with a hypochlorite solution healed significantly more slowly than a matched group of wounds treated with a hydrocolloid dressing.[13] In the light of all the available evidence, it is difficult to justify the continued use of hypochlorite solutions in wound management, save in exceptional circumstances.

OTHER WOUND CLEANSING AGENTS

Hydrogen peroxide

Hydrogen Peroxide Solution (6 per cent) BP, another commonly used 'desloughing' agent, contains 5–7% w/v of hydrogen peroxide. Sometimes known as '20-volume' solution, it liberates twenty times its own volume of oxygen upon decomposition. Hydrogen peroxide has very limited antibacterial properties *in vivo*, as it is rapidly broken down by the enzyme catalase which is present in all living tissue. The solution appears to be relatively non-toxic in animal studies, but any beneficial properties it may possess are limited to a mechanical detergent action due to the rapid liberation of bubbles of oxygen gas. Hydrogen peroxide solution should be used with care: it has been reported, that if it is used to irrigate wounds under pressure or instilled into closed body cavities, oxygen bubbles can pass into the blood stream and form a life-threatening embolus.[14,15] Hioxyl™ (Quinoderm) contains 1.5% w/v of a stabilised form of hydrogen peroxide in the form of a non-greasy cream, which is used as an antiseptic and cleansing agent.

Proflavine

Proflavine, an acridine derivative, is mildly bacteriostatic against Gram-positive bacteria but almost totally ineffective against Gram-negative organisms. It is generally supplied as a simple solution or as a water-in-oil cream (Proflavine Cream BPC 1973), which is often used in conjunction with ribbon gauze for packing wounds. It has been shown in laboratory studies that the proflavine is concentrated in the aqueous phase of the cream, and is, therefore, not available to exert any significant antimicrobial activity. As the cream contains wool fat, a known sensitising agent, there is a possibility that a skin reaction may develop as a result of the use of this particular preparation[16] (Plate 8). Some hospitals produce modified formulations of proflavine cream (based on polyethylene glycol), which do permit the release of the active ingredient, and which do not contain wool fat.

Cetrimide

Cetrimide BP is a quaternary ammonium compound, very soluble in water, with the properties and uses typical of a cationic surfactant. Solutions have pronounced emulsifying and detergent properties, and have bactericidal activity against Gram-positive and some Gram-negative organisms.[17] The combined detergent and antibacterial properties of cetrimide solutions are of value for cleaning dirty or infected wounds and burns, where they may be used alone or in combination with chlorhexidine (see below). Cetrimide in solution, even in very low concentrations, has marked cytotoxic or cytostatic properties, and, as a consequence, should probably not be used for the routine and repeated cleansing of non-infected wounds.

Chlorhexidine

Chlorhexidine is available in several forms, but the most commonly used salt is the gluconate, which forms the basis of a range of antiseptic solutions. It is active against a wide range of micro-organisms, including both Gram-positive and Gram-negative bacteria. Probably the most familiar preparation containing chlorhexidine is Savlon™ (ICI), which also contains cetrimide. Savlon is available as a concentrate containing chlorhexidine gluconate 1.5% w/v and cetrimide 15% w/v; it should be diluted before use. A 1 in 30 dilution is sometimes used in first aid, when a wound is physically contaminated with gravel, oil or other foreign material. In these situations, the detergent properties of the cetrimide are of great value and assist in the cleansing process. For the management of dirty or sloughy wounds, sachets containing a 1 in 100 dilution of Savlon are available. If a wound is clean and granulating with no evidence of infection, the detergent properties

of the cetrimide may not be required and it may be preferable to use a solution of chlorhexidine alone. This is also available in sterile sachets. Alternatively, it might be considered more appropriate to use a sterile solution of isotonic saline for gentle cleaning between dressing changes.

Miscellaneous cleansing and antiseptic solutions

Other solutions that are used to cleanse and debride wounds include Benoxyl™ (Stiefel), a solution containing up to 10% benzoyl peroxide, and Aserbine™ (Bencard) and Malatex™ (Norton), which are proprietary lotions containing benzoic acid, malic acid, salicylic acid, and propylene glycol. Potassium permanganate solution, which possesses mild disinfectant and deodorising properties, has been used as a wet dressing or soak in the treatment of eczematous conditions and acute dermatoses.

A number of solutions have been used in the past to control wound infections. A 5% solution of acetic acid was shown in one study[18] to be reasonably effective in eliminating *Pseudomonas aeruginosa* from infected wounds, but unfortunately, during the treatment, the number of *Staph. aureus* and *Proteus* species present increased significantly. Application of the solution was also said to cause significant pain or discomfort. Solutions of dyes such as brilliant green, eosin, mercurochrome and crystal violet (gentian violet) have also been used for minor wound infections and skin disorders, and at least one commercial preparation containing brilliant green is available: Variclene™ (Dermal) contains 0.5% w/w brilliant green and 0.5% w/w lactic acid in the form of an aqueous hydrogel, which is said to 'normalise skin healing' – presumably by combating infection and reducing the pH of the wound. In 1979 it was reported that a patient developed aplastic anaemia as a result of mercury intoxication caused by the local application of merbromin (mercurochrome);[19] and in 1987, the Department of Health suggested that crystal violet should no longer be applied to broken skin or mucous membranes, because of possible problems of toxicity.

A range of antiseptic products is also available that contains povidone-iodine, a potent antimicrobial agent with a wide spectrum of activity although its action is greatly reduced in the presence of pus or wound exudate. These include aqueous and alcoholic lotions, a paint and a dry powder spray. As with all preparations containing iodine, there is a possibility that some individuals may experience an adverse reaction to the use of povidone-iodine; in one recent paper it was reported that antiseptic agents containing iodine caused severe disturbances to thyroid function in very low-birthweight infants, leading to hypothyroidism during a critical period of their development.[20]

ENZYME PREPARATIONS

Enzyme preparations such as Tryptar™ (Armour), Trypure Novo™ (Novo) and Varidase™ (Lederle) are also used for cleansing wounds. Tryptar and Trypure Novo contain stabilised crystalline trypsin, a proteolytic enzyme, and Varidase contains a mixture of streptokinase and streptodornase. Streptokinase is an extracellular enzyme produced by Lancefield group A and C haemolytic streptococci, which reacts with plasminogen in human serum to transform it into plasmin, an active proteolytic enzyme which is able to degrade fibrin and fibrinogen. The enzyme is also able to activate peptidases, which, in turn, break down bradykinin-like polypeptides. Streptodornase consists of a group of enzymes (deoxyribonucleases) that liquefy and facilitate the removal of DNA derived from cell nuclei. DNA constitutes some 30–70% of the solid component of purulent exudate, and is the material that is largely responsible for the viscosity and stickiness of wet slough.[21] Laboratory[21] and clinical studies[22] have suggested that although all the enzyme preparations were able to dissolve pus and debris, Varidase was significantly more effective than the products that contain trypsin. It was also recorded that Varidase was much less likely to induce side-effects or pain.

The wound cleansing properties of Varidase have also been compared with those of other treatments. Eighty-four patients with infected wounds, many of which were necrotic, were treated with either Varidase or dextranomer beads (Debrisan™). Although both agents were said to have a beneficial effect upon the healing process, the dextranomer seemed to act faster and to stimulate more effective growth of granulation tissue.[23] Other workers compared Varidase with Eusol in a limited study involving 13 patients, but the results were inconclusive and suggested there was little to choose between the two treatments.[24]

In a further study, Varidase was compared with Betadine™ (povidone-iodine) antiseptic solution in a trial involving 33 patients with chronic venous leg ulcers. Over a three-week period, it was found that Varidase was a more effective cleanser than Betadine and had a more rapid onset of action with respect to granulation tissue formation. It was also reported that all the patients in the Varidase group improved during the study, but six of the Betadine group (35%) deteriorated or remained static.[25]

The enzyme preparations are ineffective if applied externally to wounds covered with a thick dry crust.[26] In order to overcome the barrier properties of this necrotic layer, some workers advocate the injection of an enzyme solution into the dead tissue immediately beneath, but this procedure should only be carried out by experienced personnel using extreme caution.

ADVERSE EFFECTS OF WOUND CLEANSING AGENTS

In recent years, there has been a considerable interest in the effect of hypochlorites and other antiseptic solutions on wound healing. A number of papers have been published, which demonstrate that – in in-vitro studies[27–29] using cell culture systems and in-vivo experiments with animals – hypochlorites have a marked, and in some cases irreversible, effect upon the viability of the test system used. In a rabbit ear chamber preparation, Eusol and chloramine have been shown permanently to disrupt capillary circulation in granulation tissue and thus cause a significant delay in wound healing.[30] Further evidence of the adverse effects of chloramine on the healing process was obtained in a second study, in which the antiseptic was applied to a series of standard wounds on the backs of rats.[27] Biochemical and histological examination of the wound site revealed that, compared with the saline control, wounds treated with the hypochlorite solution showed a significant increase in DNA levels, owing to the presence of elevated numbers of polymorphonuclear leucocytes (indicative of an increased inflammatory response). Collagen development was also retarded, as measured by the concentration of hydroxyproline. When chlorhexidine was tested in a similar fashion, these toxic effects were not detected.

In 1985, Lineweaver et al.[31] applied dilutions of

four commonly used antiseptics to human fibroblast cells *in vitro*. All the solutions tested − 1% povidone-iodine, 0.25% acetic acid, 3% hydrogen peroxide and 0.5% sodium hypochlorite − were found to have marked cytotoxic properties, and, with the exception of hydrogen peroxide, were also found to delay wound healing in an animal model. The action of povidone-iodine was particularly marked in this respect. In an additional series of animal studies, it was demonstrated that wounds irrigated with povidone-iodine were significantly weaker than comparable wounds irrigated with saline or the other antiseptic agents examined.[31] In a more recent and detailed study, Kozol *et al.*[29] investigated the effects of dilute solutions of sodium hypochlorite (Dakin's solution) on the viability of neutrophils, fibroblasts and endothelial cells, and found that concentrations of hypochlorite as low as 0.0025% caused marked changes in their morphology, when examined by electron microscopy. In a second series of *in-vitro* experiments, the same workers determined the effect of the solution upon random neutrophil migration, and migration in the presence of a known chemo-attractant. They demonstrated that hypochlorite concentrations as low as 0.0002% inhibited cell migration in the presence of the chemotactic agent, and random migration was inhibited by concentrations as low as 0.00002%. When examined by electron microscopy, both groups of cells revealed the normal morphological features of neutrophils, indicating that the observed reduction in migration was due to inhibition of function rather than structural cell damage. These findings may have important implications for the wound healing process. As described in chapter 1, neutrophils play an important role in the removal of bacteria and debris, assisting macrophages in wound debridement by the release of proteolytic and fibrinolyic enzymes. If this process is inhibited by the application of extremely low concentrations of hypochlorites (which are too dilute to dissolve slough or necrotic tissue, or have any bactericidal activity), then the use of, for example, out-of-date Eusol could delay wound debridement and even *increase* the possibility of a wound infection occurring, by inhibiting the natural defence mechanisms of the body.

Work carried out by the author (unpublished data) on a small range of antiseptic agents suggests that, in normal concentrations, solutions of cetrimide are also cytotoxic. Indeed, solutions have been used to irrigate wounds to prevent local tumour regrowth as a result of accidental seeding after surgery for the removal of cancerous tissue.[32,33] The presence of cetrimide in Savlon calls into question the wisdom of using this material for the routine management of clean non-infected wounds, although there is no doubt that the solution can be of value for cleansing dirty or infected lesions. Tissue culture results suggest that chlorhexidine, the other component of Savlon, is relatively free of toxicity; these findings are in agreement with the results observed in animals by Brennan *et al.*[27]

The role of antiseptics and topical agents in wound management has been reviewed previously by Leaper and Simpson,[34] who concluded that the prolonged use of antiseptics and topical antibiotics may delay healing. In particular, it was suggested that the hypochlorites could lengthen an in-patient's stay or delay return to normal life. It follows that, for routine cleansing of non-infected wounds, a sterile solution of 0.9% sodium chloride is probably all that is required. Any benefits that might be derived from the use of antiseptic agents must be weighed against their possible detrimental effects upon the healing process.

REFERENCES

1. Haury B. *et al.*, Debridement: an essential component of traumatic wound care, in *Wound Healing and Wound Infection*, Hunt T.K. (ed.), New York, Appleton-Century-Crofts, 1980, 229−240.
2. Hohn D.C., Host resistance to infection: established and emerging concepts, in Ref.1, 264−279.
3. *An Introduction to Milton Sterilizing Fluid and its Use*, Richardson-Merrell, (undated).
4. Bloomfield S.F. and Sizer T.J., Eusol BPC and other hypochlorite formulations used in hospitals, *Pharm. J.*, 1985, **235**, 153−157.
5. Dakin H.D., On the the use of certain antiseptic substances in the treatment of infected wounds, *Br. med. J.*, 1915, **2**, 318−320.
6. Taylor H.D. and Austin J.H., The solvent action of antiseptics on necrotic tissue, *J. exp. Med.*, 1918, **27**, 155−164.
7. Austin J.H. and Taylor H.D. Behavior of hypochlorite and of chloramine-T solutions in contact with necrotic and normal tissues *in vivo*, *ibid.*, 627−633.
8. Barton A. and Barton M., *The Management and Prevention of Pressure Sores*, London, Faber and Faber, 1981.

9. Thomas S., Milton and the treatment of burns, (letter), *Pharm. J.,* 1986, **236**, 128–129.

10. Tudhope M., Management of pressure ulcers with a hydrocolloid occlusive dressing; results in twenty three patients, *J. enterostom. Ther.,* 1984, **11**, 102–105.

11. Johnson A., Towards rapid tissue healing, *Nurs. Times,* 1984, **80**, 39–43.

12. Thomas S., Pressure points, *Nurs. Times, Community Outlook Suppl.,* 1988, **84**, 20–22.

13. Gorse G.J. and Messner R.L., Improved pressure sore healing with hydrocolloid dressings, *Arch. Derm.,* 1987, **123**, 766–771.

14. Bassan M.M. *et al.,* Near fatal systemic oxygen embolism due to wound irrigation with hydrogen peroxide, *Postgrad. med. J.,* 1982, **58**, 448–451.

15. Sleigh J.W. and Linter S.P.K., Hazards of hydrogen peroxide, *Br. med. J.,* 1985, **291**, 1706.

16. *Martindale, The Extra Pharmacopoeia,* 27th edn, Wade A. (ed.), London, Pharmaceutical Press, 1977, 532.

17. *ICI Antiseptics in Practice,* Macclesfield, ICI, 1978.

18. Phillips I. *et al.,* Acetic acid in the treatment of superficial wounds infected by *Pseudomonas aeruginosa, Lancet,* 1968, **1**, 11–14.

19. Slee P.H.Th.J., *et al.,* A case of merbromin (Mercurochrome™) intoxication possibly resulting in aplastic anemia, *Acta med Scand.,* 1979, **205**, 463–466.

20. Smerdely P. *et al.,* Topical iodine-containing antiseptics and neonatal hypothyroidism in very-low-birthweight infants, *Lancet,* 1989, **2**, 661–664.

21. Hellgren L. and Vincent J., Degradation and liquefaction effect of streptokinase-streptodornase and stabilized trypsin on necroses, crusts of fibrinoid, purulent exudate and clotted blood from leg ulcers, *J. int. med. Res.,* 1977, **5**, 334–337.

22. Suomalainen O., Evaluation of two enzyme preparations – Trypure and Varidase in traumatic ulcers, *Ann. Chir. Gynaec.,* 1983, **72**, 62–65.

23. Hulkko A. *et al.,* Comparison of dextranomer and streptokinase-streptodornase in the treatment of venous leg ulcers and other infected wounds, *Ann. Chir. Gynaec.,* 1981, **70**, 65–70.

24. Smith M. *et al.,* Report of a comparative study of the efficacy of Varidase topical versus Eusol in the cleaning of leg ulcers, in *A Biological Approach to the Wound Healing Process,* Rue Y. (ed.), Proceedings of a Symposium, Royal College of Physicians, London, 5 June, 1987, Andover, Medifax, 1987, 3–7.

25. Graham-Brown R.A.C. *et al.,* A comparative study of the safety and efficacy of topical enzymatic therapy *vs* standard antiseptic dressings in the cleansing of leg ulcers, in Ref. 22, 43–48.

26. Hellgren L., Cleansing properties of stabilized trypsin and streptokinase-streptodornase in necrotic leg ulcers, *Eur. J. clin. Pharmac.,* 1983, **24**, 623–628.

27. Brennan S.S. *et al.,* Antiseptic toxicity in wounds healing by secondary intention, *J. Hosp. Infect.,* 1986, **8**, 263–267.

28. Thomas S. and Hay N.P., Wound cleansing, (letter), *Pharm. J.,* 1985, **235**, 206.

29. Kozol R.A. *et al.,* Effects of sodium hypochlorite (Dakin's Solution) on cells of the wound module, *Arch. Surg.,* 1988, **123**, 420–423.

30. Brennan S.S. and Leaper D.J., The effect of antiseptics on the healing wound: a study using the rabbit ear chamber, *Br. J. Surg.,* 1985, **72**, 780–782.

31. Lineweaver W. *et al.,* Topical antimicrobial toxicity, *Arch. Surg.,* 1985, **120**, 267–271.

32. Gibson G.R. and Stephens F.O., Experimental use of cetrimide in the prevention of wound implantation with cancer cells, *Lancet,* 1966, **2**, 678–680.

33. Umpleby H.C. and Williamson R.C.N., The efficacy of agents employed to prevent anastomotic recurrence in colorectal carcinoma, *Ann. R. Coll. Surg.,* 1984, **66**, 192–194.

34. Leaper D.J. and Simpson R.A., The effect of antiseptics and topical antimicrobials on wound healing. *J. antimicrob. Chemother.,* 1986, **2**, 135–137.

Chapter 12

The Selection and Use of Wound Management Materials

As described in earlier chapters, many new surgical dressings and wound management materials have been introduced in recent years. Unlike traditional products, which have a simple absorptive or protective function, some of these new dressings react chemically with exudate, or change their physical state to form a gel or viscous semi-solid covering the surface of the wound. These so-called 'interactive' materials produce changes in the micro-environment at the wound surface that can have a dramatic effect upon the healing process.

As dressings become more sophisticated, they also tend to become more 'wound-specific'. For example, a product that is ideally suited for application to a moist or heavily exuding wound may be totally unsuitable for application to a dry or lightly exuding lesion.

The introduction of so many new and varied products has led to a certain amount of confusion in the minds of some users, who find themselves faced with an array of different dressings that are claimed by the manufacturers to be indicated for a similar range of clinical conditions. As no single dressing is suitable for the management of all types of wound, and few dressings are ideally suited for the treatment of a single wound during all stages of the healing process, the selection of the most appropriate product for use in any given situation can be extremely difficult. Medical and nursing staff receive very little formal training in the use of surgical dressings, and consequently their experience in wound management techniques is gained from older and more senior colleagues — who may not be fully aware of the properties and advantages of some of the newer materials available to them. As a result, progress in this important area is sometimes unnecessarily slow.

In order to provide simple guidelines for the use of some of the new materials, a classification system has been adopted, based upon the physical appearance and nature of the wound. Using this classification and a knowledge of the properties of the individual dressings, it is possible to identify those products that are likely to be best suited for the management of a given wound *at any particular stage in the healing process*. It should always be remembered that healing is a dynamic process, and therefore, the properties and performance that are required of a dressing may change as healing progresses.

CLASSIFICATION OF WOUNDS BY APPEARANCE

For the purposes of dressing selection, wounds may be classified as follows:

- black and necrotic — covered with a hard, dry black necrotic layer,

- yellow and sloughy — covered (or filled) with a soft yellow slough,

- clean with significant tissue loss (granulating)

- clean and superficial (epithelialising).

It will be recognised that this simple classification represents not only different *types* of wound, but also the various stages through which a single wound may pass as it heals. It follows, therefore, that as the condition of the wound changes, it may be necessary to change the type of dressing that is applied to it. Similarly, the presence of infection may influence the choice of wound dressing.

STAGES OF HEALING

The mechanisms of wound healing have been described in chapter 1, but, for the purposes of dressing selection, the principal stages of the process (which relate to the wound types outlined above) are as follows:

- cleansing and removal of debris,

- granulation and vascularisation,

- epithelialisation.

In addition to the above, wound contraction is also important; this may begin almost as soon as the wound is clean, and will continue until healing is complete.

Stage 1: Cleansing and removal of debris

Given favourable conditions, tissue that has become anoxic and non-viable, for example as a result of the sustained application of high levels of pressure, will often separate spontaneously from the healthy layer beneath. This occurs as a result of autolysis, and is presumably due to macrophage activity and the action of proteolytic enzymes. However, if such an area is exposed to the atmosphere for extended periods, the epidermis, which is unable to control the loss of moisture vapour, becomes dehydrated and hard and may take on a black leathery appearance. As this process continues, it becomes progressively more difficult for autolysis to take place, and the separation of the dead tissue or slough may be delayed indefinitely. It follows, therefore, that any product that reverses this process of dehydration will assist in the removal of the necrotic tissue. Depending upon the severity of the condition, the necrotic layer may be relatively superficial or extremely deep. Often, large cavities develop beneath the surface of the black eschar, which are filled with dead or partially liquified tissue; in exceptional cases, these can extend right down to the bone.

In the past, rehydration was usually achieved by the frequent application of wet packs of Eusol or normal saline, but these can be irritant or cause maceration of the surrounding area. Recently, however, it has been found that dry necrotic wounds of this type can be treated very effectively by the use of an occlusive dressing, which rehydrates the necrotic skin by retaining the moisture that would otherwise be lost as vapour. Granuflex™ was the first dressing to be employed in this way, although any of the hydrocolloid dressings may be used, as most of these materials are relatively occlusive in the dry state. The dressing is simply placed in position and left undisturbed for a number of days, after which the black area will be found to have softened and changed to a dark brown or olive green colour on the outer surface (Plates 9 to 12). The speed at which this occurs depends upon the depth of the wound and the blood supply to the area, but some change in the condition of the necrotic skin is usually evident within a few days.

On superficial wounds, the autolytic process may be allowed to continue undisturbed, apart from an occasional change of dressing; in these situations, the necrotic layer will eventually separate to reveal a healthy granulating wound surface beneath. On deeper or more extensive injuries, however, once the dead tissue starts to soften or loosen, it is advisable to remove it as quickly as possible using scissors or a scalpel.

If, for some reason, a hydrocolloid dressing cannot be used, similar beneficial results may usually be achieved by the application of one of the amorphous hydrogels, such as Scherisorb™ or Bard™ Absorption Dressing. Both of these materials contain a significant proportion of water; when they are placed on the necrotic epidermis, some of this water is taken up by the dead tissue, which becomes rehydrated (thereby facilitating autolysis). Hydrogels have a tendency to dry out if left exposed to the air, and, therefore, for this particular application, they should be covered with a secondary dressing that will prevent or reduce the loss of moisture vapour. Perforated plastic film absorbent dressings (such as Melolin™ or Telfa™) have been found to be particularly useful for this purpose, but semipermeable films (such as Opsite™, Tegaderm™ or Bioclusive™) have also been used. Despite their different modes of action, there is probably little to choose between the hydrocolloid dressings and the hydrogels, in terms of their ability to rehydrate necrotic tissue, although for relatively small areas on heels or buttocks the hydrocolloids are more convenient to use. The gel dressings are to be preferred on more extensive wounds or areas that are hard to dress with the hydrocolloid sheets (Plate 13 to 16).

It has been suggested that preparations containing proteolytic enzymes, or other agents that can break down fibrin and slough, may be used to debride necrotic areas that have first been scarified with a scalpel. Alternatively, it has been said that these solutions can be injected beneath the eschar with a hypodermic syringe. There is little published evidence to support this use of these materials and they are probably best reserved for the treatment of wounds containing soft yellow slough, or necrotic wounds from which the epidermal layer has been removed. Some clinicians add the enzyme preparations to starch pastes or hydrogels which are then applied in the usual way, although in these situations it is not clear whether it is the enzyme or the gel that is mainly responsible for any debriding effect.

In particularly deep or extensive wounds on the buttocks or sacrum, the cavity that is sometimes found beneath the dead skin may be full of foul-smelling necrotic material (Plate 17), which may contain oily yellow fat droplets. Once again, surgery is the best and most rapid method of debridement, but, if this is not possible, dressing the wound with an amorphous hydrogel, or a hydrocolloid paste or granules can facilitate the cleansing process. Sugar pastes have also been found to be of value in these situations.

Generally these dressings are inserted into the wound, covered with an absorbent pad, and changed at least daily. For moist sloughy lesions, the polysaccharide bead dressings (Iodosorb™ and Debrisan™) are also claimed to be effective, either alone or in the form of a paste made with polyethylene glycol. Iodosorb has the additional advantage that it liberates iodine, which imparts antibacterial properties to the dressing. For practical reasons, however, the bead dressings are best reserved for use in smaller wounds.

A different form of slough can develop upon the surface of a previously clean wound, such as a burn, as a result of the accumulation of fibrin, leucocytes and DNA protein. The application of a hydrocolloid, or an amorphous hydrogel covered with a semi-occlusive dressing, may prevent the formation of this layer, or speed its removal if already present. Relatively shallow sloughy wounds that produce limited amounts of exudate can be dressed with hydrocolloids, which facilitate autolysis by the mechanisms described previously. In addition, pectin, one of the ingredients found in certain of the hydrocolloid products, may confer additional benefits: recent studies have shown that Granuflex is able to lyse human fibrin clots *in vitro* (chapter 8), and it is possible that this effect may contribute to the wound cleansing process.

Hydrocolloid sheets should be applied with caution over deep cavity wounds, although the pastes or granules produced by some manufacturers may often be used with advantage in these situations, since they can be introduced directly into the cavity. Alternatively, an amorphous hydrogel may be used in a similar fashion and covered with a secondary dressing: if the wound is producing large volumes of exudate, a moisture-retaining dressing will not be required – a simple absorbent pad may be a more appropriate secondary dressing.

Large exuding wounds that bear isolated sloughy or necrotic areas may be dressed with alginates, provided that sufficient moisture is present for the dressing to form a gel, and thus provide a moist covering over the affected area (Plates 18, 19).

Pressure areas and other sloughy wounds, particularly those in the sacral region, are prone to colonisation and infection by bacteria. This frequently results in the production of a most offensive odour, which can be unpleasant for staff and relatives and embarrassing to the patient. Topical or systemic antibacterial therapy may be appropriate, and the use of a medicated dressing such as Iodosorb, Iodosorb Ointment, or Inadine™ may be of value in controlling the infection. It has been the experience of the author that the application of Scherisorb gel containing 0.8% metronidazole powder can be an extremely effective method of controlling infections, and hence the odour caused by some anaerobic micro-organisms, in wounds such as pressure areas, fungating carcinomas and some leg ulcers. This treatment should only be carried out under medical supervision.

Metrotop™ (Tillots), a preparation containing metronidazole 0.8% w/v in an aqueous gel, is available commercially on a named patient basis.

The application of a dressing containing activated charcoal may also help to reduce the smell from an infected wound, and a number of these materials are now available (chapter 10).

Stage 2: Granulation and vascularisation

For the granulation stage of healing, it is generally agreed that a dressing is required that provides a moist environment, good thermal insulation and a reasonable fluid-handling capability. It has also been suggested (chapter 2) that an acidic environment and low oxygen tension may accelerate the formation of granulation tissue.

In practical terms, the management of wounds with significant tissue loss depends upon a number of factors, including the size, site, shape and origin of the lesion. Surgical wounds, such as those resulting from the excision of a pilonidal sinus or the dissection of the axillae or groins as a treatment for hidradenitis suppurativa, have been shown to respond well to the use of a Silastic™ Foam stent. In these situations, the patient can often be discharged from hospital at an early stage to manage the wound at home with only minimal professional help, returning at intervals to a hospital clinic where progress is monitored and a new stent is prepared as required. Similarly, good results can be obtained when Silastic Foam is used in the treatment of large abdominal wall wounds that are left to heal by secondary intention (Plate 20). The evidence for the use of Silastic Foam in the treatment of chronic exuding wounds (such as leg ulcers) is less convincing, however, and in these situations it may be more appropriate to use an alternative treatment. Silastic Foam should not be used in wounds containing small sinuses or tracks because pieces of the dressing may become trapped in the wound causing problems at a later date.

On rare occasions, wounds that are being dressed with Silastic Foam may produce a degree of slough. In these situations, coating the stent with a layer of Scherisorb may help to overcome the problem.

Recently, a new dressing for cavity wounds has been introduced. Intrasite™ Cavity Wound Dressing is available in a number of shapes and sizes, and although it lacks the exceptional conformability of Silastic Foam it is somewhat easier to use.

As a cavity wound heals and decreases in depth, the dressings described above may no longer be appropriate, and a change in therapy may be indicated for the final stages of healing.

Heavily exuding wounds with a significant degree of tissue loss (including leg ulcers and some infected surgical or traumatic wounds) frequently respond well to treatment with an alginate dressing, such as Sorbsan™. If the wound is relatively deep, compared with its diameter, the rope or ribbon form may be used, but this must not be packed in too tightly. Hydrocolloid dressings may also be used, in conjunction with granules or paste to provide additional absorbent capacity. The polyurethane foam dressing Lyofoam™ has similarly proved to be of value, not only in the treatment of exuding wounds such as leg ulcers and pressure sores, but also in the management of shallow, more superficial injuries in the later stages of healing.

Wounds that show evidence of clinical infection

may be dressed with a medicated product such as Inadine, but tulles containing antibiotics should *not* be used, unless specifically indicated, because of the possibility of bacterial resistance and the development of sensitivity reactions. There is some evidence to suggest that the use of Actisorb Plus™ can help to control infection, as bacterial cells become firmly bound onto the dressing, which also exerts an antimicrobial effect (owing to the presence of silver ions).

Plain unmedicated tulle gras, once the mainstay of treatment for leg ulcers and similar conditions, has been shown in recent studies to be considerably less effective than some of the newer wound management materials.

Some pressure areas become flask shaped, with a narrow entrance opening into a large cavity beneath the surface of the skin. Most practitioners would agree that a patient with such a wound should be referred for surgery to open up the wound and make it a better shape for healing. If this is not done, some form of packing is essential to keep the entrance of the wound open whilst granulation tissue forms from below. Alginate ribbon or rope may be suitable, provided care is taken to remove all residues each time the dressing is changed. Ribbon gauze that has been thoroughly impregnated with Scherisorb may also be effective, probably more so than the Eusol or proflavine packs that have been used in the past.

Provided that the full extent of the injury is known, a relatively deep wound of limited size may be filled with an amorphous hydrogel or hydrocolloid granules or paste. The opening should be covered with an absorbent pad and the dressing changed daily. The gel can be removed by irrigation with normal saline using a syringe and quill.

Stage 3: Epithelialisation

Once a defect has become filled with granulation tissue, epithelialisation takes place. For this, the final stage of the process, a dressing is required that provides a moist environment and will not adhere to the surface of the wound (causing trauma upon removal). As in the granulation stage, an acidic pH may be an advantage. It has also been demonstrated that in the management of clean, low exudate wounds, the oxygen permeability of the dressing can influence the rate of epithelial cell growth.

Many different types of material are available

for use in this situation. The older products, such as the perforated film absorbent dressings (Melolin and Telfa) have been joined by polyurethane foams, such as Lyofoam and Allevyn™; and the so-called 'non-adherent' paraffin tulle has been challenged by N-A™ Dressing and Transite™. Adhesive semipermeable films (Opsite, Tegaderm, Bioclusive, etc.) are still widely used, but second and third generation products have become available, such as the Tegaderm Pouch Dressing and the new hydrophilic non-adhesive material Omiderm™, all of which are intended for use on high exudate wounds such as burns and donor sites.

As a group, the alginates are not the treatment of choice if a wound is exuding lightly; the hydrocolloid dressings can be used, despite their relatively impermeable nature, provided there is no evidence of the production of hypergranulation tissue.

SUMMARY OF DRESSING FUNCTIONS

The functions required of a dressing in the various stages of healing are summarised on the right.

From these general requirements and a knowledge of the properties of the various dressings, a list has been compiled of products that may be suitable for the treatment of different types of wound. This is reproduced below. It should be stressed, however, that these recommendations are based upon the personal experience of the author with the materials concerned, and are not intended to be fully comprehensive or exclusive.

At the present time, there is an almost complete lack of comparative clinical data on the use of different wound management products. Until this becomes available, medical and nursing staff have little option but to develop their own local wound management policies and procedures. It is hoped that this simple wound classification system and product guide may form a useful starting point in the production of such a policy.

Wound type	Dressing function
Dry, necrotic wounds	Moisture retention
Slough-covered wounds	Moisture retention Fluid absorption Odour absorption* Antimicrobial properties*
Clean, exuding wounds	Fluid absorption Odour absorption* Antimicrobial properties* Thermal insulation
Dry, low exudate wounds	Moisture retention Low adherence Thermal insulation

*Not always required

DRESSING SELECTION GUIDE

Wound type	Recommended dressings	Proprietary examples
Black necrotic wounds		
Small and superficial	Hydrocolloid sheet	Granuflex, Biofilm, Intrasite, Tegasorb, Comfeel
Extensive and deep	Amorphous hydrogel (with moisture-retaining dressing)	Scherisorb, Bard Absorption Dressing
Wounds covered or filled with yellow/brown slough		
Small and dry	Hydrocolloid sheet	Granuflex, Biofilm, Intrasite, Tegasorb, Comfeel
	Amorphous hydrogel (with moisture-retaining dressing)	Scherisorb, Bard Absorption Dressing
Small and moist	Polysaccharide beads or paste	Debrisan, Debrisan Paste, Iodosorb, Iodosorb Ointment
	Hydrocolloid sheet (with paste or granules, if appropriate)	Granuflex, Biofilm, Intrasite, Tegasorb, Comfeel
	Amorphous hydrogel	Scherisorb, Bard Absorption Dressing
	Polyurethane foam	Lyofoam
Large deep cavities containing semi-liquid necrotic material	Amorphous hydrogel (with absorbent pad)	Scherisorb, Bard Absorption Dressing
	Hydrocolloid granules or paste (with absorbent pad)	Granuflex, Comfeel
	Sugar paste	
Granulating wounds		
Clean surgical wounds with significant tissue loss	Cavity foam dressing	Silastic Foam, Intrasite Cavity Wound Dressing
Chronic wounds with low to moderate exudate	Hydrocolloid sheet	Granuflex, Biofilm, Intrasite, Tegasorb, Comfeel
	Alginate island dressing	Sorbsan SA, Kaltoclude
	Alginate sheet	Sorbsan, Kaltostat, Tegagel
	Polyurethane foam	Lyofoam
Chronic open wounds with moderate to high exudate	Alginate sheet, rope, or ribbon	Sorbsan, Kaltostat, Tegagel
	Alginate with integral absorbent pad	Sorbsan Plus
	Polyurethane foam	Lyofoam
	Hydrophilic polyurethane foam	Allevyn

Wound type	Recommended dressings	Proprietary examples
Chronic flask-shaped wounds	Alginate ribbon or rope	Sorbsan, Kaltostat
	Amorphous hydrogel (with ribbon gauze)	Scherisorb
	Hydrocolloid granules or paste	Granuflex, Comfeel
	Sugar paste	
Epithelialising wounds		
Clean, low exudate wounds	Semipermeable film	Opsite, Tegaderm, Bioclusive
	Hydrocolloid sheet	Granuflex, Biofilm, Intrasite, Tegasorb, Comfeel
	Alginate island dressing	Sorbsan SA, Kaltoclude
Clean wounds with medium to high exudate (e.g. burns, donor sites)	Alginate sheet	Sorbsan, Kaltostat, Tegagel
	Alginate with integral absorbent pad	Sorbsan Plus
	Hydrocolloid sheet (extra absorbent)	Granuflex E
	Pouch dressing made from semipermeable film	Tegaderm Pouch Dressing
	Hydrophilic polyurethane foam	Allevyn
	Hydrophilic polyurethane film	Omiderm
	Knitted viscose primary dressing	N-A Dressing, Tricotex
	Paraffin tulle	Jelonet, Paratulle
Clinically infected wounds		
Extensive or heavily exuding wounds	Alginate sheet or rope*	Sorbsan, Kaltostat, Tegagel
Small cavities or craters	Beads/pastes containing iodine	Iodosorb, Iodosorb Ointment
	Amorphous hydrogel containing metronidazole**	Metrotop***
	Sugar paste	
Shallow open wounds	Povidone-iodine tulle	Inadine
	Alginate sheet*	Sorbsan, Kaltostat, Tegagel
	Chlorhexidine tulle	Bactigras, Clorhexitulle
	Activated charcoal dressing containing silver	Actisorb Plus
	Amorphous hydrogel containing metronidazole**	Metrotop***
	Sugar paste	
Malodorous wounds		
Infected pressure sores, fungating carcinomas, etc.	Activated charcoal dressing	Actisorb Plus, Lyofoam C, Kaltocarb, Carbonet
	Amorphous hydrogel containing metronidazole**	Metrotop***
	Sugar paste	

* Changed daily and used in conjunction with systemic antibiotics (see chapter 6)
** Only where specifically indicated
*** Available on a named patient basis

Chapter 13

Bandages and Bandaging

There is little doubt that the art and therapeutic importance of bandaging are often under-rated. It is not generally appreciated that the selection of an inappropriate bandage, or the incorrect application of a suitable product, can have an adverse effect upon the outcome of a course of treatment or a surgical procedure.

Bandages have a history stretching back thousands of years. The ancient Egyptians, in particular, were skilled in their use, often coating simple woven fabrics with adhesives, resins and other medicaments to aid wound healing. Simple cloth bandages (not dissimilar to those used by the Egyptians) continued to be used until well into the 19th century, but, because of their high cost, they were frequently washed and reused many times — a practice that was soundly condemned by Davidson in a letter to the *Lancet* in 1875.

The first elastic bandages — containing natural rubber — were produced around the middle of the 19th century, and, in 1878, Callender published an article in the *Lancet* describing their use in the management of ulcers and varicose veins.

An early specification for roller bandages was laid down in 1718, by Lorenz Heister, the great German surgeon, who insisted that they should be made from suitable pieces of clean linen cloth, softened by wearing, and free from seams and large ends. The first official British specifications for bandages appeared in the second supplement to the 1911 British Pharmaceutical Codex, which included monographs on calico, crêpe, domette, flannel, muslin and open-wove bandages. Additional products were added in subsequent editions, but, with the demise of the BPC, monographic standards for bandages and other surgical dressings were transferred to the British Pharmacopoeia.

In recent years, several factors have led to a huge increase in the number and variety of bandages available. On the positive side, improvements in manufacturing and fibre technology have resulted in the widespread use of polyamide and polyurethane yarns, and the production of knitted bandages (which have largely replaced woven cotton-based materials for some applications). It has also been recognised that a number of bandages that have been used for

many years to provide support and compression are totally unsuitable for this purpose, and, as a result, a number of highly effective alternatives have been developed. Sadly, however, as these are generally much more expensive than traditional products, they have not become widely used. A range of tubular bandages have also been produced, which have the advantage that — for the application of low levels of pressure — they are easy to apply and less dependent upon the skill of the user.

Less desirable aspects of bandage development have been brought about by financial constraints within the health service, which have forced manufacturers to produce cheaper and less effective materials in order to secure hospital contracts.

Bandages can be divided into six basic groups, as follows:

- non-extensible bandages,
- extensible bandages,
- adhesive/cohesive bandages,
- tubular bandages,
- medicated paste bandages,
- orthopaedic casting materials.

These different groups are described below, with the exception of the orthopaedic casting materials, which are the subject of chapter 14.

NON-EXTENSIBLE BANDAGES

Until the relatively recent past, most bandaging needs were met by the use of products made from non-extensible woven fabrics; but, by their very nature, these materials were not particularly conformable, and, as a result, were difficult to apply correctly. This problem was recognised as early as 600 BC by Sushruta, who suggested that bandaging techniques should be practised upon full-sized dolls or mannikins made of stuffed linen. In the first half of this century, the techniques of bandaging formed an important part of a nurse's training, and a number of texts were produced that described in precise terms how bandages should be applied. However, with the development of more conformable and extensible products, much of this expertise has been lost.

Although flannel, domette and calico bandages are still available, their use is extremely limited, and the only non-extensible roller bandage that is still purchased today in any quantity is Open-wove Bandage BP, more familiarly known as White Open Wove (WOW). As its name suggests, this consists of a loosely woven cloth made from cotton or cotton and viscose. Three types are described in the BP, which differ in the number of threads in the warp and weft, and, therefore, the weight per unit area. Once used for almost all bandaging applications, WOW has largely been replaced by more extensible products, although a significant quantity is still used in theatres for tying anaesthetic tubes and drains in position during operations, and holding up surgeons' trousers!

EXTENSIBLE BANDAGES

Extensible bandages vary in structure and performance, ranging from heavyweight highly elastic products, like Elastic Web Bandage (Blue Line Webbing), to lightweight relatively inextensible materials, such as Cotton Conforming Bandage. Depending upon the nature of the product concerned, they have traditionally been classified into three basic groups, which have the following functions:

- dressing retention,
- support,
- compression.

Dressing retention

The first product to be produced specifically for this purpose was the Cotton Conforming Bandage of the BP. Two types are available, Kling™ (Johnson & Johnson) and Crinx™ (Smith &

Nephew). Both are made from lightweight cotton fabrics that have been treated to impart a degree of extensibility to the warp and weft. More recently, a new group of retention bandages has been developed, which are sometimes called conforming-stretch or contour bandages. Examples include Stayform™ (Robinsons) and Slinky™ (Cuxson Gerrard). These are lightweight and conformable and possess good elastic properties to ensure that the dressing is held in close proximity to the wound. In use, they should not inhibit movement, apply significant pressure or restrict blood flow (unless required to achieve haemostasis).

Support

Support may be defined as the retention and control of tissue without the application of compression. It is usually provided to prevent the development of a deformity, or a change in shape of a mass of tissue due to swelling or sagging. Although non-extensible bandages are sometimes used for this purpose, a product that has a degree of extensibility is generally easier to apply.

Compression

Compression implies the deliberate application of pressure, which is usually achieved by the use of elasticated stockings or an appropriate bandage, and is most commonly used to control oedema and reduce swelling in the treatment of venous disorders of the lower limb.

THE ROLE OF COMPRESSION

In order to appreciate the clinical importance of compression, it is first necessary to understand a little of the anatomy and physiology of the circulatory system of the leg.

The veins of the leg are subdivided into two systems, superficial and deep, according to their relationship to the deep fascia. The major superficial veins are the long saphenous vein, which runs from toe to groin on the inner aspect of the leg, and the short saphenous vein, which runs along the rear and outer aspect from the foot to the back of the knee. These are linked to the deep veins by other vessels called perforators. Like the rest of the veins in the leg, these connecting vessels contain valves that only permit the flow of blood in one direction, from the outer or superficial system to the deep veins.

In a supine subject, the pressure in the veins in the ankle region is around 10 mmHg. When the subject stands upright, this pressure is increased by an amount equivalent to the weight of a column of blood stretching from the point of measurement to the right auricle of the heart. In an individual of average height, this distance will be around 110 cm, giving rise to an additional pressure of 80 mmHg.

When a subject is at rest, blood passes through the calf muscles at the rate of 1–2 mL per 100 mL of tissue per minute, but when walking at a moderate pace, the blood flow through the same tissue may increase to about 20–30 mL per 100mL of tissue per minute, due to the action of the calf muscle pump.[1] During walking, as the foot is flexed dorsally, the contraction of the calf muscle compresses the deep veins to the point at which they become almost totally collapsed, producing internal pressures of up to 250 mmHg and emptying them of blood. In a normal leg, the distal valves of the deep veins and the valves of the perforators will ensure that the blood that is expelled can go in only one direction – upwards, back to the heart. As the foot is plantar flexed, the pressure in the veins falls, the proximal valves close, and the veins are refilled by blood passing through the perforators from the superficial system. If this cycle is repeated, the venous pressure in the ankle region will gradually fall until it reaches a steady state, usually about 30 mmHg in the deep veins and 40 mmHg in the superficial veins. If the subject then stands still, the pressure in both systems will slowly return to a stable value of about 90 mmHg, a process that usually takes about 20–30 seconds.

If the function of the venous system is impaired, for example by a thrombosis, normal blood flow will be affected, resulting in the formation of varicosities (varicose veins), swelling, or even ulceration. The severity of these symptoms will depend upon the site and extent of the damage. In patients who have sustained damage to the valves in the perforators, the contraction of the calf muscle forces some blood outwards into the superficial system, resulting in the formation of varicosities. In such individuals, the pressure in the superficial system can be as high as 70% of the pressure in the deep veins (compared with a maximum of 30% in normal subjects). If a thrombus has blocked or partially occluded one of the deep vessels, however, the action of the calf muscle pump will simply serve to force the blood in the deep venous system out through the superficial system into the capillaries. In time, this will produce distention of the dermal capillary bed, causing venous flare and oedema. As a result of this increased capillary pressure, fluid containing protein and red cells may leak into the surrounding tissue; if this occurs, the red cells will break down and form haemosiderin, a pigment, which causes staining of the skin. Fibrin may also be deposited around the dermal capillaries, which will lead to subcutaneous lipodermatosclerosis and tissue hypoxia, major contributory factors to the development of leg ulcers.[2,3]

In order to prevent or minimise these effects, it is generally agreed that conservative treatment for all forms of chronic swollen legs should be directed at increasing the transfer of tissue fluid from the interstitial spaces back into the vascular and lymphatic compartments, and achieving a maximal increase in deep venous velocity in order to reduce pooling of blood in the calf veins. Both of these aims may be met by the application of external compression.

The degree of pressure required depends upon the condition to be treated, and remains a matter of some debate, although it is accepted that a pressure gradient should be produced along the leg, with the highest pressure being exerted at the ankle. In a study using recumbent volunteers without overt vascular disease, Lawrence and Kakkar[4] examined the effects of a range of pressures on three parameters – deep venous velocity, and blood flow in calf muscle and subcutaneous tissue. They found that a pressure gradient of 18 mmHg at the ankle to 14 mmHg at the calf to 8 mmHg on the upper thigh produced a mean increase in deep venous velocity of about 75%, compared with resting values. Higher pressure profiles produced a greater increase in some patients, but others showed a *reduction* in blood flow. Similar improvements were also noted in relation to flow in muscle and subcutaneous tissue. Further studies showed that equally beneficial results were obtained when only the lower part of the leg was compressed, suggesting that compression below the knee contributed most to the increased velocity of blood in the femoral vein. The pressure gradient used (18 mmHg at the ankle to 14 mmHg at the calf) is identical to that previously recommended by Sigel *et al.*,[5] and is also in agreement with the findings of Chant,[6] some years earlier, who showed that intracapillary pressure varied with posture and was exceeded by 15 – 20 mmHg of compression in the recumbent patient.

Jones et al.[7] compared the effects of the different levels of pressure applied by two brands of compression stocking on three groups of patients – normal subjects, patients with varicose veins and others with post-phlebitic limbs. Using foot volumetry and sodium ([24]Na) subcutaneous tissue clearance, they found that, in patients with superficial varicose veins, pressures of the order of 30 – 40 mmHg applied to the ankle improved the rate of clearance of tissue fluid and resulted in a significant increase in the time taken for a limb to refill after exercise. In contrast, a lower level of pressure (20 mmHg) was found to be almost totally ineffective. Although patients with post-phlebitic limbs also derived significant benefits from the application of pressures of 30 – 40 mmHg, in most instances, further benefits were obtained by the use of still higher levels, of the order of 40 – 50 mmHg.

Most of the information that has been generated on the effects of compression has been obtained using elasticated hosiery. One type of stocking (the so-called 'anti-embolism' stocking) has been designed specifically to prevent the formation of thrombosis in hospitalised patients,[8] particularly those undergoing major surgery,[9,10] using the levels of pressure suggested originally by Sigel et al.[5]

A group of products described as Graduated Compression Hosiery has recently become the subject of a British Standard specification (BS 6612:1985), and three different classes of stocking, providing levels of support ranging from 14 to 35 mmHg at the ankle are now included in the Drug Tariff. The medical reasons for using the new products have been discussed by Scurr,[11] whilst McCreedy[12] reviewed the amendments that had to be made to the Drug Tariff to enable these stockings to be supplied upon a GP's prescription, and also provided a useful guide to their clinical usage.

The German Association of Manufacturers of Medical Elastic Stockings (GZG), in cooperation with the German Society for Phlebology and Proctology, have established four categories of compression hosiery, which have been described by Stemmer et al.[1] The pressure values they have chosen, however, tend to be significantly higher than those specified in the British Standard, and it

has been suggested in a recent review that these higher levels are likely to be of more value clinically.[13]

One major Swiss manufacturer of compression hosiery (Sigvaris) recommends the use of even higher pressures although the need for these has been questioned in the past.[14] The levels of pressure that are recommended for use in a range of clinical conditions by each of the three sources identified above are summarised in the table below.

Indications	Recommended pressures (mmHg)		
	BS	GZG	Sigvaris
Superficial varices Varicosis during pregnancy	14 – 17	18.4 – 21.2	20 – 30
Varicosis during pregnancy Varices of medium severity Ulcer treatment and prevention Mild oedema After stripping or sclerotherapy	18 – 24 *	25.1 – 32.1	30 – 40
Gross varices Gross oedema Ulcer treatment and prevention Post-venous insufficiency Lymphoedema	25 – 35 *	36.4 – 46.5	40 – 50
Severe lymphoedema	*	59	50 – 60

* Not mentioned specifically

The consequences of the inappropriate or excessive application of pressure have been described by Callam et al.,[15] who recorded that the injudicious use of compression – by the use of bandages, compression hosiery or anti-embolism stockings – in limbs with occult arterial disease had apparently led to severe skin necrosis and, in a few instances, amputation. As a result, they recommended that, unless distal pulses of good volume could be detected, Doppler pressures should be measured in the ankle before treatment with compression.

The ability of a bandage to provide dressing retention, support or compression is largely determined by its elastic properties, although the thickness, weight and conformability of the fabric are also important. Sub-bandage pressure is a function of the tension induced in the fabric during application and the radius of curvature of the limb, and can be calculated from Laplace's Law as follows:

$$P = \frac{T}{RW}$$

where P = pressure (in Pa)
     T = bandage tension (in N)
     R = radius of curvature of the limb (in m)
     W = bandage width (in m)

In more practical units, this equation may be rewritten as:

$$P = \frac{T \times 4630}{CW}$$

where P = pressure (in mmHg)
     T = bandage tension (in kgf)
     C = circumference of the limb (in cm)
     W = bandage width (in cm)

As the effects of additional layers of bandage are additive, two turns applied at a constant tension will give virtually twice the pressure of a single turn.

The extensibility of a bandage may be determined by using a constant rate of traverse machine, which extends a sample of the material at a constant rate, whilst recording the tension that is developed within it. Typical load-extension curves for three different types of bandage are shown in Fig.13-1.

Each of these curves was produced by loading a sample of bandage to a predetermined tension, and then allowing it to return to its original unstretched length. It may be seen that, in each case, the extension and regain curves cannot be superimposed, but form a typical hysteresis loop.

The slope and shape of the curves provide information on the elasticity and power inherent in the bandages, and hence useful information on their likely clinical application. For example, a dressing retention bandage (Fig.13-1a) should have a long, shallow extensibility curve, which allows the bandage to stretch and conform, without restricting movement, when applied over a joint. In such products, the additional extension of the bandage during normal movement or flexing should not result in a significant increase in tension or sub-bandage pressure – which, in any event, should not exceed a few millimetres of mercury.

In contrast, bandages that are required to apply significant levels of pressure should have good regain characteristics, and a load-extension curve that rises smoothly but not too rapidly over the useful working range (Fig.13-1c). It is important to ensure, however, that a bandage is not applied at full extension, or at a point where the slope of the extension curve begins to rise steeply. In these situations, a small change in extension could result in a massive rise in tension (and, therefore, sub-bandage pressure).

Because sub-bandage pressure is inversely proportional to the radius of curvature of the limb, it follows that a bandage applied with constant tension will exert different levels of pressure at various points on the leg. In the main, this will help to provide the required pressure gradient along the leg, as the average pressure on the calf will be lower than that produced at the ankle region; but over the tibia, for example, where the radius of curvature is relatively small, very high pressure may be generated. It is possible to make use of this effect when local areas of high pressure are required after the injection of a sclerosing agent as a treatment for varicose veins. A small foam wedge or cylinder – placed under a bandage directly over the injection site – will effectively transmit additional pressure to the skin and tissues beneath, preventing the veins from recanalising.

Bandages whose primary function is one of support should have a degree of extensibility, to facilitate application, but should resist excessive extension when subjected to further tension (Fig.13-1b). Such bandages are not suitable for the application of pressure to swollen limbs.

As it is generally accepted that, for ease of application, a bandage should be applied at between 20% and 100% extension, it is possible to determine from the extensibility curves the range of tension that will develop in each product under normal conditions of use. For example, using the Laplace formula, it is possible to calculate that, in order to achieve a pressure of 50 mmHg on a swollen ankle 30 cm in circumference, two layers of a bandage 7.5 cm wide must be applied with a tension of 1.22 kgf. By reference to the curves

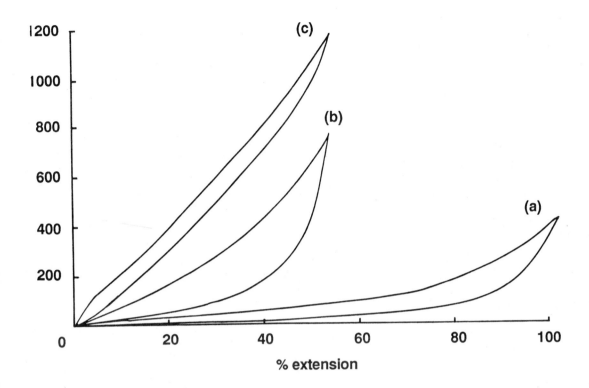

Figure 13-1 Load extension curves of three different types of bandages.

shown in Fig.13-1, it will be seen that this tension can only be achieved and maintained by one of the three bandage types, the others falling far short of this figure. Any attempt to use an all-cotton or crêpe-type bandage for this purpose is bound to meet with failure. This has been demonstrated in the past both in the laboratory[16] and in the clinical situation: in one study, it was found that cotton bandages had to be reapplied every 6−8 hours if they were to achieve and maintain therapeutically active levels of pressure.[17] In a further study, it was found that over a four-hour period, the pressure recorded beneath a crêpe-type bandage fell by some 63%, compared with a 10% drop beneath a competent compression bandage.[18]

The technique of the operator is also very important, as sub-bandage pressure is controlled by both the tension produced in the bandage during application, and the number of turns applied. Most medical and nursing staff apply a compression bandage at the tension that they consider to be appropriate to the size and

condition of the limb. However, this value varies from one person to another and, as a result, the levels of pressure applied by different individuals can be very different. A number of attempts have been made to overcome this problem by manufacturers who have printed geometrical designs upon their bandages which change shape when a predetermined level of tension is achieved. In this way it is possible to exert some control over the application tension and thus the sub-bandage pressure that is produced.

The importance of compression in the treatment of chronic venous ulcers was demonstrated by Backhouse et al.,[19] who described a study in which they compared an occlusive dressing (Granuflex™) with a simple fabric dressing (N-A™) in the treatment of fifty-six patients with chronic venous ulcers. A standard bandaging technique was used for both groups of patients, as follows. A layer of orthopaedic wadding (Velband™ − Johnson & Johnson) was applied over the primary dressing, to act as an absorbent layer and distribute the pressure from the bandages that were applied subsequently. A layer of crêpe bandage was used to compress the Velband, and this was followed by a layer of Elset™ bandage (Seton) and a final layer of a cohesive bandage (Coban™ – 3M). The pressure under these bandages was measured at four points between the medial malleolus and the knee, in 16 volunteers. In each case, a gradual fall in pressure was recorded – from 42 mmHg at the ankle to 17 mmHg just below the knee.

As the healing rates in the two groups of patients were not significantly different, the authors stated that there was little benefit to be gained from the use of the occlusive dressing and concluded that 'careful graduated compression bandaging achieves healing even in the majority of so-called resistant chronic venous ulcers'.

It is interesting to note that none of the bandages used by Backhouse *et al.* would normally be considered to be a compression bandage when applied individually, but in combination they appear to be able to achieve the desired levels of pressure. However, the same result could have been achieved at lower cost by the use of a single competent compression bandage.

CLASSIFICATION OF EXTENSIBLE BANDAGES

A working party consisting of members of the surgical dressings industry together with interested parties in the NHS has recently reclassified extensible bandages into groups, according to their performance and ability to produce and sustain predetermined levels of pressure under normal conditions of use. A laboratory method has also been devised, which may be used to help characterise the various products and predict their clinical performance, although final limits for this test are still to be agreed.

The various product groups are described below together with examples of the different types of bandage.

Type 1: Lightweight conforming stretch bandages

These are products that have a simple dressing retention function; they usually incorporate lightweight elastomeric threads, which impart a high degree of elasticity, but little power, to the bandage. Examples of bandages in this group are:

- Stayform™ – Robinsons,
- J Fast™ – Johnson & Johnson,
- Transelast™ – Lohmann,
- Lastotel™ – Hartmann,
- Slinky™ – Cuxson Gerrard,
- Peha-Crep™ – Hartmann,
- Gauzelast™ – BDF.

Type 2: Light support bandages

These bandages, which include the familiar crêpe-type products of the British Pharmacopoeia, may be used to prevent the formation of oedema, and give support in the management of mild sprains and strains. In contrast to the products in Groups 3–6, these materials have limited extensibility and elasticity, and tend to 'lock out' at relatively low levels of extension. It is this feature that enables the bandages to be applied firmly over a joint to give support without generating significant levels of pressure. It follows, therefore, that such products are *not* suitable for applying pressure or for reducing existing oedema.

The official bandages of this type are Crêpe Bandage BP, Cotton Stretch Bandage BP, and Cotton Crêpe Bandage BP. In addition to these there are numerous 'non-official' variations of these bandages, which are manufactured from cotton or cotton and viscose, and which vary quite significantly in their performance.

Type 3a: Light compression bandages

These bandages, which are equivalent in performance terms to Class 1 compression hosiery of the Drug Tariff, are designed to provide *and maintain* low levels of pressure, of the order of 14–17 mmHg on an ankle of average dimensions. The clinical indications for products of this type include the management of superficial or early varices, and varicosis formed during pregnancy. In general, they are not suitable for controlling or reducing existing oedema, or for applying even low levels of pressure to very large limbs. At the present time, the number of products that fit into this group is somewhat limited, although it is known that several manufacturers have new bandages under development. Existing products include:

- K-Crepe – Parema,
- Tensolastic – Smith & Nephew.

ADHESIVE BANDAGES

Type 3b: Moderate compression bandages

These products, which are equivalent in performance terms to Class 2 compression hosiery of the Drug Tariff, may be used to apply moderate to high levels of compression, of the order of 18 – 24 mmHg on an ankle of average dimensions. They are indicated for the treatment of varicosis during pregnancy, varices of medium severity, the prevention and treatment of ulcers and the control of mild oedema. An example of a product which falls into this group is Veinopress™ (Steriseal).

Type 3c: High compression bandages

These products, which are equivalent in performance terms to Class 3 compression hosiery of the Drug Tariff, may be used to apply high levels of compression, of the order of 25 – 35 mmHg on an ankle of average dimensions. Indications for these bandages include the treatment of gross varices, post-thrombotic venous insufficiency, and the management of leg ulcers and gross oedema in limbs of average circumference. Products in this category are not necessarily able to achieve these levels of pressure on very large limbs that have been further enlarged by the presence of oedema. Examples of bandages that fall into this group include:

- Tensopress™ – Smith & Nephew,
- Bilastic Medium™ – Steriseal,
- Setopress™ – Seton.

Type 3d: Extra-high performance compression bandages

These bandages are capable of applying pressures in the range 35 – 50 mmHg, or even higher, and their power is such that they can be expected to apply and sustain these pressures on even the largest and most oedematous limbs for extended periods of time. This group includes:

- Elastic Web Bandage BP (Blue Line Webbing),
- Bilastic Forte™ – Molinier.

(All the pressures referred to above are based on the assumption that the bandage has been applied in the form of a spiral with a 50% overlap between turns, effectively producing a double layer of bandage at any point on the limb.)

The elastic adhesive bandages of the BP are made from a woven cotton or cotton and viscose fabric, coated with a suitable adhesive mass (which contains zinc oxide, rubber, and natural resins). Crêpe-twisted cotton yarns in the warp impart a degree of elasticity to the bandage, which is used to provide compression in the treatment of varicose veins, and support for fractured ribs, clavicles, injured joints and sports injuries. The adhesive may be applied uniformly over the surface of the bandage ('plain spread'), perforated by holes ('porous spread'), or applied to only specific parts of the cloth (in which case the bandage is described as 'half-spread' or 'ventilated').

The ability of an elastic adhesive bandage to maintain compression was investigated by Blair *et al.*,[20] who compared the pressure profiles obtained beneath one such product (Elastoplast™) with those obtained under the four-component bandaging system used by Backhouse[19] and described previously. In all cases, the pressures measured beneath the elastic adhesive bandage were significantly lower than those recorded beneath the four-component system. It was also reported that 74% of ulcers that had failed to heal when dressed with a zinc paste bandage and an adhesive bandage healed within 12 weeks of the application of the alternative bandaging system.

Examples of the various adhesive products that are available are given below.

- Elastoplast (Smith & Nephew) is available in the porous spread form, and also half spread (where the adhesive is applied to one half of the bandage only).

- Flexoplast™ (Robinsons) is available both plain spread and ventilated (where the adhesive is applied as strips along the length of the bandage).

- Zopla-Band™ (Hinders-Leslies) is available in the plain spread form.

For many years, the combination of an elastic adhesive bandage and a zinc paste bandage has been one of the standard forms of treatment for venous ulcers, but, unfortunately, one or more components of the adhesive system are known to cause skin reactions in some patients. In order to overcome this problem, a number of products that bear synthetic adhesives have been developed. These tend to be based upon lighter fabrics than the official bandages and contain nylon or other synthetic yarns. They include Hapla-Band™ (Hinders-Leslies), Lite-Flex™ (Johnson & Johnson) and Veinoplast™ (Steriseal). In the main, these lightweight bandages do not have the same adhesive properties or tack characteristics as the zinc oxide materials, and have yet to reach their full potential in terms of sales and usage.

Two other alternatives are available for patients who are sensitive to traditional adhesive bandages. Lestreflex™ (Seton) consists of a cosmetically coloured bandage spread with strips of an adhesive mass consisting of lead oleate and resin. The bandage should be warmed prior to application or stored in a warm room. Also available is Poroplast™ (Scholl), which has an adhesive mass containing titanium dioxide but free from rubber and zinc oxide. This bandage complies with the monograph in the BP for Titanium Dioxide Elastic Adhesive Bandage.

Elastoplast Extension Plaster (Smith & Nephew) also complies with an official monograph (for Extension Plaster BP). It is similar in appearance to standard Elastoplast Elastic Adhesive Bandage, but is extensible across the width. It is designed to secure traction equipment to a limb, and, in these situations, the sideways stretch inherent in the bandage is said to be an advantage.

COHESIVE BANDAGES

Cohesive bandages combine some of the characteristics of ordinary stretch bandages with those of the adhesive products. Whilst they do not adhere to the skin, a special coating on their surface enables the bandages to adhere to themselves, which prevents overlapping turns slipping or becoming undone, under normal conditions of use. When using cohesive bandages, care must be taken to ensure that they are not applied with excessive tension, particularly over joints or bony areas. Unlike ordinary fabric products, the turns of the bandage will be unable to move relative to each other to equalise local areas of high tension, and, as a result, may cause a tourniquet effect. Cohesive bandages may be used in place of the adhesive products for many applications, but they are particularly useful for providing support in sports situations, as they tend to remain in place even during exercise; unlike the adhesive products they can be removed without causing pain or trauma.

The cohesive bandages currently on the market are Secure™ and Secure Forte™ (Johnson & Johnson), Cohepress™ (Steriseal) and Coban (3M).

TUBULAR BANDAGES

Tubular bandages, like ordinary roller bandages, are available in a number of different forms, each of which is intended to perform a different function. The simplest form, sometimes known as stockinette, consists of a knitted tube of a lightweight fabric made from cotton or viscose, and manufactured in both plain and ribbed versions. Stockinettes are used under orthopaedic casts, or placed over arms or legs that are covered with cream or other medication, where they serve a simple protective function. For situations where a non-absorbent material is required, stockinettes coated with paraffin or made from polypropylene are available. Proprietary tubular bandages of this type include the following products.

- Tubiton™ (Seton) is manufactured from a mix of viscose rayon and unbleached cotton, which gives the dressing limited water-repellant properties.

- Tubinette™ (Seton) is manufactured from 100% rayon. It is the cheapest product in the range and is used where dressings require frequent replacement.

- Tubegauz™ (Seton) is produced from bleached cotton and is claimed to be well suited for dermatological use, being comfortable against the skin.

Seton also produce a lightweight elasticated tubular bandage called Tubifast™. Similar in appearance to a stockinette, it has fine elastic threads incorporated into its structure, which makes the material highly conformable. The bandage is available in a range of sizes to fit most parts of the body and can be used for most of the applications for which a stockinette is indicated. In addition, it has the advantage that it will not go baggy or sag in use.

One of the most versatile tubular products available is tubular net bandage, which consists of an open net in the form of a tube manufactured from elasticated yarns. Produced in a range of sizes, the net may be used as supplied, or cut and formed into garments for retaining dressings on the head, shoulders, groin regions and other areas that are difficult to dress.

The products available include:

- Netelast™ – Roussel,
- Netgrip™ – BDF,
- Setonet™ – Seton,
- Surgifix™ – Hospital Management & Supplies.

The final member of the tubular bandage family (and probably the most familiar, yet most abused) is Elasticated Tubular Bandage BP. First developed by Seton, a number of brands are now available, which include:

- Rediform™ – Salt,
- Tensogrip™ – Smith & Nephew,
- Tricodur™ – BDF,
- Tubigrip™ – Seton.

The bandages are quick and easy to apply, and are often used as an alternative to roller bandages to provide pressure and support in the treatment of swollen legs. Unfortunately, the levels of pressure that these materials generate are considerably lower than most experienced medical and nursing staff would anticipate. For example, work carried out by the author (unpublished data) has shown that a single layer of Tubigrip size C (or the equivalent size from any other manufacturer), when applied to a small leg with an ankle circumference of 24 cm and a calf size of about 35 cm, will apply a pressure of the order of 6 mmHg at the ankle and 7 mmHg at the calf. If two layers are applied, in accordance with the manufacturer's instructions, this will result in pressures of 12 mmHg at the ankle and 14 mmHg at the calf – causing a reversed pressure gradient on the leg. (These figures do not agree with the information provided on the tension guide produced by Seton, which suggests that the pressures beneath the bandages in these circumstances would be of the order of 10–20 mmHg at the ankle and 20–30 mmHg at the calf.) Clearly, this is not in accord with the recommendations of Sigel et al.[5] and others, as described earlier.

It is obvious from these results that elasticated tubular bandage is of very limited value for anything other than the application of the lowest levels of pressure. It cannot be used as a substitute for a good compression bandage, and should not be used as the sole means of applying pressure to an oedematous limb. In the community, large amounts of elasticated tubular bandage are used in the treatment of varicose ulcers, a procedure that is of extremely questionable value. If the product is to be used, it would probably be advantageous to apply it in three separate pieces, of decreasing length, one from the toes to the knee, a second over the foot and lower calf, and a third over the ankle only. In this way, it might at least be possible to achieve a reasonable pressure gradient along the leg, with the highest level at the ankle region where it is required. In an attempt to overcome the shortcomings of the plain tubular bandages, a number of manufacturers also produce shaped elasticated tubular stockinettes, which are claimed to give a degree of graduated compression. However, the pressures produced by these bandages still fall short of the values that are required clinically.

MEDICATED PASTE BANDAGES

The medicated paste bandages share a common basic structure, consisting of a cotton fabric of plain weave impregnated with a medicated paste or cream. A number of different formulations are available, most of which contain zinc oxide. Details of the formulation of each may be found in the Drug Tariff Technical Specifications. It might be expected that the introduction of new dressings such as the alginates and the hydrocolloids would cause the market share of the paste bandages to decrease but at the time of writing there is no evidence that this is the case and the plain zinc paste bandage in particular remains a standard treatment for leg ulcers.

- Zinc Paste Bandage BP is available as Zincaband™ (Seton) or Viscopaste PB7™ (Smith & Nephew). The bandage is impregnated with a simple zinc oxide paste, which has been used extensively for the treatment for leg ulcers and other chronic wounds. Once applied, the bandage may be left undisturbed for up to a week in some instances. Zinc paste bandage, in conjunction with compression therapy, is often used as a yardstick when assessing the performance of other leg ulcer treatments.

- Zinc Paste and Coal Tar Bandage BP, available as Tarband™ (Seton) and

Coltapaste™ (Smith & Nephew), is sometimes used for the treatment of chronic eczema, lichenification (lichen simplex), infantile eczema and atopic dermatitis.

- Zinc Paste and Ichthammol Bandage BP, available as Icthaband™ (Seton) and Ichthopaste™ (Smith & Nephew), is used for the treatment of chronic eczema where tar cannot be tolerated, and for subacute gravitational eczema.

- Zinc Paste and Calamine Bandage (Drug Tariff), available as Calaband™ (Seton), is used for the non-exudative stages of acute and subacute eczema, erythema, and dermatitis after plaster removal.

- Zinc Paste, Calamine, and Clioquinol Bandage BP, available as Quinaband™ (Seton), has mild antibacterial activity and is used to combat infection and odour in the treatment of leg ulcers.

REFERENCES

1. Stemmer R. *et al.*, Compression treatment of the lower extremities particularly with compression stockings, *Dermatologist*, 1980, **31**, 355–365.
2. Browse N.L. and Burnand K.G., The cause of venous ulceration, *Lancet*, 1982, **2**, 243–245.
3. Burnand K. *et al.*, Venous lipodermatosclerosis: treatment by fibrinolytic enhancement and elastic compression, *Br. med. J.*, 1980, **280**, 7–11.
4. Lawrence D. and Kakkar V.V., Graduated, static, external compression of the lower limb; a physiological assessment, *Br. J. Surg.*, 1980, **67**, 119–121.
5. Sigel B. *et al.*, Types of compression for reducing venous stasis, *Arch. Surg.*, 1975, **110**, 171–175.
6. Chant A.D., The effects of posture, exercise, and bandage pressure on the clearance of ^{24}Na from the subcutaneous tissues of the foot, *Br. J. Surg.*, 1972, **59**, 552–555.
7. Jones N.A.G. *et al.*, A physiological study of elastic compression stockings in venous disorders of the leg, *ibid.*, 1980, **67**, 569–572.
8. Wilkins R.W. *et al.*, Elastic stockings in the prevention of pulmonary embolism; a preliminary report, *New Engl. J. Med.*, 1952, **246**, 360–364.
9. Holford C.P., Graded compression for preventing deep venous thrombosis, *Br. med. J.*, 1976, **2**, 969–970.
10. Magdy A. *et al.*, Deep venous thrombosis after total hip arthroplasty; a prospective controlled study to determine the prophylactic effect of graded pressure stockings, *Br. J. Surg.*, 1981, **68**, 429–432.
11. Scurr J., Why use elastic hosiery?, *Pharm. J.*, 1988, **240**, 410–411.
12. McCreedy C., Elastic hosiery on the NHS, *ibid.*, 412–413.
13. Burnand K.G. and Layer G.T., Graduated elastic stockings, *Br. med. J.*, 1986, **293**, 224–225.
14. Fentem P.H., Claims about compression treatment for venous disease, (letter), *ibid.* 1982, **285**, 61.
15. Callam M.J. *et al.*, Hazards of compression treatment of the leg: an estimate from Scottish surgeons, *ibid.*, 1987, **295**, 1382.
16. Thomas S. *et al.*, Performance profiles of extensible bandages, in *Phlebology 85*, Negus D. and Jantet G. (eds), Proceedings of a Symposium, Union Internationale de Phlebologie, London, 16–20 September 1985, London, John Libbey, 1986, 667–670.
17. Raj T.B *et al.*, How long do compression bandages maintain their pressure during ambulatory treatment of varicose veins?, *Br. J. Surg.*, 1980, **67**, 122–124.
18. Tennant W.G., Testing compression bandages, *Phlebology*, 1988, **3**, 55–61.
19. Backhouse C.M. *et al.*, Controlled trial of occlusive dressings in healing chronic venous ulcers, *Br. J. Surg.*, 1987, **74**, 626–627.
20. Blair S.D. *et al.*, Sustained compression and healing of chronic venous ulcers, *Br. med. J.*, 1988, **297**, 1159–1161.

Orthopaedic Casting Materials

But if thou make thine apparatus with lime and white of egg it will be much handsomer and still more useful; in fact, it will become as hard as stone and will not need to be removed until the healing is complete.

Rhazes, AD 860

THE DEVELOPMENT OF CASTING MATERIALS

Throughout the ages, many different resinous and adhesive materials have been used, in conjunction with suitable cloth, to immobilise an injured limb.[1-5] As early as 1600 BC, the Edwin Smith papyrus describes the treatment of 48 cases of wounds, dislocations and fractures resulting from accidents, and records the use of splints made from padded wood and plastered or glued linen. In 350 BC, Hippocrates described the use of bandages containing waxes, resins and similar substances, while Celsus (AD 30) wrote of bandages stiffened with starch to treat fractures and dislocations. The use of a lime-based material, similar to that mentioned by Rhazes (above), was described by Abu Mansur Muwaffaq, a Persian pharmacist (c. AD 975).

In Europe, from the Middle Ages until well into the 19th century, surgeons continued to bind injured limbs with rags soaked in mixtures made from a variety of materials (such as flour and albumen) before applying splints and bandages (Fig. 14-1). These materials were far from satisfactory, as they took so long to dry that it was difficult to maintain the initial reduction of the fracture. In 1834, Baron Seutin, Senior Medical Officer of the Belgian army, introduced a bandage impregnated with a starch paste — similar to that first described by Celsus nearly two thousand years earlier — which he used in conjunction with soaked cardboard splints. Once set (a process that could take up to two days), the bandage could be divided along its length and hinged, thus giving access to the limb for the application of local treatments. The starch bandage became very widely used and remained popular for many years, as it allowed the patient a degree of mobility not previously possible.

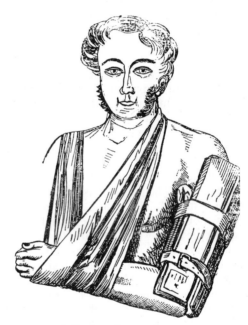

A BROKEN ARM IN POSITION.

Figure 14-1 Splinting a broken arm (*circa* 1851).

Probably the first references to the orthopaedic use of plaster of Paris may be found in Arabian writings of the tenth century AD, which referred to a combination of materials including slaked lime and gypsum. Abu'l Qassim, a Moorish surgeon of the 11th century, described the use of a padded plaster with an aperture over the wound for compound fractures — possibly the first recorded use of the technique of 'windowing'. Eastern expertise in the methods of fracture reduction was referred to in a letter written in 1794 by W. Eaton, the British Consul at Basra, to a Dr Guthrie of Peterborough. He described the use of plaster of Paris as follows:

'I saw in the eastern parts of the Empire a method of setting bones practised which appears to me worthy of the attention of surgeons in Europe. It is by enclosing the broken limb, after the bones are put in their places, in a case of plaster-of-Paris (or gypsum) which takes exactly the form of the limb, without any pressure, and in a few minutes the mass is solid and strong.'

In his letter, he went on to describe the successful treatment of a 'most terrible fracture of the leg and thigh' (caused by cannon fire), in which the victim's leg was encased in plaster from below the heel to the upper part of the thigh.

Western surgeons, however, were slow to adopt this new technique. Many remained largely unaware of the potential value of plaster of Paris for orthopaedic purposes, despite the fact that the material was used to make models and casts of deformities – both to provide a pattern for the construction of an appliance, and also to provide a record of the condition for comparison after corrective treatment. However, in the early part of the 19th century, a splinting method was developed in which the injured limb was placed inside a box, and plaster (in the form of a creamy liquid) was poured over it. The plaster was allowed to set and the box removed. This method was not generally very popular, because the weight and thickness of the cast were difficult to control. These problems were largely overcome by Pirogoff, a Russian surgeon, who brushed a slurry of plaster onto strips of bandage, or other materials (such as stockings or underwear) previously applied to the limb. During the Crimean War, between January and April 1855, this technique was used to treat some 600 fracture cases in the Russian hospital in Sebastopol, this being the first large-scale use of plaster of Paris in military surgery.

It was not until 1851 that a convenient method of utilising the useful properties of plaster of Paris became available, when Mathysen, a Dutch army surgeon, produced a plaster of Paris bandage by rubbing the finely divided powder into a coarse cotton cloth. It is interesting to note that Mathysen was responsible for laying down one of the earliest manufacturing standards for plaster of Paris bandages, as he insisted that the cloth used 'be free from starch and dressing'. Using this material, the surgeon was able, for the first time, to produce a quick-setting, strong cast, which was not excessively heavy. It was this development that

eventually led to the widespread use of plaster of Paris for medical applications. The first walking cast was introduced in 1887 by Krause, who applied it from groin to toes. Once it was set, the patient was able to walk directly on the cast, although a special lace boot was applied for outdoor use.

In 1900, Johnson & Johnson developed the world's first commercial plaster bandage, using a crinoline fabric impregnated with the dry plaster powder. This material, Orthoplast™, remained available until 1952 although many hospitals continued to produce their own plaster of Paris bandages (Fig. 14-2). For almost 80 years, all bandages had to be produced by a method similar to that originally described by Mathysen; but, in 1927, an entirely new process was developed, in which the plaster was applied to the fabric in combination with a suitable binder, using a water-based coating process. Bandages produced in this way were much less likely to lose plaster during handling or wetting than those made by the simple dry impregnation method. In a further advance, in 1931, Lohmann developed a non-aqueous solvent-based coating process, which was licensed to Smith & Nephew shortly afterwards, both companies selling under the Cellona™ brand name. Smith & Nephew modified the product by

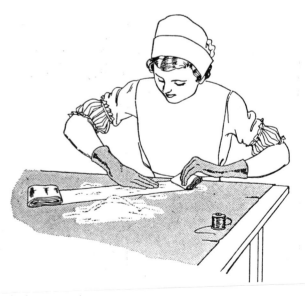

Figure 14-2 A nurse producing a plaster of Paris bandage, from Mary Farnworth, *Roller and Triangular Bandaging Illustrated*, 1939, (*courtesy of Faber and Faber*).

COLOUR PLATES

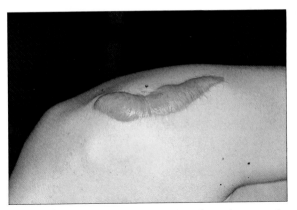

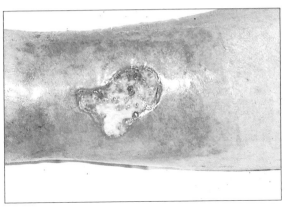

Plate 1   A keloid scar that developed on the arm of a young man following a vaccination.

Plate 2   Area of inflammation formed around a leg ulcer dressed with a perforated plastic film dressing.

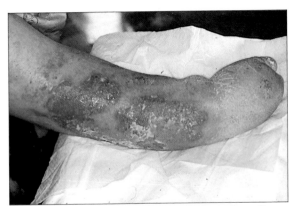

Plate 3   A sensitivity reaction to the use of a tulle dressing containing framycetin.

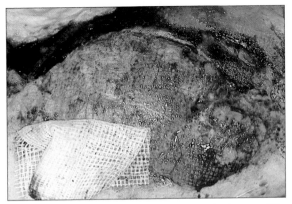

Plate 4   Trauma caused during removal of a paraffin gauze dressing.

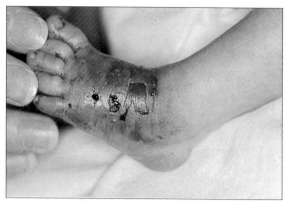

Plate 5 Extravasation injury with severe bruising

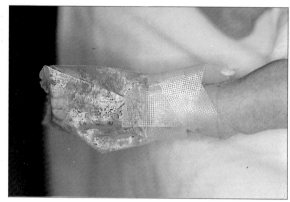

Plate 6 Foot enclosed in plastic bag containing Scherisorb™ gel.

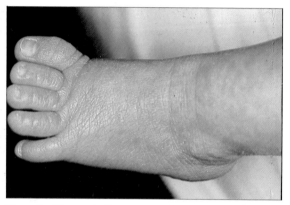

Plate 7 The healed wound.

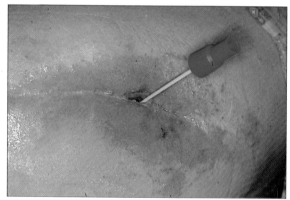

Plate 8 Sensitivity reaction on the skin surrounding a sinus packed with proflavine cream.

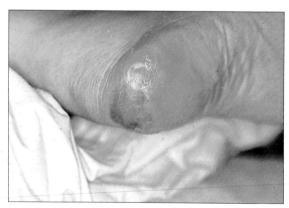

Plate 9 An early stage in the formation of a serious pressure sore showing purple discoloration of the skin.

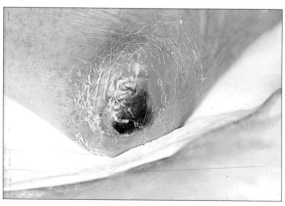

Plate 10 A later stage in which a similar area has become dehydrated and taken on a black leathery appearance.

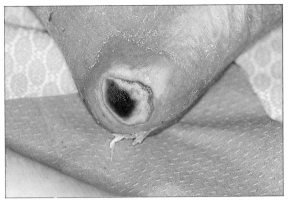

Plate 11 A black necrotic area that has been dressed with a hydrocolloid dressing (Granuflex™); note the moist condition of both the slough and the surrounding skin.

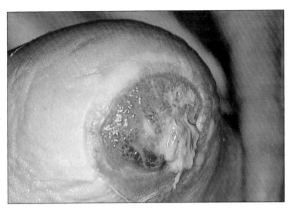

Plate 12 Following autolysis, the necrotic tissue is now almost completely detached.

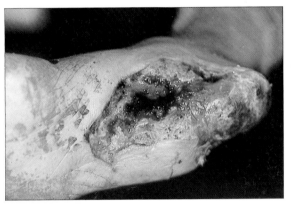

Plate 13 A large sloughy area on the foot of a diabetic patient which developed following surgical debridement.

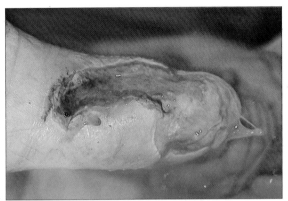

Plate 14 After a period of treatment with Scherisorb Gel, the slough has started to liquify.

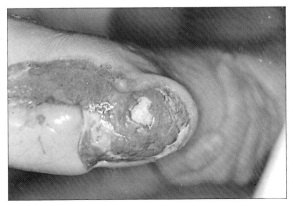

Plate 15 The wound, now almost completely clear of slough, showing granulation tissue forming over the exposed bone.

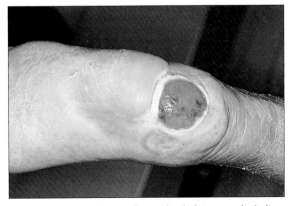

Plate 16 Wound now almost healed, currently being dressed with Granuflex sheets.

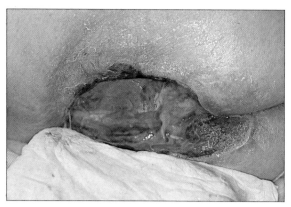

Plate 17 A large, foul-smelling, sacral pressure sore filled with yellow slough.

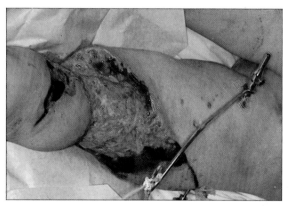

Plate 18 A large necrotic area on the lower leg; dressed with a calcium alginate dressing (Sorbsan™).

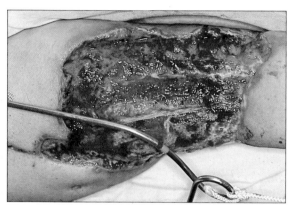

Plate 19 The same wound two weeks later.

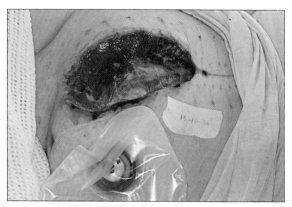

Plate 20 A large abdominal wound suitable for treatment with Silastic Foam™.

the introduction of a leno-weave gauze, and, in 1947, changed the brand name to Gypsona™.

With minor modifications and improvements the plaster of Paris bandage remained the material of choice for most orthopaedic applications for over 50 years, but its position is now being challenged by a variety of synthetic materials which have very different properties and performance characteristics. One of the earliest attempts to improve the properties of plaster of Paris was reported by Bennett et al.,[6] who painted plaster of Paris casts with cellulose acetate solution, to improve their water resistance. In the late 1940s, melamine-formaldehyde adhesives were developed for use in the manufacture of waterproof plywood, and Cobey,[7] Spittler et al.,[8] and Harvey and Lastrapes[9] used this technology in the USA to make significant improvements to ordinary plaster of Paris casts. They immersed standard plaster bandages in an aqueous solution of melamine resin containing ammonium chloride as a catalyst. They found that the resultant resin plaster casts were more water-resistant, stronger, and lighter than those made from ordinary plaster. These findings were subsequently confirmed during early clinical use of the material in the UK.[10–14]

Resin plasters manufactured using this technology were developed commercially in the mid-1950s by Johnson & Johnson (Specialist™ Orthopaedic Resin, and later Zoroc™), Smith & Nephew (Gypsona Extra™), and Lohmann (Cellamin™), of which Cellamin is the only product still available. As these new casting materials became more widely used, there were occasional reports that the formaldehyde in the resin was causing contact dermatitis in plaster room staff,[15–17] but this could be avoided by the use of gloves.

In another type of casting tape, cellulose acetate fibres were knitted or woven into a bandage. The material was activated by immersion in acetone, which partially dissolved the cellulose acetate fibres, allowing them to stick together. The solvent then evaporated. In 1955, Smith & Nephew introduced a product called Glassona™, which was composed of glass and cellulose acetate fibres knitted together for extra strength, but the flammable nature of the solvent, a 15-minute setting time, and the significant incidence of skin reactions to the solvent severely limited its acceptance in plaster rooms.

In the late 1960s, a novel system for making casts was patented, based on a knitted fibreglass substrate coated with a photo-sensitive resin that polymerised after exposure to ultraviolet light. This product was marketed by Merck Sharp & Dohme as Lightcast I™, and required two separate wrapping and curing stages to make a satisfactory weight-bearing cast. An improved version, Lightcast II™, which needed only a single wrapping and curing cycle, was introduced by 3M in 1973. However, despite the fast setting and weight-bearing time, excellent cast strength, durability, and water resistance,[18,19] the need for an expensive specialised UV lamp limited its use in the UK.

Around 1975, in the FRG, Bayer began investigating new uses for their moisture-curing polyurethane resin system. Although prototype bandages based on a knitted fibreglass substrate were produced, they decided instead to market a product based on a woven bleached cotton bandage, coated with a pre-polymer resin. This bandage was used clinically in the FRG (where it was known as Baycast™) in 1977, and in the USA (as Cuttercast™) in 1978. The rolls of tape were simply immersed in water before use and required no lamps or solvents. The casts were strong, lightweight, and water-resistant, and were thus readily accepted by plaster room staff, once the new bandage-wrapping technique had been learned.

In 1978, Hexcel adopted a fresh approach, using a thermoplastic polymer – poly (caprolactone) – coated onto a knitted cotton mesh fabric. The rolls of the product, Hexcelite™, were immersed in water at 80°C to soften the plastic before use. Although Hexcelite was rather bulky in use, it produced casts that were lightweight, very porous, durable, and strong.[20] The finished casts could also be remoulded, with care. The main disadvantage of the product was the interliner (which prevented the layers sticking together when the roll was immersed in hot water). The interliner had to be torn away as the tape was wrapped onto the limb, and was thus rather inconvenient.

In 1979, Smith & Nephew brought out a new product called Crystona™, which was based on the ioner cement technology that had recently been developed by the Laboratory of the Government Chemist – known as ASPA, alumino-silicate poly(alkenoic acid).[21] Crystona used conventional application techniques, and casts were water-resistant and early weight-bearing.

In 1982, Johnson & Johnson introduced Baycast Plus™, which was an improved version of Baycast in which the resin was applied to a cotton bandage that was extensible across its width. Baycast Plus was subsequently renamed Delta-Cast™.

In 1980, 3M introduced a product called Scotchcast™, based upon a polyurethane resin applied to a fibreglass fabric. This rapidly gained acceptance, and was swiftly followed by new products from Johnson & Johnson, Hexcel, Smith & Nephew, Zimmer, and Lohmann, with the result that a wide range of polyurethane-based casting tapes is currently available.

Over the years, advances have been made both in tape conformability (by utilising fabrics with length and widthways stretch) and in the resin systems used (which now have improved handling characteristics, reduced setting and weight-bearing times, and, more recently, a virtual elimination of resin tack). However, all these new products still use the same basic resin chemistry, based on moisture-curing urethane pre-polymers. Advances within this area are so rapid that the dressings on the market are constantly changing, as old formulations are improved and new ones are developed in an attempt to improve the stability and handling characteristics of the products. These changes, coupled with the aggressive marketing techniques of some of the manufacturers, have led to some confusion about the differences between the various brands, and the most appropriate product for use in any given situation. Rowley *et al.*,[22] in the course of a comparative study into the properties of plaster and plaster substitutes, suggested that the ideal casting material should:

- be strong, relative to its weight and bulk;

- be sufficiently rigid to act as a splint, but flexible enough not to be susceptible to brittle failure during normal use;

- be easy to work and mould, causing minimal mess;

- allow examination by X-ray and other imaging techniques without removal;

- be waterproof, but porous enough to prevent skin maceration;

- be simple to handle;

- require no gross capital expenditure and cost as little as possible.

By its very nature, the application of an orthopaedic cast is a process that requires considerable manual skill and expertise; there is little doubt that slight differences in the individual techniques of plaster room staff, combined with minor differences in the properties of the bandages, can result in the rejection by an individual operator of a product that may be well accepted and widely used elsewhere.

PLASTER OF PARIS BANDAGES

Plaster of Paris is produced by dehydrating gypsum (calcium sulphate), a mineral that occurs naturally,[23] and also as a by-product of phosphoric acid production or power station flue gas desulphurisation. When heated, gypsum loses water to form the hemihydrate. The process may be carried out at atmospheric pressure in an open pan or kettle at approximately 160°C, or by an alternative process in which the raw material is treated in an autoclave at 130°C. In the latter method, excess water is removed by filtration and the resultant paste is rapidly dried at high temperature. The dry hemihydrate is reduced to a fine powder by milling.

The crystalline form of the calcium sulphate hemihydrate depends upon its method of manufacture: the material produced in an autoclave consists of alpha crystals, which are small and squat, whilst the beta crystals produced by the dry heat method are thinner and more irregular. These different crystalline structures have important effects upon the setting process and handling characteristics of the plasters produced from them. Because of their regular shape, the alpha crystals are able to pack together closely to form a dense cast, taking up only a small amount of excess water. The more irregularly shaped beta crystals do not set so closely together, and, therefore, take up a larger amount of excess water, producing a less dense final cast. These differences have important implications for the strength and drying properties of the cast. An increase in the alpha plaster content will result in a stronger but more brittle cast, whilst an increase in the beta plaster content is said to result in a bandage with improved handling properties, having a smoother creamier consistency when wet.

Whilst the alpha and beta forms liberate similar amounts of heat on rehydration, the lower water excess associated with the alpha plaster results in greater heat build-up; therefore, lower water immersion temperatures are usually indicated for plasters with a high content of the alpha form. When water is added to the dry plaster of Paris powder, the hexahydrate reverts back to the dihydrate, according to the equation:

$$2CaSO_4.\tfrac{1}{2}H_2O + 3H_2O \leftrightarrow 2CaSO_4.2H_2O + Heat\uparrow$$

The reaction starts immediately in an unmodified plaster, and the plaster sets in about 10–15 minutes. The resultant material then gains about 40% of its final dry strength in the first two hours.

In order to produce a material with a workable consistency, more water is added to the plaster than is actually required to enable the reaction to take place. As a cast sets, it passes through a series of stages, during which small quantities of the plaster progressively dissolve in the water to form a supersaturated solution of the dihydrate. This then precipitates out, leaving the residual water available to dissolve more plaster and so continue the process. Because of this unique mechanism, the resultant cast consists of a mass of interlocking crystals, which are responsible for the strength of the final material. Any water remaining in the cast is lost by simple evaporation, partly aided by the heat that is given off during the reaction. Until all the water is removed, the plaster does not achieve its full final strength. In very large thick casts, this drying process may take up to 72 hours, and it is important that during this time the cast is not subjected to excessive stress or damaged in any way. For this reason, patients should be warned that plaster casts applied to the lower limbs may not be capable of bearing their full weight for up to two days.

For orthopaedic purposes, the setting time of plaster of Paris can be modified by the addition of various chemicals to the water used to soak the bandages. Potassium sulphate will speed up the setting process, and borax will slow it down – a 1% solution of borax will effectively increase the setting time by up to 15 minutes. A more efficient retarder is trisodium citrate – a 1% solution will increase the setting time by as much as three hours, but, in practice, a 0.1% solution is more commonly used, retarding a '15-minute setting' plaster by about 15–30 minutes. The setting process is temperature-dependent and will take place faster if the water is warm. Conversely, setting is retarded if cold water is used. For this reason, it is important to ensure that the manufacturer's directions are carefully followed in this respect: the recommended temperature of the water used for the immersion of the Lohmann products (20–25°C) tends to be lower than that suggested for the Smith & Nephew bandages (25–30°C).

In general, all the plaster-based products sold in Britain share a common structure, consisting of a cellulose fabric (generally cotton), impregnated with a mass that consists of calcium sulphate hemihydrate blended with binders and accelerators. During manufacture, the mass is applied to the cloth in the form of a slurry, suspended in a volatile organic solvent (which is removed from the bandage by evaporation at the end of the process, condensed, and reused). Commercial plaster of Paris bandages are manufactured from a blend of the alpha and beta forms, and it is primarily this blending process that is responsible for the strength build-up and handling characteristics of the finished product.

The plaster of Paris bandages currently available on the UK market are:

- Gypsona – Smith & Nephew,
- Gypsona S™ – Smith & Nephew,
- Cellona SR™ – Lohmann,
- Cellona Elastic™ – Lohmann,
- Orthoflex™ – Johnson & Johnson.

As might be expected, coming from the same manufacturer, Gypsona and Gypsona S are virtually identical in terms of the composition of the plaster mass, but they differ in the structure of the base fabric. Gypsona, which complies with the BP monograph for Plaster of Paris Bandage, is based upon a leno-weave gauze fabric – which is claimed to impart extra stability to the bandage and reduce creasing, when compared with the plain-weave gauze that is used in the manufacture of the non-BP products. However, the use of a leno-weave gauze inevitably adds to the manufacturing costs of the product, and Gypsona S was introduced as a cheaper alternative to compete on economic terms with other non-BP products of continental origin. The Cellona products, manufactured by Lohmann of the FRG, are currently making significant inroads into the UK market. Like Gypsona S, they are made from a plain-weave cotton gauze fabric, impregnated with a mixture of calcium sulphate hemihydrate and accelerators and binders. Cellona SR has a higher proportion of alpha crystals than Gypsona, and, as a result, requires a shorter dip time to activate the plaster. In contrast, Cellona Elastic contains only beta crystals. This is to provide a longer setting time, which is sometimes required when producing prosthetic moulds and casts for amputation stumps.

Cellona SR has an initial setting time of the order of 2–2.5 minutes, slightly longer than the 2 minutes recorded for the Smith & Nephew products. However, these times are subject to significant variability, depending upon the temperature of the water and the thickness of the final cast. The differences in the recommended temperature of the water, the method and duration of immersion of the bandage, and the setting time mean that users may need to adjust their technique when changing from one brand to another.

Modifications to the structure of the base fabric have resulted in the production of bandages that are claimed to have advantages over the more traditional materials for certain applications.

Orthoflex consists of a standard plaster of Paris mass applied to a slightly pre-tensioned elasticated gauze fabric. When the bandage is dipped into warm water (29°C), the tension is released, and thus, it is claimed, the bandage is able to form itself more closely to the contours of the limb. A similar approach has been adopted in the design of Cellona Elastic. Both materials are intended for use as a first layer in the production of a standard orthopaedic cast, which may be completed using Cellona SR, Gypsona, or any other suitable material. Because they conform so closely to the limb, the elasticated products are thought to be particularly useful for mould making, fresh fractures, holding manipulations, and as slabs for splinting soft tissue repairs. The use of either of these materials requires a minor modification in technique, as the additional conformability of the product means that it should not be necessary to use tucks or folds during application. The bandage is simply rolled on, taking care not to impart any additional tension.

In general, plaster of Paris bandages are reasonably conformable, easy to apply, and significantly cheaper than the synthetic materials. The rapid setting time is also of value in immobilising unstable fractures. The disadvantages of plaster of Paris are, principally, the weight of the final cast, its tendency to break down or crack, and its susceptibility to damage by moisture. In addition, the material is relatively opaque to X-rays, and the prolonged drying time before the bandage is fully weight-bearing can also be a significant disadvantage.

PLASTER OF PARIS AND RESIN BANDAGES

Cellamin (Lohmann) is the only product of this type remaining on the UK market. It consists of a plain-weave gauze, impregnated with a combination of plaster of Paris and a synthetic resin made from melamine and formaldehyde. During setting, the plaster crystals, which are largely responsible for the strength of the cast, are encased by the plastic resin. This structure leads to the formation of a water-resistant cast that is thinner and lighter than one made from plaster alone, and with cost advantages over the polyurethane materials. Cellamin casts require 30% less material than plain plaster ones, and are weight-bearing after one hour. Cellamin may be used as an alternative to plaster of Paris bandage for most casting applications, or as a waterproofing or strengthening layer over plaster walking casts. It is particularly useful in the formation of frog plasters, where resistance to urine may be important.

Because of the risk of formaldehyde sensitisation, plaster room staff should wear gloves when using this material.

POLYURETHANE-BASED CASTING MATERIALS

In general terms, the majority of the polyurethane casting materials share the same basic structure and chemistry. Each consists of a warp-knitted bandage substrate covered with a moisture-curing polyurethane pre-polymer coating, rolled around a plastic core and packaged in a laminate pouch. When the products are exposed to moisture, isocyanate groups on the resin react with water to produce amine groups, which, in turn, react with further isocyanate groups, producing urea crosslinks within the structure. It is this cross-linking that is responsible for the bandage setting and solidifying. Other reactions may occur in the absence of water – terminal isocyanate groups reacting with active hydrogens in the main chain. This leads to an increase in the viscosity of the resin, and hence determines the shelf life of the bandage.

The chemical reactions of the resin are accompanied by several physical changes. Before contact with water, the resin is only slightly sticky, being viscous enough not to drip off the bandage. After immersion in water, the resin rapidly increases in tack as the reaction proceeds. This allows good lamination between the layers. The escaping bubbles of carbon dioxide gas produced as a by-product of the reaction can often be heard at this stage. As the tack begins to diminish, the material enters a plastic phase, during which it may be moulded to shape. Finally, the cast becomes hard and tough as complete curing and cross-linking of the resin takes place. Recent developments have masked the changes in stickiness by incorporating slip agents into the resin, which virtually eliminate the tack, but the underlying physical changes still occur within the resin.

The principal advantages of the synthetic products lie in their weight, as casts produced from them are many times lighter than equivalent casts made from plaster of Paris. They are also highly resistant to damage and stress, water-resistant, transparent to X-rays, porous, and early weight-bearing. Polyurethane casts are also of value where incontinence is likely to be problem, as the cast will not disintegrate in contact with urine, and can be washed if required. Although the synthetic materials can be used to replace plaster of Paris for many applications, their major disadvantage is simply one of cost − they can be 4−8 times more expensive than plaster of Paris, when calculated on a cast-for-cast basis. Mainly for financial reasons, therefore, they are not generally used for the production of primary casts that may need to be replaced after a relatively short period.

The handling characteristics and techniques required for the application of the polyurethane bandages are very different from those of plaster of Paris bandages, as working and curing times vary significantly. It is generally recommended that gloves be worn when handling polyurethane-based casting tapes, to prevent resin adhering to the skin, and to protect the user from the slight risk of sensitisation to the uncured resin. Casts made from materials based on fibreglass fabrics are generally removed using a reciprocating cast saw; in these situations, the use of dust extraction equipment is desirable. Recently, cutters designed specifically for fibreglass casts have been developed, which should overcome some of the problems of dust formation associated with the use of cast saws.

Although polyurethane casts are generally weight-bearing in about 30 minutes or less, compared with up to 48 hours for plaster of Paris, the setting times for these materials are generally longer than those experienced with plaster of Paris. For this reason, most practitioners prefer plaster of Paris bandages for routine use, particularly for application to fresh or unstable fractures. Some manufacturers specifically state that their polyurethane products should not be applied to fresh fractures, as, in the event of the limb swelling, the cast cannot be readily removed without the use of specialised equipment.

The products currently available in the UK are as follows:

- Cellacast™ − Lohmann,
- Delta-Cast™ − Johnson & Johnson,
- Delta-Cast Plus™ − Johnson & Johnson,
- Delta-Lite S™ − Johnson & Johnson,
- Delta-Lite Conformable™ − Johnson & Johnson,
- Dynacast™ − Smith & Nephew,
- Dynacast Extra™ − Smith & Nephew,
- Scotchcast 2™ − 3M,
- Scotchcast Plus™ − 3M,
- Scotchflex™ − 3M,
- Zim-flex™ − Zimmer.

These are described briefly below.

The setting and weight-bearing times quoted below are taken from the manufacturer's literature.

Cellacast is based upon an extensible fibreglass fabric, which is coated with a polyurethane pre-polymer. The bandage is very conformable, and sets in approximately 3−4 minutes to form a strong cast, which is weight-bearing in about 20−30 minutes. Cellacast is available in four colours − white, blue, green, and pink − which allows the casts to be coded by department or stage of healing.

Delta-Cast is a lightweight, low-cost casting tape made from a cotton fabric impregnated with a catalysed urethane pre-polymer. The tape is activated by immersion in cold water and sets in 5−7 minutes. Because Delta-Cast is lighter though less strong than the fibreglass tapes, it is widely used for paediatric and geriatric applications, as well as upper limb casts where the applied stresses are lower and overall cast weight may be important.

Delta-Cast Plus is a light/mediumweight casting tape, which is particularly recommended for children and old people. It is not the product of choice for the manufacture of weight-bearing casts for large adults. It is made from a knitted polyester fabric impregnated with a catalysed urethane pre-polymer. As the fabric is extensible in all directions, it is highly conformable in use. The bandage sets in 5–6 minutes from immersion in water, to form a cast that is weight-bearing after 30 minutes. Delta-Cast Plus is easier to remove than fibreglass-based products as it can be cut with shears.

Delta-Lite S is a knitted, highly conformable fibreglass tape with multi-directional stretch, impregnated with a catalysed urethane pre-polymer. The resin has been modified by the inclusion of silicone – which reduces the tack and improves the handling characteristics of the bandage during application, allowing the production of a cast with a significantly smoother surface than that obtained with most other polyurethane-based products. Once activated by immersion in water, the material will set in approximately seven minutes and be weight-bearing about 20 minutes later. Once fully set, Delta-Lite S forms an extremely strong impact-resistant cast.

Delta-Lite Conformable consists of a highly extensible, elasticated, knitted fibreglass bandage, impregnated with a low-tack resin system similar to that found in Delta-Lite S. The nature of the fabric is such that it is claimed to be the most conformable synthetic casting tape available, rivalling plaster of Paris in its ease of application.

Dynacast consists of a catalysed urethane pre-polymer applied to a wide-meshed polyester fabric. Once activated with water, the bandage sets in around five minutes, depending upon the temperature of the water, and is load-bearing in about 30 minutes.

Dynacast Extra has evolved in a series of stages from Dynacast. The original product was modified by the inclusion of a base fabric manufactured from knitted fibreglass, which was extensible in all directions, making the bandage highly conformable. Called Dynacast XR™, this, in turn, was replaced by Dynacast Extra, which contains a surface-modifying agent in the resin to reduce the tack in the uncured bandage.

Scotchcast 2 is a development of the original Scotchcast casting tape. It consists of the same catalysed urethane pre-polymers, which are applied to a fibreglass fabric that is extensible in all directions. The new substrate makes the bandage much more conformable than the original material.

Scotchcast Plus is made from a light extensible fibreglass fabric, impregnated with a resin system that has been modified to reduce tack and provide a self-lubricating surface. The result is a conforming bandage that handles well during unwind and holding, producing a moulded cast with a smooth surface.

Scotchflex is a lightweight highly conformable casting tape, which, in weight-bearing situations, should be strengthened by the addition of a second stronger material, such as Scotchcast 2.

Zim-flex is a development of an earlier product, Zimcast™. Zim-flex consists of a polyurethane resin applied to an extensible fibreglass fabric. The highly conformable bandage sets in approximately five minutes to form a strong cast, which is weight-bearing in about 30 minutes.

In the laboratory, it is possible to demonstrate differences between the physical properties of the products concerned, and a number of studies (both published and unpublished) have compared various aspects of their performance.[22,24–27] However, clinical usage would suggest that some of these differences may be of limited relevance – making the interpretation of the laboratory data difficult.

An excellent review of the properties of seven polyurethane bandages was published by Martin et al.,[28] who described a series of useful tests that may be used to assess various aspects of the performance of orthopaedic casting materials.

In the past, much has been made of the relative strengths of the casts prepared from the various materials, but – when applied in accordance with the manufacturer's instructions – virtually all the products are significantly stronger than plaster of Paris; therefore, such differences as do exist are probably not highly significant. The properties of a polyurethane bandage that are generally agreed to be of major importance include its:

- conformability,
- tack characteristics,
- setting and moulding time,
- weight-bearing time,
- strength (by diametral compression),

- impact resistance,
- moisture permeability,
- ability to resist delamination,
- cost (on a cast-for-cast basis).

Most workers would agree that, based upon the tests of Martin *et al.* and the requirements outlined above, it is not possible to identify any single product as being significantly better than the others in every aspect of its performance, for all applications. It is, however, possible to group the products according to their handling characteristics, and the nature and strength of the casts that they produce. Such a classification is shown below.

CLASSIFICATION OF POLYURETHANE BANDAGES

Group 1: Delta-Cast and Scotchflex

These represent the older casting tapes, which do not have the strength of the materials described below. Delta-Cast is unique amongst the polyurethane products in that it has a cotton fabric base. Both Delta-Cast and Scotchflex tend to be significantly less expensive than the other polyurethane-based materials, and, although they do not have the same load-bearing capabilities, they can be used for most casting applications. Both products are particularly suitable for paediatric and geriatric patients, as well as upper limb applications where very lightweight casts are indicated.

Group 2: Delta-Cast Plus

Based upon a polyester substrate, Delta-Cast Plus is a development of the older products in group 1. The bandage has improved conformability and strength, but remains lightweight and easy to remove. It also tends to be less expensive than the fibreglass-based materials, but is strong enough for most casting applications.

Group 3: Dynacast

Based upon a synthetic substrate, Dynacast is the last of the early polyurethane casting materials to remain commercially available. It is significantly stronger than the products in group 1, but

the structure is such that it lacks some of the conformability of the products in groups 4 and 5.

Group 4: Cellacast, Scotchcast 2, and Zim-flex

Broadly similar to Dynacast in terms of setting time and cast strength, these bandages are more conformable, and are generally recognised as being improved versions of the products that preceded them.

Group 5: Delta-Lite S, Delta-Lite Conformable, Dynacast Extra, and Scotchcast Plus

The enhanced handling characteristics of the resin, together with the conformability of the fabric, mean that these materials together probably represent the current 'state of the art' in the manufacture of synthetic casting tapes. However, in view of the rapid pace of product development, and the number of new materials introduced onto the market in recent years, it is likely that even these products will be further developed and improved in the future.

CRYSTONA

Crystona (Smith & Nephew) consists of an open-weave cotton cloth, evenly spread with a mass consisting of alumino-silicate with poly(acrylic acid). Once activated by immersion in water, the bandage has a working time of up to two minutes, after which it enters a rubbery phase. During this stage, the cast begins to exude drops of water and should no longer be worked. The cast then takes a further 20 minutes to harden.

Crystona is used in conjunction with standard plaster of Paris bandages to provide a hard waterproof shell, which makes the cast less liable to accidental damage or breakdown. When used as directed, combination casts made from Crystona and plaster are weight-bearing in about one hour.

The handling characteristics and the method of use of the material are not dissimilar to those of plaster of Paris, although operators should wear gloves to prevent the bandage sticking to their hands. If the gloves are kept wet, a cast with a smooth finish may be achieved.

NEOFRACT

Neofract™ (Johnson and Johnson) is a unique material which can be used to form casts or braces that can be easily removed and replaced as required. It consists of a polyurethane foam formed by the reaction between a di-isocyanate pre-polymer and a polyhydroxyl (polyol). The two components are mixed with a mechanical mixer immediately prior to use, poured into a pre-shaped cotton pattern and rolled to obtain a uniform thickness. The pattern is then applied to the patient. Bubbles of carbon dioxide, produced by the chemical reaction that takes place, cause the liquid to form a foam. This expands within the pattern, which in turn moulds itself to the contours of the body. The foam hardens within 10 minutes and is weight-bearing 30 minutes after mixing. Each pattern has one or more zips built into it so the cast can be easily and quickly removed and replaced.

SELECTION AND USE OF ORTHOPAEDIC CASTING MATERIALS

Because it is recognised that plaster room staff will have preferences for specific products, based upon their experience and individual techniques, it is not appropriate to attempt to recommend which products should be used for any particular application in other than the very general terms outlined below.

Primary casts used in the management of acute fractures, particularly those that are likely to be replaced after a short period of time, and subsequent secondary casts:

- Plaster of Paris bandage.

Secondary casts in low-load situations, upper limb casts, and casts for children and elderly patients where cast weight is a primary consideration:

- Any of the polyurethane-based materials — products in groups 1 and 2 are likely to be cheaper and lighter than the remainder.

Secondary casts for use in high load-bearing situations, functional braces, and difficult applications such as hip spicas:

- Plaster of Paris bandage,

- Cellamin,

- Crystona — used in conjunction with plaster of Paris bandage,

- Any of the polyurethane products in groups 2, 3, 4 or 5 — if maximum strength and conformability are particularly important, the bandages in groups 4 and 5 are likely to be the most acceptable.

Where casts or jackets need to be removed for treatment or exercise:

- Neofract.

REFERENCES

1. Elliott I.M.Z., *A Short History of Surgical Dressings,* London, Pharmaceutical Press, 1964.
2. Bishop W.J., *A History of Surgical Dressings,* Chesterfield, Robinson and Sons., 1959.
3. Monro J.K., The history of plaster of Paris in the treatment of fractures, *Br. J. Surg.,* 1935, **23**, 257–266.
4. Roy D.K., History of plaster bandages, *Fracture,* 1986, **8**, Hull, Smith & Nephew, 8–10.
5. Cameron D.M., Plaster of Paris — a history, *Am. J. Orthop.,* 1961, **3**, 8–11.
6. Bennett G.E. *et al.,* Molded plaster shells for the rest and protection treatment of infantile paralysis, *J. Am. med. Ass.,* 1937, **109**, 1120.
7. Cobey M.C., Waterproof plaster, *Am. Surg.,* 1952, **18**, 413–415.
8. Spittler A.W. *et al.,* The use of melamine formaldehyde in the application of casts, *U.S. Armed Forces med. J.,* 1953, **4**, 373–381.
9. Harvey J.P. and Lastrapes T., Experiences with resin-containing plaster of Paris, *J. Bone Jt Surg. (Am.),* 1954, **36A**, 822–824.
10. Morrison J.B., Melamine resin in the making of plaster casts, *Lancet,* 1953, **2**, 1317–1318.
11. Maudsley R.H., Melamine resin in the making of plaster casts, *ibid.,* 1954, **1**, 106.
12. Maudsley R.H., Resin-impregnated plasters, *Lancet,* 1955, **1**, 847.
13. Arden G.P. and Ward F.G., Experiences with experimental plaster bandages containing resin, *J. Bone Jt Surg. (Br.),* 1955, **37B**, 639.
14. Sayle-Creer W., Experimental plaster bandages, *ibid.,* 640–641.
15. Conrad A.H. and Ford L.T., Allergic contact dermatitis caused by Melmac Orthopedic Composition, *J. Am. med. Ass.,* 1953, **153**, 557.
16. Logan W.S. and Perry H.O., Cast dermatitis due to formaldehyde sensitivity, *Arch. Derm.,* 1972, **106**, 717–721.
17. Logan W.S. and Perry H.O., Contact dermatitis to resin-containing casts, *Clin. Orthop.,* 1973, **90**, 150–152.

18. Leach R.E., New fiber glass casting system, *ibid.*, 1974, **103**, 109–117.

19. Dockery G.L. *et al.*, A fiberglass casting material for use in podiatry, *J. Am. Podiatry Ass.*, 1977, **67**, 436–440.

20. Dockery G.L. *et al.*, A new thermoplastic casting system, *ibid.*, 1978, **68**, 194–200.

21. Wilson A.D. and Prosser H.J., Polyelectrolyte cements, in *Developments in Ionic Polymers – 1*, Wilson A.D. and Prosser H.J. (eds), London, Applied Science Publishers, 1983, 217–267.

22. Rowley D.I. *et al.*, The comparative properties of plaster of Paris and plaster of Paris substitutes, *Archs orthop. traum. Surg.*, 1985, **103**, 402–407.

23. *Plaster of Paris Technique,* Hull, Smith & Nephew, 1986.

24. Gill J.M. and Bowker P., A comparative study of the properties of bandage-form splinting materials, *Eng. Med.*, 1982, **11**, 125–134.

25. Goldberg L.A., Determination of the flammability of commercial splinting bandages, *Pharm. J.*, 1980, **275**, 528.

26. Oser Z. *et al.*, New predictive methods for evaluating the stability characteristics of polyurethane resin orthopaedic casting tapes, Paper presented to the Tenth Annual Meeting of the Society for Biomaterials, Washington DC, 27 April–1 May 1984.

27. Oser Z. *et al.*, New methods for evaluating the application characteristics of polyurethane resin orthopaedic casting tapes, *ibid.*

28. Martin P.J. *et al.*, A comparative evaluation of modern fracture casting materials, *Eng. Med.*, 1988, **17**, 63–70.

Chapter 15

Dressings Monographs

ACTISORB PLUS™

Classification Name
Dressing Activated Charcoal Cloth with Silver

Manufacturer
Johnson & Johnson

Product Description

Actisorb Plus incorporates a woven cloth consisting of 95–98% carbon, produced by carbonising and activating a knitted viscose rayon fabric. The charcoal cloth is enclosed in a sleeve of spun-bonded non-woven nylon fabric, which is sealed along all four edges to facilitate handling and reduce particle and fibre loss.

Activated charcoal has the property of adsorbing odour and noxious materials such as toxins and degradation products from the wound, and this forms the basis of its use as a dressing. It has been shown that, in the laboratory, certain micro-organisms are taken up by the dressing and removed from aqueous suspensions. It has been suggested that this effect may occur *in vivo*, reducing the level of contamination in a wound and thus improving the healing environment. The charcoal cloth contains silver residues, chemically and physically bound onto the carbon. These impart antimicrobial properties to the fabric, in addition to the adsorptive characteristics described above.

Indications

Actisorb Plus is recommended for use in the management of a range of malodorous wounds, including fungating breast cancers, faecal fistulae, infected decubitus ulcers, and heavily exuding varicose ulcers.

Contra-indications

Actisorb Plus should not be used on patients who are sensitive to nylon, and should be used with care as a primary dressing on wounds that have a tendency to dry out, where adherence is likely to become a problem.

Method of Use

Actisorb Plus is intended for use as a primary wound dressing. In use, the product is applied directly to the surface of the wound and covered with a secondary dressing, held in position with tape or a bandage, as appropriate. The secondary dressing chosen will depend upon the nature of the wound, but in general a simple absorbent pad will be sufficient. There may be circumstances where it is not considered appropriate to place Actisorb Plus directly onto the surface of a malodorous wound. In these instances, the dressing may be placed between the selected wound contact material and the secondary dressing.

Frequency of Dressing Changes

The frequency of dressing changes will depend entirely upon the nature and condition of the wound: on heavily exuding wounds, daily changes will be required; but on drier wounds, this interval may be extended at the discretion of the nurse in charge.

Warnings and Precautions

Actisorb Plus should be used in the intact state, and not cut to shape prior to application to the wound.

Presentation

Actisorb Plus is presented in a waterproof peel pouch, sterilised by gamma irradiation.

10.5 cm × 10.5 cm	NSV No. ELV 031
19.0 cm × 10.5 cm	NSV No. ELV 033

ALLEVYN™

Classification Name
Dressing Polyurethane Foam Hydrophilic

Manufacturer
Smith & Nephew

Product Description

Allevyn consists of a layer of soft, hydrophilic polyurethane foam, 4 mm thick, bonded onto a polyurethane film. The film, which is permeable to moisture vapour, provides a barrier to the passage of water or wound exudate, and also prevents the passage of micro-organisms in to or out of the dressing. The surface of the dressing to be placed in contact with the wound is covered with an apertured three-dimensional plastic net, which is claimed to reduce adherence to granulating tissue. The dressing has a high absorbent capacity, and strike-through is prevented by the semipermeable backing. By virtue of these characteristics, the dressing provides a micro-environment at the surface of the wound that is conducive to moist wound healing, and, within limits, independent of the rate of exudate formation.

Indications

Allevyn may be applied to a variety of heavily exuding wounds, including leg ulcers, minor burns, and donor sites.

Contra-indications

No absolute contra-indications to the use of Allevyn have been reported, but the dressing will be of limited use if applied to wounds covered with a dry scab or hard black necrotic tissue. This should first be removed surgically or by some other means.

Method of Use

A size of Allevyn is chosen that will overlap the edges of the wound by 2–3 cm, and it is placed with the patterned side next to the skin. The dressing may be secured with tape or a piece of a dressing retention sheet (such as Hypafix™ or Mefix™), or held in position with a suitable compression bandage, as appropriate. If necessary, Allevyn may be cut to shape with a pair of sterile scissors.

Frequency of Dressing Changes

The frequency with which the dressing should be changed depends upon the nature of the wound, but on a clean non-infected wound, it is possible to leave Allevyn in position for up to four days, although this will depend upon the amount of exudate produced.

Presentation

Allevyn is presented double-wrapped in a paper peel pouch, sterilised by irradiation.

10 cm × 10 cm   NSV No. ELA 131
20 cm × 20 cm   NSV No. ELA 133

BIOCLUSIVE™

Classification Name
Dressing Semipermeable Adhesive BP

Manufacturer
Johnson & Johnson

Product Description

Bioclusive consists of a thin polyurethane membrane coated with a layer of an acrylic adhesive. The dressing, which is permeable to both water vapour and oxygen, is impermeable to micro-organisms. Once in position, it provides an effective barrier to external contamination, whilst producing a moist environment at the surface of the wound by reducing water vapour loss from the exposed tissue. Under these conditions in shallow wounds, scab formation is prevented and epidermal regeneration takes place at an enhanced rate, compared with that which occurs in wounds treated with traditional dry dressings.

Indications

Bioclusive may be used in the treatment of minor burns, pressure areas, donor sites, post-operative wounds, and a variety of minor injuries including abrasions and lacerations. It may also be used as a dressing for peripheral and central intravenous catheters, and as a protective cover to prevent skin breakdown due to friction or continuous exposure to moisture.

Contra-indications

Although there are no absolute contra-indications to the use of Bioclusive, it is not recommended that the material be applied over deep cavity wounds, third degree burns, or wounds that show evidence of clinical infection.

Method of Use

Bioclusive is applied in the same manner as an adhesive plaster. An appropriately sized dressing is selected, the central part of the backing paper is removed, and the dressing is placed in direct contact with the wound whilst being held at both ends. The two end pieces of backing paper are removed and the dressing is lightly smoothed into position.

In order to ensure good adhesion, the dressing should be allowed a minimum overlap of 4–5 cm from the margin of the wound onto the surrounding skin.

On clean heavily exuding wounds, such as donor sites, large quantities of fluid sometimes accumulate beneath the film. This should be left undisturbed as far as possible, but if the accumulation becomes excessive, it may be aspirated off with a syringe using an aseptic technique. A small patch of Bioclusive should be applied over the puncture to prevent leakage or contamination.

Frequency of Dressing Changes

In general, Bioclusive dressings should not be left in position for longer than seven days to avoid the possibility of bacterial colonisation occurring. This is particularly important where the dressing is being used to retain an IV catheter in position.

Presentation

Bioclusive is presented individually wrapped in a peel pouch, sterilised by ethylene oxide.

5.1 cm × 7.6 cm	NSV No. ELW 111
10.2 cm × 12.7 cm	NSV No. ELW 113
10.2 cm × 25.4 cm	NSV No. ELW 115
20.3 cm × 25.4 cm	NSV No. ELW 117
12.7 cm × 17.8 cm	NSV No. ELW 119

Bioclusive is available on Drug Tariff.

BIOFILM™

Classification Name
Dressing Hydrocolloid Permeable

Manufacturer
Biotrol, distributed by CliniMed

Product Description

Biofilm incorporates a non-woven polyester fabric sheet, which is permeable to water vapour and gases. The fabric is hydrophobic and will resist penetration by aqueous solutions, or bacteria, under normal conditions of use. The side of the dressing in contact with the wound is coated with an adhesive mass composed of polyisobutylene and hydrophilic particles composed of gelatin, pectin and carboxymethylcellulose. When the dressing comes into contact with wound exudate, these particles absorb water and swell to form a hydrophilic gel. In the dry state, the dressing is virtually impermeable to water vapour, but as it takes up fluid and a gel is produced, the permeability increases until a steady state is reached.

Indications

Biofilm may be used in the treatment of leg ulcers, pressure areas, and many types of granulating wound. It can also be of value in the treatment of wounds covered with dry black necrotic skin, such as the 'black heels' that occur on bedridden patients.

Contra-indications

It is not recommended that Biofilm be used in the treatment of clinically or grossly infected wounds, and it is probably not the product of choice for application to very heavily exuding wounds, at least in the initial stages of treatment (as the dressing would require replacing too frequently).

Method of Use

An appropriately sized dressing is removed from its paper backing and lightly pressed into position over the wound. In order to ensure good adhesion to the surrounding skin, a minimum overlap of 2–3 cm from the margin of the wound should be allowed. Because Biofilm is adhesive, no additional dressings are usually required, but on areas such as the sacral region, where the edges of the product are likely to be disturbed by movement, it may be necessary to cover the dressing and surrounding area with a piece of an adhesive dressing retention sheet (such as Hypafix™ or Mefix™). The use of such secondary dressings should be kept to a minimum, as they will effectively reduce the permeabilty of Biofilm and thus prevent the loss of water vapour. Upon removal of the dressing, a viscous gel with a characteristic odour may be found on the surface of the wound. This is normal, and consists of the partially liquefied adhesive base. It is not pus and does not indicate the presence of infection. The wound should be gently cleansed with sterile normal saline before the application of the next dressing.

The absorbent base material is also available in the form of a powder, which may be used in conjunction with the sheet dressing to provide an increase in absorbent capacity for use on heavily exuding wounds.

Frequency of Dressing Changes

The frequency of dressing changes will be governed by the state of the wound. If large volumes of exudate are produced, daily changes may be required; but on some wounds the dressing may be left in place for up to seven days before it must be changed. Because Biofilm is highly permeable when hydrated, it will allow the removal of significant volumes of exudate by evaporation through the non-woven fabric backing, and less frequent dressing changes may be required than would be the case with a less permeable product.

Presentation

Biofilm is presented individually wrapped in a peel pouch, sterilised by ethylene oxide.

Sheets

10 cm × 10 cm	NSV No. ELM 051
20 cm × 20 cm	NSV No. ELM 053

Powder

5 g sachet†	NSV No. ELO 031

†Sterilised by gamma irradiation

BLUE LINE WEBBING

Classification Name
Bandage Elastic Web BP

Manufacturer
Seton

Product Description

Blue Line Webbing consists of a characteristic fabric woven in ribbon fashion, in which the warp threads are composed of cotton and rubber and the weft threads are of cotton or combined cotton and viscose yarns. The mid-line warp threads are coloured blue. The fabric, which is extensible along its length, is highly elastic by virtue of the rubber threads, which also impart considerable power to the bandage. Blue Line Webbing may be washed repeatedly, if required, without affecting its performance significantly. The product is available in bulk rolls and pre-cut lengths, which may also have a foot loop stitched at one end to facilitate application.

Indications

Blue Line Webbing, which is one of the most powerful extensible bandages currently available, may be used to apply and maintain very high levels of sub-bandage pressure. The maximum pressure that the product is able to achieve on an average leg is well in excess of 60 mmHg, which is probably much higher than would ever be required clinically. The primary indication for the use of Blue Line Webbing is in the management of large, grossly oedematous limbs and other conditions where compression therapy is required (such as before and after stripping of varicose veins), and other situations where the traditional crêpe-type products fail to achieve the desired levels of sub-bandage pressure.

Contra-indications

Because of the power inherent in the bandage, care must be taken to ensure that it is not applied with excessive tension. The pressure that is produced beneath Blue Line Webbing will not decrease significantly with time, unlike that beneath a cotton bandage.

All extensible bandages should be used with caution on patients who have marked ischaemia or impaired arterial blood supply, but the incorrect use of Blue Line Webbing in these situations could have very serious consequences.

Method of Use

When used to apply support or compression, the bandage should be held with the bulk roll facing upwards. Working from the inner aspect of the leg, a single turn should be made over the top of the foot around the base of the toes to secure the bandage, and a second turn taken up to the base of the heel. After making a figure-of-eight around the ankle, the bandage should be applied up the leg, with each turn overlapping the previous one by 50% (using the line in the centre of the bandage as a guide). Once in place, the bandage may be fastened with clips or pins, as appropriate. Care should be taken to ensure that the bandage does not cause a tourniquet effect at the knee, and the operator should ensure that a pressure gradient exists beneath the bandage, with the highest levels of pressure at the ankle.

Frequency of Dressing Changes

Provided the bandage has been correctly applied and does not become displaced, it will continue to apply the desired levels of compression over an extended period. However, the characteristics of the fabric of the bandage are such that it has a tendency to become loose as the various overlapping turns slip and slide over one another. The fabric also tends to be heavy and abrasive and some patients cannot tolerate its use for extended periods of time. It is sometimes recommended that high performance products such as Blue Line Webbing should be removed at night and re-applied before the patient gets out of bed in the morning.

Presentation

Blue Line Webbing is presented individually shrink-wrapped.

7.5 cm × 2.25 m*†	NSV No. EBA 031
7.5 cm × 25 m	NSV No. EBA 011
10.0 cm × 25 m	NSV No. EBA 013

*Available on Drug Tariff.

†Also available with foot loop.

CELLACAST™

Classification Name
Bandage Orthopaedic Resin

Manufacturer
Lohmann

Product Description

Cellacast consists of a knitted fibreglass substrate impregnated with a polyurethane resin. The fabric is extensible in all directions, which makes the bandage very conformable in use. When exposed to moisture vapour or immersed in water, the resin undergoes a polymerisation reaction, which causes the tape to harden and become rigid. A cast made from Cellacast will set in approximately 3–4 minutes. Once set, it can be bivalved or windowed, and will be fully weight-bearing after 20–30 minutes. The resultant cast is lightweight, strong, porous, and translucent to X-rays.

Cellacast is available in a choice of four colours, white, pink, green, and blue, to facilitate coding by department, technician, or stage of fracture.

Indications

Cellacast may be used in most situations where rigid immobilisation is required. This includes the formation of standard orthopaedic casts and specialised prosthetic appliances.

Contra-indications

In common with all polyurethane casting tapes, Cellacast should be applied with caution on fresh fractures where swelling of the injured limb may be anticipated (which could make rapid removal of the cast necessary).

Method of Use

Cellacast should be applied over a layer of stockinette and orthopaedic padding. Although any suitable product may be used, some workers prefer to use non-absorbent materials based upon synthetic fibres such as polyester, rather than the rayon- or cotton-based materials often used in conjunction with plaster of Paris (which will retain moisture, should the final cast become wet). Before the foil pouch is opened, disposable gloves should be put on. Prior to application, the bandage should be immersed in water at 21–25°C, and firmly squeezed 1–3 times under the surface to ensure complete penetration of water into the body of the bandage. After removal from the dip water, it should not be squeezed further, although any excess water may be removed by vigorous shaking.

The tape should be applied in the form of a spiral, each turn overlapping the previous one by about one-third to one-half of the width of the tape. Three layers of bandage are usually sufficient in most non-weight-bearing situations, but four or five layers may be required for a weight-bearing cast. If splints are needed, these may be produced from three or four layers of Cellacast. The cast may be moulded to its final shape during the last minute of its setting cycle, after which time it may be windowed or trimmed with shears or a standard cast saw. A cast made from Cellacast may be repaired or reinforced by the application of additional tape. Although this will adhere successfully to the existing cast, a complete layer should be applied, if possible, to achieve the maximum adhesive bond.

Warnings and Precautions

Prior to setting, the polyurethane resin will adhere firmly to unprotected skin and clothing. Operators should always wear gloves when handling Cellacast, and care should be taken to ensure that the uncured tape it does not come into contact with the patient's skin. Any uncured resin may be removed from the skin by gently swabbing with acetone or ethanol. The temperature of the water used for dipping must not exceed 27°C.

Once set, Cellacast is not adversely affected by moisture, but immersion of the cast in water is not recommended, as it may prove very difficult to dry the underlying padding. This in turn may lead to maceration and irritation of the skin.

If the cast is removed with a reciprocating cast saw, the use of dust extraction apparatus is advisable.

Shelf Life and Storage Precautions

Cellacast has a shelf life of two years from the date of manufacture. The unopened rolls of casting tape should be stored in a cool dry atmosphere below 24°C. Above this temperature, the shelf life will be decreased.

Presentation

Cellacast is presented as a roll, wrapped around a hollow plastic core, and heat-sealed in a plastic-coated pouch.

5.0 cm × 3.6 m	NSV No. EAF 511
7.5 cm × 3.6 m	NSV No. EAF 513
10.0 cm × 3.6 m	NSV No. EAF 515
12.5 cm × 3.6 m	NSV No. EAF 517

CELLAMIN™

Classification Name
Bandage Plaster of Paris Resin Reinforced

Manufacturer
Lohmann

Product Description

Cellamin consists of a plain-weave gauze fabric that is coated with a blend of the alpha and beta forms of calcium sulphate hemihydrate (plaster of Paris), together with a plastic resin based upon melamine-formaldehyde. The bandage is supplied wrapped around a plastic spool, which is designed to allow rapid, even wetting of the bandage upon immersion. Once wet, the calcium sulphate hemi-hydrate is converted to the dihydrate, and the bandage sets to form a hard rigid structure. The crystals are encased by the plastic resin during the setting process, providing additional strength and water resistance to the cast. The rate of setting is largely governed by the temperature of the water, but if the bandage is used in accordance with the manufacturer's intructions, a cast made from Cellamin may be bivalved or windowed 15 minutes after application, and will be load-bearing after one hour, although it may not gain its maximum strength for up to 24 hours. Casts made from Cellamin require 30% less material than those made from standard plaster of Paris and are therefore significantly lighter. They also have the advantage that they are water-resistant and therefore more durable in use. The principal disadvantages of Cellamin, in common with other plaster of Paris bandages, are its weight and opacity to X-rays.

Indications

Cellamin bandages may be used for most orthopaedic applications, and other situations in which rigid immobilisation is required. It is particularly suitable for making scoliosis jackets, and for the young and elderly, where the reduced weight is important; for the formation of frog plasters, where water resistance is a major factor; and as a protective waterproofing layer over standard plaster casts to enhance strength and durability.

Contra-indications

Cellamin should not be used on patients who are known to be sensitive to formaldehyde.

Method of use

Cellamin should be applied over a layer of stockinette and orthopaedic padding. Prior to application, the first 10–15 cm of the bandage should be unrolled to enable the rapid location of the end after dipping. The bandage is held lightly in one hand, and immersed in a suitable container of water at a temperature of 20–25°C, at an angle of 45°, for two seconds. For 8-ply back slabs (used to hold reductions), a higher temperature – maximum 35°C – is recommended, and the dip time reduced to one second. After the bandage is removed from the container, any excess water is gently squeezed out. The bandage is then rolled evenly around the limb, without tension, avoiding the formation of wrinkles but producing pleats or tucks where necessary. As each successive bandage is applied, it should be constantly moulded and smoothed with wet hands to ensure the formation of a homogeneous cast. Any areas of potential weakness may be strengthened by the addition of five or six layers of bandage, previously formed into a slab.

Warnings and Precautions

Users should apply barrier cream or wear gloves before using Cellamin because of the risk of formaldehyde sensitisation.

When applying a cast, it is important to ensure that all bony prominences are adequately padded, and operators should take care to ensure that no indentations are made in the soft plaster that could lead to the application of local areas of high pressure and the formation of plaster sores. Rough finishes on the edges of the cast should also be avoided. If the bandage is applied to a fresh fracture, sufficient padding should be used to accomodate any swelling of the limb.

Shelf Life and Storage Precautions

The unopened rolls of Cellamin should be stored in a cool dry atmosphere.

Presentation

Cellamin is presented as a roll, wrapped around a plastic core, and sealed in a paper pouch.

6 cm × 2 m	NSV No.	EAB 111
8 cm × 2 m	NSV No.	EAB 113
10 cm × 2 m	NSV No.	EAB 115
12 cm × 2 m	NSV No.	EAB 117
15 cm × 2 m	NSV No.	EAB 119
20 cm × 2 m	NSV No.	EAB 121
60 cm × 5 m	NSV No.	EAB 123

CELLONA SR™
CELLONA ELASTIC™

Classification Name

Cellona SR – Bandage Plaster of Paris
Cellona Elastic – Bandage Plaster of Paris
  Elasticated

Manufacturer

Lohmann

Product Description

Cellona SR consists of a plain-weave gauze fabric that is coated with a blend of the alpha and beta forms of calcium sulphate hemihydrate (plaster of Paris), together with binders and accelerators. A predominance of alpha crystals means that less water at a lower temperature is required to ensure full even saturation and activation of the plaster mass, compared with bandages that have a high content of beta crystals. The high proportion of alpha crystals is also said to increase cast strength, both during setting and subsequently.

Cellona Elastic differs from Cellona SR in two respects: the base fabric is an elasticated gauze, and the crystals of calcium sulphate hemihydrate are entirely of the beta form. Beta crystals provide a slightly longer moulding time, which is sometimes required when producing prosthetic moulds and casts for amputation stumps. The fabric is held in a slightly pre-tensioned condition by the plaster mass; when the bandage is dipped into water, the tension is released and the elasticity that is inherent in the bandage ensures the formation of a close-fitting cast. Cellona Elastic is intended for use as an initial conforming layer in the production of a cast, which may be completed using a standard plaster of Paris bandage or a resin reinforced plaster bandage.

Cellona SR and Cellona Elastic are supplied wrapped around plastic spools which are designed to allow rapid, even wetting of the bandage upon immersion. Once wet, the calcium sulphate hemihydrate is converted to the dihydrate, and the bandage sets to form a hard rigid structure, which is both porous and absorbent. The rate of setting is largely governed by the temperature of the water, but if the bandage is used in accordance with the manufacturer's intructions, an initial set will take place in about 2–2.5 minutes for Cellona SR, 2–3 minutes for Cellona Elastic. After about 3–5 minutes, the cast should be fully set, although it may not achieve its maximum strength and become weight-bearing for up to 24 hours, depending upon its thickness. Casts made from Cellona SR or Cellona Elastic may be bivalved or windowed about ten minutes after dipping.

The principal disadvantages of Cellona SR and Cellona Elastic lie in their weight and opacity to X-rays. Once set, they are also susceptible to damage by moisture.

Indications

Cellona SR and Cellona Elastic may be used for most orthopaedic applications, and other situations in which rigid immobilisation is required, including the management of fresh or unstable fractures. The enhanced conformability of Cellona Elastic is said to make it particularly suitable for use in prosthetics and mould making, and for holding manipulations and splinting soft tissue repairs.

Method of Use

Cellona SR and Cellona Elastic should be applied over a layer of stockinette and orthopaedic padding. Prior to application, the first 10–15 cm of the bandage should be unrolled to enable the rapid location of the end after dipping. The bandage is held lightly in one hand, and immersed in a suitable container of water at a temperature of 20–25°C, at an angle of 45°, for 3 seconds for Cellona SR, 3–5 seconds for Cellona Elastic. For 8-ply back slabs of Cellona SR (used to hold reductions), a higher temperature – maximum 35°C – is recommended, and the dip time reduced to one second. After the bandage is removed from the container, any excess water is gently squeezed out. The bandage is then rolled evenly around the limb, without tension, avoiding the formation of wrinkles. With Cellona SR, pleats or tucks should be produced where necessary; the need for this is reduced with Cellona Elastic, because of its conformability. As each successive bandage is applied, it should be constantly moulded and smoothed with wet hands to ensure the formation of a homogeneous cast. Any areas of potential weakness may be strengthened by the addition of five or six layers of Cellona SR, previously formed into a slab.

Warnings and Precautions

When applying a cast, it is important to ensure that all bony prominences are adequately padded, and operators should take care to ensure that no indentations are made in the soft plaster that could lead to the application of local areas of high pressure and the formation of plaster sores. Rough finishes on the edges of the cast should also be avoided. If Cellona SR or Cellona Elastic is applied to a fresh fracture, sufficient padding should be used to accommodate any swelling of the limb.

Shelf Life and Storage Precautions

The unopened rolls of Cellona SR or Cellona Elastic should be stored in a cool dry atmosphere.

Presentation

Both Cellona SR and Cellona Elastic are available in the form of a roll, wrapped around a plastic core, and sealed in a plastic pack. Cellona SR is also available as a slab, in a sealed plastic bag.

Cellona SR rolls

5.0 cm × 2.7 m	NSV No. EAA 111
7.5 cm × 2.7 m	NSV No. EAA 113
10.0 cm × 2.7 m	NSV No. EAA 115
15.0 cm × 2.7 m	NSV No. EAA 117
20.0 cm × 2.7 m	NSV No. EAA 119

Cellona SR slabs

10 cm × 20 m	NSV No. EAA 131
15 cm × 20 m	NSV No. EAA 133
20 cm × 20 m	NSV No. EAA 135

Cellona Elastic rolls

10 cm × 2m	NSV No. EAA 141
12 cm × 2m	NSV No. EAA 143

CREVIC™

Classification Name

Bandage Cotton Crêpe BP

Manufacturer

Grout

Product Description

Crevic consists of a pink-coloured cotton fabric of plain weave with a characteristic appearance. The fabric is extensible along its length, having a degree of elasticity that is imparted by the presence of crêpe-twisted cotton yarns. The bandage may be washed if required; when allowed to dry naturally, loosely folded, it will regain some of its original elasticity.

Indications

Crevic is widely used for the application of light pressure and support in the treatment of sprains and strains, and varicose veins; and as a support to aid rehabilitation following orthopaedic surgery. It is also used in the treatment of varicose ulcers – in conjunction with a suitable primary dressing, such as a zinc paste bandage – although other more elastic products are more suitable for this application.

Contra-indications

As with other bandages manufactured from cotton and other non-elastomeric fibres, the sub-bandage pressures that can be achieved and maintained by Crevic are limited. Such products are unlikely to be suitable for the sustained application of pressures in excess of 8 – 10 mmHg at the calf of an average-sized leg.

Because cotton bandages do not have the ability to 'follow in' (thereby maintaining compression on limbs that decrease in circumference as a result of the application of surface pressure), they are of little value in reducing existing gross oedema. For this application and other situations where high levels of pressure are required, alternative products containing elastomeric threads of rubber, nylon or polyurethane are available.

All extensible bandages should be used with caution on patients who have marked ischaemia or impaired arterial blood supply.

Method of Use

When used to apply support or compression, the bandage should be held with the bulk roll facing upwards. Working from the inner aspect of the leg, a single turn should be made over the top of the foot around the base of the toes to secure the bandage, and a second turn taken up to the base of the heel. After making a figure-of-eight around the ankle, the bandage should be applied up the leg, with each turn overlapping the previous one by 50%. Once in place, the bandage may be fastened with safety pins or tape, as appropriate. Care should be taken to ensure that the bandage does not cause a tourniquet effect at the knee, and the operator should ensure that a pressure gradient exists beneath the bandage, with the highest levels of pressure at the ankle.

Frequency of Dressing Changes

In critical applications where the control of sub-bandage pressure is important, the bandage should be reapplied or replaced as frequently as practicable. In other situations, it is not uncommon for a bandage to be left undisturbed for up to 5 – 7 days, although there is little doubt that, at the end of this time, the residual pressure beneath the bandage will be only a fraction of the original application pressure.

Presentation

Crevic is presented individually shrink-wrapped.

5.0 cm × 4.5 m (stretched) NSV No. ECA 031
7.5 cm × 4.5 m (stretched)*NSV No. ECA 033
10.0 cm × 4.5 m (stretched)*NSV No. ECA 035
15.0 cm × 4.5 m (stretched) NSV No. ECA 037

*Available on Drug Tariff.

DEBRISAN™
DEBRISAN™ PASTE
DEBRISAN™ ABSORBENT PAD

Classification Name

Debrisan – Dressing Polysaccharide Bead
Debrisan Paste – Dressing Polysaccharide
    Bead Paste

Debrisan Absorbent Pad – Dressing
  Polysaccharide Bead Paste Pad

Manufacturer

Pharmacia

Product Description

Debrisan consists of sterile, pale yellow dextranomer beads, 0.1–0.3 mm in diameter. When introduced into an exuding wound, one gram of the dressing will absorb up to four grams of exudate. Any bacteria or cellular debris present in the wound may be taken up by capillary action and become trapped in the spaces between the beads. When the dressing is changed, this debris will be washed away. The beads, which have a high suction pressure (up to 200 mmHg), have been claimed to reduce local tissue oedema and control odour formation.

Debrisan Paste is a sterile, granular semi-solid prepared from Debrisan beads 64%, with polyethylene glycol 600 and water.

Debrisan Absorbent Pad contains a sterile, off-white granular paste prepared from Debrisan beads 90%, with polyethylene glycol and water. The paste is enclosed in a textile bag, 6 cm × 4 cm, which is divided in half.

Debrisan, Debrisan Paste, and Debrisan Absorbent Pad are intended for use in the treatment of infected, yellow sloughy wounds, including surgical or post-traumatic wounds, decubitus ulcers, and leg ulcers.

Indications

All three Debrisan products are intended for use in the treatment of moist, yellow sloughy wounds. Debrisan Paste and Debrisan Absorbent Pad are particularly useful for the treatment of shallow wounds or other areas that are difficult to dress with the free-flowing beads.

Contra-indications

Debrisan should not be used on dry or lightly exuding wounds. In these situations, there is a danger that the beads may dry out and form a crust, which may be difficult to remove.

Debrisan, Debrisan Paste, and Debrisan Absorbent Pad should not be used in the treatment of deep narrow wounds or sinuses from which removal may be difficult. Debrisan and Debrisan Paste should not be applied near the eye.

Debrisan Absorbent Pad may be used with caution.

Method of Use

A layer of Debrisan or Debrisan Paste, not less than 3 mm thick, is applied to the wound and covered with a suitable pad or dressing retention material – a semipermeable film dressing has been found to be particularly well suited for this purpose. Exudate from the wound is drawn up into the beads or paste, which should be changed before they become fully saturated. This is best accomplished by irrigating the wound with sterile water or normal saline, using a syringe. Once the wound has been cleansed, a new layer is applied while the area is still moist.

Debrisan Absorbent Pad is placed directly in contact with the surface of the wound and covered with a suitable dressing, such as a semipermeable film. Wound exudate and cellular debris are drawn up into the pad, which should be changed before it is entirely saturated or discoloured with secretions. The pad should not adhere to the surface of the wound, but if this is found to be a problem, irrigation with sterile normal saline should aid its removal. Once the wound has been cleansed, a new pad is applied whilst the area is still moist.

Frequency of Dressing Changes

The frequency of dressing changes will depend entirely upon the nature of the wound. Initially, twice daily changes may be required; but after the first two days, a change of dressing every other day may be sufficient.

Warnings and Precautions

Occasionally, transient pain in the area of the wound has been reported soon after application of Debrisan, Debrisan Paste, or Debrisan Absorbent Pad. This may be avoided by ensuring that the wound is moistened well before the dressing is applied.

Debrisan, Debrisan Paste, and Debrisan Absorbent Pad should not be applied to dry wounds; their use in the management of more heavily exuding wounds should be discontinued as granulation takes place and exudate production decreases.

In order to prevent the possibility of cross-infection, a drum of Debrisan beads should be reserved for the treatment of a single patient. Spillage of the beads can render surfaces very slippery. Any that are spilt should be cleared up immediately.

The use of an occlusive dressing with Debrisan is not recommended, as this may lead to maceration of the skin around the wound.

Shelf Life and Storage Precautions

Debrisan should be stored in a dry place in well-closed containers. Debrisan Paste has a shelf life of two years when stored at room temperature.

Presentation

Debrisan is available in a foil sachet and a plastic drum (castor). Debrisan Paste and Debrisan Absorbent Pad are presented in foil/plastic laminate sachets.

Debrisan sachet
4g   NSV No. ELT 011
        (PL No. 0009/0021)

Debrisan castor
60g   NSV No. ELT 015
        (PL No. 0009/0021)

Debrisan Paste sachet
10g   NSV No. ELT 11
        (PL No. 0009/0044)

Debrisan Absorbent Pad
3g   NSV No. ELT 131
        (PL No. 0009/0048)

Legal Category
Debrisan – Pharmacy Only [P]
Debrisan Paste and Debrisan Absorbent Pad – Prescription Only Medicine [POM]

DELTA-CAST™
DELTA-CAST PLUS™

Classification Name
Bandage Orthopaedic Resin

Manufacturer
Johnson & Johnson Orthopaedics

Product Description
Delta-Cast bandage consists of a lightweight knitted cotton fabric, impregnated with a polyurethane resin. A Delta-Cast splint consists of four layers of a woven bleached cotton fabric, stitched together and impregnated with the same resin. Delta-Cast Plus consists of a knitted polyester fabric, also impregnated with a clear polyurethane resin. The fabric used in the construction of Delta-Cast Plus is extensible in all directions, which makes it very conformable in use.

When Delta-Cast or Delta-Cast Plus is exposed to moisture vapour or immersed in water, the resin undergoes a polymerisation reaction, which causes the tape to harden and become rigid. The setting time depends upon the temperature of the dip water, but will be about 5–7 minutes for Delta-Cast, and 5–6 minutes for Delta-Cast Plus. Once set, the cast can be bivalved or windowed, and will be weight-bearing after 30 minutes. A cast made from Delta-Cast is lightweight, 98% transparent to X-rays, and has a water vapour permeability similar to that of plaster of Paris. A Delta-Cast Plus cast is lightweight, strong, porous, and translucent to X-rays.

Indications

Although Delta-Cast may be used in most situations where rigid immobilisation is required, it does not have the same strength and load-bearing capabilities as the fibreglass-based bandages. For this reason, it is often reserved for use on paediatric and geriatric patients, and for the formation of upper limb casts (where low weight is of primary importance). Delta-Cast Plus has a high strength-to-weight ratio, and may be used for most secondary casting applications. It is intermediate in strength between Delta-Cast and the fibreglass-based products, and is probably not the product of choice for the formation of weight-bearing casts in very heavy individuals.

Contra-indications

In common with all polyurethane casting tapes, Delta-Cast and Delta-Cast Plus should be applied with caution on fresh fractures where swelling of the injured limb may be anticipated (which could make rapid removal of the cast necessary).

Method of Use

Delta-Cast and Delta-Cast Plus should be applied over a layer of stockinette and orthopaedic padding. Although any suitable product may be used, some workers prefer to use non-absorbent materials based upon synthetic fibres such as polyester, rather than the rayon- or cotton-based materials usually used in conjunction with plaster of Paris (which will retain moisture, should the final cast become wet).

Before the foil pouch is opened, disposable gloves should be put on. Prior to application, the bandage should be immersed in water at 20°C, and firmly squeezed four or five times under the surface to ensure complete penetration of water into the body of the bandage. After removal from the dip water, the bandage should not be squeezed further.

The tape should be applied in the form of a spiral, each turn overlapping the previous one by about one-third to one-half of the width of the tape. With Delta-Cast, 6–8 layers of bandage are usually sufficient in non-weight-bearing situations, but 8–10 layers may be required for a weight-bearing cast. With Delta-Cast Plus, 3–5 layers and 5–7 layers would be required, respectively. Prefabricated Delta-Cast splints are available; if splints are needed for use with Delta-Cast Plus, they may be produced from 3–4 layers of the bandage.

The cast may be moulded to its final shape during the last 30 seconds of its setting cycle, after which time it may be windowed or trimmed with shears or a standard cast saw. A cast made from Delta-Cast or Delta-Cast Plus may be repaired or reinforced by the application of additional tape. Although this will adhere successfully to the existing cast, a complete layer should be applied, if possible, to achieve the maximum adhesive bond.

A cast made from Delta-Cast or Delta-Cast Plus may usually be removed with plaster shears. A plaster saw is not generally required.

Warnings and Precautions

Prior to setting, the polyurethane resin will adhere firmly to unprotected skin and clothing. Operators should always wear gloves when handling Delta-Cast or Delta-Cast Plus, and care should be taken to ensure that the uncured tape does not come into contact with the patient's skin. Any uncured resin may be removed from the skin by gently swabbing with acetone or ethanol.

Once set, Delta-Cast and Delta-Cast Plus are not adversely affected by moisture, but immersion of the cast in water is not recommended, as it may prove very difficult to dry the underlying padding. This in turn may lead to maceration and irritation of the skin.

Shelf Life and Storage Precautions

Delta-Cast and Delta-Cast Plus have a shelf life of two years from the date of manufacture given on the carton. The unopened rolls of casting tape should be stored in a cool dry atmosphere below 25°C. Above this temperature, the shelf life will be decreased.

Presentation

Both Delta-Cast and Delta-Cast Plus are available in the form of a roll, wrapped around a hollow core, and heat-sealed in a poly/foil/poly laminate pouch.

Delta–Cast rolls

5.0 cm × 3 m	NSV No. EAF 251
7.5 cm × 3 m	NSV No. EAF 253
10.0 cm × 3 m	NSV No. EAF 255
15.0 cm × 3 m	NSV No. EAF 257

Delta–Cast splints

10 cm × 75 cm	NSV No. EAF 259
15 cm × 75 cm	NSV No. EAF 261

Delta–Cast Plus rolls

5.0 cm × 3.6 m	NSV No. EAF 431
7.5 cm × 3.6 m	NSV No. EAF 433
10.0 cm × 3.6 m	NSV No. EAF 435
12.5 cm × 3.6 m	NSV No. EAF 437

DELTA-LITE S™
DELTA-LITE CONFORMABLE™

Classification Name

Bandage Orthopaedic Resin

Manufacturer

Johnson & Johnson Orthopaedics

Product Description

Delta-Lite S and Delta-Lite Conformable consist of a knitted fibreglass substrate impregnated with a polyurethane resin. A silicone material has been added to the resin which makes the bandages less tacky to handle than conventional polyurethane bandages, and results in a cast with a smoother surface. The fabric base used in Delta-Lite S is extensible in all directions, which allows the bandage to conform well in use. The fabric used in the construction of Delta-Lite Conformable is elasticated and thus highly conformable, and the product is said to rival plaster of Paris bandage in terms of its ease of application in this respect.

When Delta-Lite S or Delta-Lite Conformable is exposed to moisture vapour or immersed in water, the resin undergoes a polymerisation reaction, which causes the tape to harden and become rigid. A cast made from Delta-Lite S will set in approximately seven minutes. Delta-Lite Conformable sets in about four and a half minutes. Once set, both products form casts that can be bivalved or windowed, and will be weight-bearing after 20 minutes. The resultant cast is lightweight, strong, porous, and translucent to X-rays.

Indications

Delta-Lite S and Delta-Lite Conformable may be used in most situations where rigid immobilisation is required. This includes the formation of standard orthopaedic casts and specialised prosthetic appliances.

Contra-indications

In common with all polyurethane casting tapes, both should be applied with caution on fresh fractures where swelling of the injured limb may be anticipated (which could make rapid removal of the cast necessary).

Method of Use

Delta-Lite S and Delta-Lite Conformable should be applied over a layer of stockinette and orthopaedic padding. Although any suitable product may be used, some workers prefer to use non-absorbent materials based upon synthetic fibres such as polyester, rather than the rayon- or cotton-based materials usually used in conjunction with plaster of Paris (which will retain moisture, should the final cast become wet). Before the foil pouch is opened, disposable gloves should be put on. Prior to application, the bandage should be immersed in water at 21–27°C, and firmly squeezed four or five times under the surface to ensure complete penetration of water into the body of the bandage. After removal from the dip water, the bandage should not be squeezed further.

The tape should be applied in the form of a spiral, each turn overlapping the previous one by about one-third to one-half of the width of the tape. Three or four layers of bandage are usually sufficient in most non-weight-bearing situations, but five or six layers may be required for a weight-bearing cast. If splints are needed, these may be produced from three or four layers of Delta-Lite S. The cast may be moulded to its final shape during the last 30 seconds of its setting cycle, after which time it may be windowed or trimmed with shears or a standard cast saw. A cast made from Delta-Lite S or Delta-Lite Conformable may be repaired or reinforced by the application of additional tape. Although this will adhere successfully to the existing cast, a complete layer should be applied, if possible, to achieve the maximum adhesive bond.

Warnings and Precautions

Prior to setting, the polyurethane resin will adhere firmly to unprotected skin and clothing. Operators should always wear gloves when handling these materials and care should be taken to ensure that the uncured tape does not come into contact with the patient's skin. Any uncured resin may be removed from the skin by gently swabbing with acetone or ethanol.

The final casts are not adversely affected by moisture, but immersion of the cast in water is not recommended, as it may prove very difficult to dry the underlying padding. This in turn may lead to maceration and irritation of the skin.

If the cast is removed with a reciprocating cast saw, the use of dust extraction apparatus is advisable.

Shelf Life and Storage Precautions

Delta-Lite S and Delta-Lite Conformable have a shelf life of four years from the date of manufacture given on the carton, and embossed on the seal of the foil pouch. The unopened rolls of casting tape should be stored in a cool dry atmosphere below 24°C. Above this temperature, the shelf life will be decreased.

Presentation

Both Delta-Lite S and Delta-Lite Conformable are available in the form of a roll, wrapped around a hollow plastic core, and heat-sealed in a poly/foil/poly laminate pouch.

Delta-Lite S

2 in × 4 yd	NSV No. EAF 411
3 in × 4 yd	NSV No. EAF 413
4 in × 4 yd	NSV No. EAF 415
5 in × 4 yd	NSV No. EAF 417

Delta-Lite Conformable

2 in × 4 yd	NSV No. EAF 551
3 in × 4 yd	NSV No. EAF 553
4 in × 4 yd	NSV No. EAF 555
5 in × 4 yd	NSV No. EAF 557

DERMIFLEX™

Classification Name
Dressing Hydrocolloid Impermeable

Manufacturer
Johnson & Johnson

Product Description

Dermiflex incorporates a PVC foam sheet bonded onto a plastic film, which is impermeable to both water vapour and micro-organisms. The side of the dressing in contact with the wound is coated with an adhesive mass composed of polyiso-butylene, in which are dispersed particles of carboxymethylcellulose, karaya gum and silica. The dressing is presented on a sheet of release paper, which extends past the edge of the dressing to facilitate removal. When Dermiflex comes into contact with wound exudate, the adhesive mass absorbs water and swells, forming a hydrophilic gel. The moist conditions produced under the dressing promote angiogenesis and wound healing, without causing maceration.

Indications

Dermiflex may be used in the prevention and management of pressure sores, and the treatment of leg ulcers, minor burns, donor sites (after haemostasis has been achieved), and many types of granulating wound. It can also be of value in the treatment of wounds covered with dry black necrotic skin, such as the 'black heels' that occur on bedridden patients. In these situations, the impermeable nature of the dressing leads to the retention of moisture vapour, rehydrating the dead tissue, which is then removed by autolysis.

Contra-indications

It is not recommended that Dermiflex be used in the treatment of clinically infected wounds, and it is probably not the product of choice for application to very heavily exuding lesions, at least in the initial stages of treatment (as the dressing would require replacing too frequently).

Method of Use

An appropriately sized dressing is removed from its paper backing and lightly pressed into position over the wound. In order to ensure good adhesion to the surrounding skin, a minimum overlap of 3–4 cm from the margin of the wound should be allowed. Because Dermiflex is adhesive and impermeable, no additional dressings are usually required. However, in situations where the edges of the product are likely to become disturbed by movement, such as on the sacral area, it is sometimes useful to cover the dressing with a piece of an adhesive dressing retention sheet (Hypafix™ or Mefix™, for example), or to stick the edges down with a suitable adhesive tape.

Upon removal of the dressing, a viscous granular gel may be found on the surface of the wound. This is normal, and consists of the partially liquefied adhesive base. It is not pus and does not indicate the presence of infection. The wound should be gently cleansed with sterile normal saline before the application of the next dressing.

Frequency of Dressing Changes

The frequency of dressing changes will be governed by the state of the wound. If large volumes of exudate are produced, daily changes may be required initially; but on drier wounds, the dressing may be left in place for 4 or 5 days before it must be changed.

Presentation

Dermiflex is presented individually wrapped in a peel pouch, sterilised by gamma irradiation.

10.2 cm × 10.2 cm	NSV No. ELM 031
16.5 cm × 16.5 cm	NSV No. ELM 032

ELASTOCREPE™

Classification Name
Bandage Cotton Crêpe BP

Manufacturer
Smith & Nephew

Product Description

Elastocrepe consists of a pink-coloured cotton fabric of plain weave with a characteristic appearance, bearing a yellow line up the centre. The fabric is extensible along its length, having a degree of elasticity that is imparted by the presence of crêpe-twisted cotton yarns. The bandage may be washed if required; when allowed to dry naturally, loosely folded, it will regain some of its original elasticity.

Indications

Elastocrepe is widely used for the application of light pressure and support in the treatment of sprains and strains, and varicose veins; and as a support to aid rehabilitation following ortho-paedic surgery. It is also used in the treatment of varicose ulcers — in conjunction with a suitable primary dressing, such as a zinc paste bandage — although other more elastic products are more suitable for this application.

Contra-indications

As with other bandages manufactured from cotton and other non-elastomeric fibres, the sub-bandage pressures that can be achieved and maintained by Elastocrepe are limited. Such products are unlikely to be suitable for the sustained application of pressures in excess of 8 – 10 mmHg at the calf of an average-sized leg.

Because cotton bandages do not have the ability to 'follow in' (thereby maintaining compression on limbs that decrease in circumference as a result of the application of surface pressure), they are of little value in reducing existing gross oedema. For this application and other situations where high levels of pressure are required, alternative products containing elastomeric threads of rubber, nylon or polyurethane are available.

All extensible bandages should be used with caution on patients who have marked ischaemia or impaired arterial blood supply.

Method of Use

When used to apply support or compression, the bandage should be held with the bulk roll facing upwards. Working from the inner aspect of the leg, a single turn should be made over the top of the foot around the base of the toes to secure the bandage, and a second turn taken up to the base of the heel. After making a figure-of-eight around the ankle, the bandage should be applied up the leg, with each turn overlapping the previous one by 50%, using the line in the centre of the bandage as a guide. Once in place, the bandage may be fastened with clips or tape, as appropriate. Care should be taken to ensure that the bandage does not cause a tourniquet effect at the knee, and the operator should ensure that a pressure gradient exists beneath the bandage, with the highest levels of pressure at the ankle.

Frequency of Dressing Changes

In critical applications where the control of sub-bandage pressure is important, the bandage should be reapplied or replaced as frequently as practicable. In other situations, it is not uncommon for a bandage to be left undisturbed for up to 5 – 7 days, although there is little doubt that, after this time, the residual pressure beneath the bandage will be only a fraction of the original application pressure.

Presentation

Elastocrepe is presented individually shrink-wrapped.

  5.0 cm × 4.5 m (stretched) NSV No. ECA 031
  7.5 cm × 4.5 m (stretched)*NSV No. ECA 033
10.0 cm × 4.5 m (stretched)*NSV No. ECA 035
15.0 cm × 4.5 m (stretched) NSV No. ECA 037

*Available on Drug Tariff.

GELIPERM™ SHEET
GELIPERM™ SHEET (DRY)
GELIPERM™ GRANULATED GEL

Classification Name
Geliperm Sheet — Dressing Hydrogel Sheet
Geliperm Sheet (Dry) — Dressing Hydrogel Sheet Dry
Geliperm Granulated Gel — Dressing Hydrogel Granulated

Manufacturer
Geistlich

Product Description

Geliperm Sheet is a strong, transparent hydrogel,

containing 96% water. The remaining 4% consists of agar (a gellable polysaccharide) and polyacrylamide (a cross-linked absorbent polymer of an acryl derivative), which together form a structure of two interwoven molecular networks. The polyacrylamide stabilises the agar, which, on its own, would be unsuitable for use as a dressing because of its low tensile strength. The porosity of the gel is such that it is permeable to water vapour, gases, and small protein molecules, but impermeable to bacteria. Geliperm Sheet provides a moist, warm, well-oxygenated environment upon the surface of the wound in which healing can take place. Provided the dressing is not allowed to dry out, it will not adhere to the underlying tissue upon removal. As the sheet has a low acoustic impedance, it may be used as a contact medium for pulsed shortwave or ultrasound treatment.

Geliperm Sheet (Dry) consists of a partially dehydrated polymer containing agar and polyacrylamide, together with approximately 35% glycerol. When immersed in an aqueous solution, the dressing absorbs water and any low molecular weight material, swells slightly, and becomes highly elastic, a process that takes about 15–30 minutes to complete. The physical characteristics and properties of Geliperm Sheet (Dry) are very similar to those of the hydrated version, but the dry sheet is more absorbent.

Geliperm Granulated Gel contains agar, polyacrylamide, and 93.5% water. It has been reduced by a milling process to an amorphous mass, which is presented in a collapsible plastic tube. In this form, the gel is able to absorb up to six times its own weight of wound exudate; cavities produced within the granular structure can also take up bacteria, pus, and cell debris, by capillary action.

Indications

Geliperm Sheet may be used in the treatment of a wide range of wounds involving skin and tissue loss, both chronic and acute in origin. These include donor and recipient graft sites, dermabrasions, burns, and superficial pressure areas. The sheet has also been used to prevent the drying-out of exposed bradytrophic tissue (such as tendon, periosteum, or bone), and in the preparation of sites prior to free skin transplantation. The dressing is cool and soothing to the touch, and is said to reduce local pain and discomfort in some types of injury. Geliperm Sheet (Dry) is particularly indicated for use where large volumes of wound exudate are expected (in burns, for example).

Geliperm Granulated Gel is used for the treatment of discharging cavities and cratered defects, such as decubitus ulcers and traumatic infected wounds. Infected surgical wounds of limited area that have been laid open to heal by secondary intention may also be treated.

All the Geliperm products may be used to deliver water-soluble topical drugs – such as antimicrobials, local anaesthetics, and haemostatics – to the surface of a wound, but Geliperm Sheet (Dry) is particularly suited for this application.

Contra-indications

Geliperm Sheet and Geliperm Sheet (Dry) should not be used as a covering for deep narrow cavities or sinuses. Geliperm Granulated Gel should only be used on deep cavities and sinuses if their full extent is known.

Geliperm products should not be applied to wounds known to be infected with *Pseudomonas* species, unless medicated with an appropriate water-soluble antimicrobial agent.

Method of Use

Geliperm Sheet or Geliperm Sheet (Dry) may be placed directly onto the surface of an exuding wound and held in place with tape or a bandage, as appropriate. On awkward areas an island dressing may be produced, using a dressing retention sheet such as Hypafix™ or Mefix™. If additional absorbency is required, an absorbent pad may be placed immediately over the hydrogel sheet. On dry wounds there is sometimes a possibility that the dressing will dry out. If this occurs, it may be readily rehydrated with sterile water or normal saline, prior to removal. As the Geliperm sheets do not cause tissue maceration, they do not have to be cut to the shape of the wound and may be allowed to overlap onto the surrounding skin.

When treating dry or infected wounds with Geliperm Sheet (Dry), it may be desirable to soak the dressing in normal saline or a solution of an antimicrobial agent for about 15–30 minutes prior to application.

When Geliperm Granulated Gel is used, the wound should first be cleansed with a suitable sterile solution (such as normal saline), and any wound debris removed – as far as possible –

either mechanically or surgically. The tip of the nozzle of the plastic tube is removed and the gel introduced into the wound, filling it to approximately one-third to one-half of its depth, depending upon the amount of exudate produced. The wound is then covered with a dry dressing held in place with tape or a bandage, as appropriate. Care should be taken to ensure that the secondary dressing will not prevent the gel swelling in the wound as it absorbs exudate, or areas of high pressure could occur, causing pain and further tissue damage. When the wound is re-dressed, the gel may be removed by irrigation with sterile normal saline (using a syringe), or washed off in the bath.

Frequency of Dressing Changes

All the Geliperm products should be changed as often as the condition of the wound dictates, but as a general rule, the dressing should be replaced after about 3–4 days, or when it has become cloudy or opaque owing to the absorption of wound exudate. In the treatment of an infected wound, it may be necessary to change the dressing more frequently, or apply further amounts of the antimicrobial agent to the hydrogel on a daily basis. If Geliperm Granulated Gel is being used as a wound cleansing agent, it may need to be changed at least daily in the early stages.

Warnings and Precautions

A Geliperm dressing should not be applied to a wound that shows evidence of clinical infection, unless the product is first soaked in a solution of an appropriate water-soluble antimicrobial agent. When Geliperm Granulated Gel is introduced into deep wounds, care should be taken to ensure that all the dressing is removed at each change.

Shelf Life and Storage Precautions

Geliperm Sheet, Geliperm Sheet (Dry), and Geliperm Granulated Gel should be stored in a cool place.

Presentation

Both Geliperm Sheet and Geliperm Sheet (Dry) are presented in a plastic tray with a transparent cover, sterilised by ethylene oxide. Geliperm Granulated Gel is presented in a soft plastic tube, sterilised by ethylene oxide.

Geliperm Sheet

130 mm × 120 mm	NSV No. ELE 031
260 mm × 120 mm	NSV No. ELE 033

Geliperm Sheet (Dry)

250 mm × 110 mm	NSV No. ELE 039

Geliperm Granulated Gel

20 g	NSV No. ELG 031
50 g	NSV No. ELG 033

GRANUFLEX™
GRANUFLEX™ EXTRA THIN
GRANUFLEX™ TRANSPARENT
GRANUFLEX™ E

Classification Name

Granuflex – Dressing Hydrocolloid Semipermeable

Granuflex Extra Thin – Dressing Hydrocolloid Semipermeable Thin

Granuflex Transparent – Dressing Hydrocolloid Semipermeable Transparent

Granuflex E – Dressing Hydrocolloid Semipermeable Extra Absorbent

Manufacturer

ConvaTec

Product Description

Granuflex incorporates a thin polyurethane foam sheet bonded onto a polyurethane film, which is impermeable to exudate and micro-organisms. The side of the dressing in contact with the wound is coated with an adhesive mass composed of polyisobutylene, within which are dispersed hydrophilic particles containing gelatin, pectin and carboxymethylcellulose. When the dressing comes into contact with wound exudate these particles absorb water and swell, forming a gel; eventually the dressing undergoes phase inversion, so that the adhesive mass becomes dispersed in the newly formed gel. The moist conditions produced under the dressing promote angiogenesis and wound healing, without causing maceration.

In addition to the sheet presentation, the hydrocolloid base itself is available in the form of paste and granules, which may be used in conjunction with the sheet to provide additional absorbent capacity in the management of wound cavities or heavily exuding wounds.

Granuflex Extra Thin and Granuflex Transparent consist of a thin layer of the hydrocolloid base applied directly to a sheet of polyurethane film. In both these presentations, there is no intervening foam layer and, as a result, the dressings are more conformable in use than the original Granuflex.

Granuflex E is significantly different from the other products in the range although it has the same basic structure, consisting of a polyurethane foam sheet backed with a polyurethane film. The principal difference lies in the composition of the adhesives and polymers which are combined with the gelatin, pectin and sodium carboxymethyl-cellulose. In the hydrated state the gel that is formed as a result of the absorption of wound exudate is not mobile and free running but is held within the structure of the dressing itself. Initial studies with this material suggest that it may be able to cope with larger volumes of exudate than traditional Granuflex when used in the management of heavily exuding wounds such as donor sites.

Indications

Granuflex may be used in the treatment of leg ulcers, pressure sores, minor burns, donor sites (after haemostasis has been achieved), and many types of granulating wound. It has also been found to be of value in the treatment of wounds covered with dry black necrotic skin, such as the 'black heels' that occur on bedridden patients. The dressing prevents the loss of water vapour from the surface of the skin, and this effectively rehydrates the dead tissue, which is then removed by autolysis.

Granuflex Extra Thin has a different range of indications. Because the absorbency of the dressing is reduced as a result of the decreased thickness of the hydrocolloid base, it is intended for use in the management of lightly exuding wounds such as abrasions, superficial pressure sores and post-operative wounds.

Granuflex Transparent, which is thinner than Granuflex Extra Thin, and consequently less absorbent, is designed to be used as a catheter dressing or incise drape.

Granuflex E is designed for the treatment of more heavily exuding wounds such as donor sites and burns. In these situations, the enhanced fluid handling properties of the dressing make dressing changes less messy than with the standard hydrocolloid dressings.

Contra-indications

It is not recommended that any of the Granuflex range be used in the treatment of clinically infected wounds and, with the possible exception of Granuflex E, they are probably not the products of choice for application to very heavily exuding wounds, at least in the initial stages of treatment (as the dressing would require replacing too frequently).

Method of Use

An appropriately sized dressing is removed from its paper backing and lightly pressed into position over the wound. In order to ensure good adhesion to the surrounding skin, a minimum overlap of 3–4 cm from the margin of the wound should be allowed. Because the Granuflex products are adhesive, and will not allow exudate to pass through the backing, no additional dressings are usually required. However, in situations where the edges of the product are likely to become disturbed by movement, such as on the sacral area, it is sometimes useful to cover the dressing with a piece of an adhesive dressing retention sheet (Hypafix™ or Mefix™, for example).

Upon removal of standard Granuflex dressings, a viscous yellow gel may be found on the surface of the wound. This is normal, and consists of the partially liquefied adhesive base. It is not pus and does not indicate the presence of infection. The wound should be gently cleansed with sterile normal saline before the application of the next dressing. Wounds dressed with Granuflex E should show less evidence of this semi-solid material.

Frequency of Dressing Changes

The frequency of dressing changes will be governed by the state of the wound. If large volumes of exudate are produced, daily changes may be required; but on some wounds the dressing may be left in place for 4 or 5 days before it must be changed. It is possible to judge when a dressing needs to be replaced, as the liquefied base becomes visible through the back of the dressing as a yellow bubble. Granuflex Extra Thin should be replaced if there is evidence of fluid accumulating beneath the dressing but for post-operative use it may usually be left in position until the sutures are to be removed. When used as a catheter dressing, Granuflex Transparent should be changed immediately if any signs of moisture are present or as often as good nursing practice dictates.

Presentation

All the Granuflex preparations are presented individually wrapped in a peel pouch, sterilised by gamma irradiation.

Granuflex Sheets

10.0 cm × 10.0 cm*	NSV No. ELM 011
20.0 cm × 20.0 cm	NSV No. ELM 013
15.0 cm × 20.0 cm**	NSV No. ELM 015
20.0 cm × 30.0 cm**	NSV No. ELM 017
7.5 cm × 7.5 cm†	NSV No. ELM 021
15.0 cm × 15.0 cm†	NSV No. ELM 023

Granules

4 g sachet	NSV No. ELO 011

Paste

30 g tube	NSV No. ELO 013

Granuflex Extra Thin

7.5 cm × 7.5 cm	NSV No. ELM 311
10.0 cm × 10.0 cm	NSV No. ELM 313
15.0 cm × 15.0 cm**	NSV No. ELM 315
5.0 cm × 10.0 cm**	NSV No. ELM 317
5.0 cm × 20.0 cm**	NSV No. ELM 319

Granuflex Transparent

5.0 cm × 7.5 cm	NSV No. ELM 331
10.0 cm × 10.0 cm	NSV No. ELM 333
15.0 cm × 20.0 cm**	NSV No. ELM 335

Granuflex E

10.0 cm × 10.0 cm	NSV No. ELM 131
15.0 cm × 15.0 cm	NSV No. ELM 133
20.0 cm × 20.0 cm**	NSV No. ELM 135
15.0 cm × 20.0 cm**	NSV No. ELM 137
15.0 cm × 30.0 cm**	NSV No. ELM 139

*Available on Drug Tarriff

**Double wrapped

†Dimensions include an adhesive foam border around the dressing

---

GYPSONA™
GYPSONA S™

Classification Name

Gypsona – Bandage Plaster of Paris BP
Gypsona S – Bandage Plaster of Paris

Manufacturer

Smith & Nephew

Product Description

Gypsona consists of a leno-weave gauze fabric that is coated with a blend of the alpha and beta forms of calcium sulphate hemihydrate (plaster of Paris), together with binders and accelerators. The use of a leno-weave gauze is claimed to provide stability to the bandage, and reduce distortion and creasing during application. In Gypsona S, the base fabric is a plain-weave gauze. The formulation of the plaster mass of Gypsona S is very similar to that of Gypsona, so the handling characteristics and setting times of the two materials are almost identical.

Gypsona and Gypsona S are supplied wrapped around plastic spools which are designed to allow rapid, even wetting of the bandage upon immersion. Once wet, the calcium sulphate hemihydrate is converted to the dihydrate, and the bandage sets to form a hard rigid structure, which is both porous and absorbent. The rate of setting is largely governed by the temperature of the water, but if the bandage is used in accordance with the manufacturer's intructions, an initial set will take place in about two minutes. The cast will be fully set in about 3–5 minutes, although it may not achieve its maximum strength and become weight-bearing for up to 24–48 hours.

The principal disavantages of Gypsona and Gypsona S lie in their weight, their opacity to X-rays, and their susceptibility to damage by moisture.

Indications

Gypsona and Gypsona S may be used for most orthopaedic applications, and other situations in which rigid immobilisation is required, including the management of fresh or unstable fractures.

Method of Use

Gypsona and Gypsona S should be applied over a layer of stockinette and orthopaedic padding. Prior to application, the first 10–15 cm of the bandage should be unrolled to enable the rapid location of the end after dipping. The bandage is held lightly in one hand, and immersed in a suitable container of water at a temperature of 20–25°C, at an angle of 45°, until bubbling ceases. After the bandage is removed from the container, any excess water is gently squeezed out. The bandage is then rolled evenly around the limb, without tension, avoiding the formation of wrinkles but producing pleats or tucks where necessary. As each successive bandage is applied, it should be constantly moulded and smoothed with wet hands to ensure the formation of a homogeneous cast. Any areas of potential weakness may be strengthened by the addition of five or six layers of bandage, previously formed into a slab.

Warning and Precautions

When applying a cast, it is important to ensure that all bony prominences are adequately padded, and operators should take care to ensure that no indentations are made in the soft plaster that could cause local areas of high pressure leading to the formation of plaster sores. Rough finishes on the edges of the cast should also be avoided. If Gypsona or Gypsona S is applied to a fresh fracture, sufficient padding should be used to accommodate any swelling of the limb.

Shelf Life and Storage Precautions

The unopened rolls of Gypsona and Gypsona S should be stored in a cool dry atmosphere.

Presentation

Both Gypsona and Gypsona S are available in the form of a roll, wrapped around a plastic core, and sealed in a paper pouch.

Gypsona rolls
5.0 cm × 2.7 m	NSV No. EAA 011
7.5 cm × 2.7 m	NSV No. EAA 013
10.0 cm × 2.7 m	NSV No. EAA 015
15.0 cm × 2.7 m	NSV No. EAA 017
20.0 cm × 2.7 m	NSV No. EAA 019
90.0 cm × 2.7 m	NSV No. EAA 021

Gypsona slabs
10 cm × 20 m	NSV No. EAA 023
15 cm × 20 m	NSV No. EAA 025
20 cm × 20 m	NSV No. EAA 027
Emergency splint	NSV No. EAA 029

Gypsona S rolls
5.0 cm × 2.7 m	NSV No. EAA 171
7.5 cm × 2.7 m	NSV No. EAA 173
10.0c m × 2.7 m	NSV No. EAA 175
15.0cm × 2.7 m	NSV No. EAA 177
20.0cm × 2.7 m	NSV No. EAA 179

Gypsona S slabs
10 cm × 20 m	NSV No. EAA 183
15 cm × 20 m	NSV No. EAA 185
20 cm × 20 m	NSV No. EAA 187
Emergency splint	NSV No. EAA 189

HYPAFIX™

Classification Name
Tape Apertured Non-woven Surgical Synthetic Adhesive

Manufacturer
Smith & Nephew

Product Description

Hypafix consists of an apertured, non-woven polyester fabric coated with a layer of an acrylic adhesive, and protected on the roll by a release paper backing. The apertured structure imparts a degree of lateral extensibility and conformability to the product, which has a high tensile strength and must be cut with scissors. Hypafix is available in a range of widths and is sometimes referred to as a 'dressing retention sheet'. Because the tape is permeable to water vapour, it is unlikely to cause tissue maceration or be adversely affected by sweating. As both the fabric and the adhesive mass are radio-transparent, Hypafix does not have to be removed if the patient is to be X-rayed.

Indications

The high tensile strength and conformability of Hypafix make it ideally suited for securing catheters and drainage tubes in position, and for the retention of dressings on joints or awkward body contours. It is particularly useful for retaining dressings on the sacral region in the management of decubitus ulcers. Hypafix can also be used to produce island dressings with absorbent pads or hydrogel sheets, and probably represents the best method for applying these types of product. As the tape is coated with an acrylic adhesive system, it may generally be used on patients who have exhibited an adverse reaction to adhesives based upon zinc oxide, rubber, or resin. The polyester fabric is very 'wear-resistant': once applied, it may be left in position for prolonged periods, if required.

Contra-indications

Hypafix should not be applied to patients who are known to be sensitive to acrylic adhesives.

Method of Use

The required length of Hypafix is cut from the roll and the backing sheet removed. Care should be taken to ensure that the tape is not applied under tension; if used over a joint, it is recommended that Hypafix be orientated so that the direction of maximum extensibility of the fabric coincides with the direction of movement of the limb.

Frequency of Dressing Changes

The frequency of dressing changes will be governed by the condition of the underlying wound.

Warnings and Precautions

Care should be taken to ensure that Hypafix is not applied under tension, to prevent shearing forces causing damage to the skin.

Shelf Life and Storage Precautions

In common with all adhesive products, Hypafix should be stored in a cool dry place, and not subjected to extremes of temperature or humidity.

Presentation

5 cm × 10 m	NSV No. EHR 111
10 cm × 10 m	NSV No. EHR 113
15 cm × 10 m	NSV No. EHR 115
20 cm × 10 m	NSV No. EHR 117
30 cm × 10 m	NSV No. EHR 119

INADINE™

Classification Name
Dressing Povidone-Iodine/Polyethylene Glycol

Manufacturer
Johnson & Johnson

Product Description

Inadine consists of a knitted viscose fabric impregnated with a macrogol (PEG) basis containing 10% povidone-iodine (equivalent to 1.0% available iodine). The dressing is yellow-brown in colour and superficially resembles paraffin tulle. Povidone-iodine, a potent bactericidal agent with a broad spectrum of activity, is readily released from the PEG base. Unlike paraffin or lanolin, the base used in the production of Inadine is water-soluble and easily removed from the skin or surface of a wound.

Indications

Inadine is a medicated wound contact layer for the prophylaxis and treatment of infection in superficial burns and superficial traumatic skin-loss injuries.

Contra-indications

Inadine should not be used on patients who are sensitive to iodine or povidone-iodine.

Method of Use

Inadine is applied directly to the surface of the wound and covered with a sterile secondary dressing held in position with tape or bandages, as appropriate. Adherence to the surface of a wound is unlikely with Inadine, but if it does become a problem, the dressing may be removed by soaking it in normal saline.

Frequency of Dressing Changes

The frequency of dressing changes depends primarily upon the condition of the wound. If large quantities of exudate are produced, daily changes will probably be required; but if the wound is relatively dry, the interval between changes may be extended. For most applications, however, it is unlikely that the dressing will retain significant levels of antibacterial activity if left in position for longer than two days.

Warnings and Precautions

Inadine is for topical use only. Not more than four dressings should be applied at any one time.

Shelf Life and Storage Precautions

The dressing should be stored in a cool place.

Presentation

Inadine is presented in a peel pouch, sterilised by gamma irradiation.

5.0 cm × 5.0 cm*   NSV No. EKB 031
                     (PL No. 0084/0022)
9.5 cm × 9.5 cm*   NSV No. EKB 033
                     (PL No. 0084/0022)
*Available on Drug Tariff.

Legal Category

General Sales List [GSL]

INTRASITE™

Classification Name
Dressing Hydrocolloid Semipermeable

Manufacturer
Smith & Nephew

Product Description

Intrasite consists of a thin polyurethane film (similar to that used in Opsite™), onto which is bonded an adhesive mass that contains gelatin, pectin and carboxymethylcellulose dispersed in a polyisobutylene base. When the dressing comes into contact with wound exudate, the base absorbs moisture and swells, eventually forming a viscous yellow gel. In its dry state, the dressing has a low moisture vapour permeability, but as the base begins to liquefy, the dressing becomes permeable to water vapour, and so a proportion of the liquid under the dressing may be lost to the environment by evaporation. The conditions that exist beneath the dressing promote wound healing without causing maceration.

Indications

Intrasite may be used in the treatment of leg ulcers, pressure areas, minor burns, donor sites (after haemostasis has been achieved), and many types of granulating wound. It may also be of value in the treatment of wounds covered with dry black necrotic skin, such as the 'black heels' that occur on bedridden patients. The dressing will prevent the loss of moisture vapour from the surface of the skin and thus effectively rehydrate the dead tissue, which is subsequently removed by autolysis.

Contra-indications

It is not recommended that Intrasite be used in the treatment of clinically infected wounds, and it is probably not the product of choice for application to very heavily exuding wounds, at least in the initial stages of treatment (as the dressing would require replacing too frequently).

Method of Use

An appropriately sized dressing is removed from its paper backing and lightly pressed into position over the wound. In order to ensure good adhesion to the surrounding skin, a minimum overlap of 3–4 cm from the margin of the wound should be allowed. Because Intrasite is adhesive and impermeable to bacteria, no additional dressings are usually required. However, in situations where the edges of the product are likely to become disturbed by movement, such as on the sacral area, it is sometimes useful to cover the dressing with a piece of an adhesive dressing retention sheet (Hypafix™ or Mefix™, for example).

Upon removal of the dressing, a viscous yellow gel may be found on the surface of the wound. This is normal, and consists of the partially liquefied adhesive base. It is not pus and does not indicate the presence of infection. The wound should be gently cleansed with sterile normal saline before the application of the next dressing.

Frequency of Dressing Changes

The frequency of dressing changes will be governed by the state of the wound. If large volumes of exudate are produced, daily changes may be required; but on some wounds, the dressing may be left in place for 4 or 5 days. As the base absorbs liquid, it becomes visible through the back of the dressing as a yellow bubble; it is recommended that the dressing be changed whenever the exudate extends more than 1 cm beyond the perimeter of the wound.

Presentation

Intrasite is presented individually wrapped in a peel pouch, sterilised by ethylene oxide.

10 cm × 10 cm   NSV No. ELM 111
20 cm × 20 cm   NSV No. ELM 113

IODOSORB™
IODOSORB™ OINTMENT

Classification Name
Iodosorb – Dressing Polysaccharide Bead
    Medicated

Iodosorb Ointment — Dressing Polysaccharide
  Bead Paste Medicated

Manufacturer

Perstorp Pharma

Product Description

Iodosorb consists of sterile, yellow-brown
microspheres, 0.1–0.3 mm in diameter formed
from a three-dimensional network of cadexomer
— a chemically modified starch. The hydrophilic
beads contain 0.9% w/w of iodine which is held
firmly within the structure of the polymer and not
liberated in the dry state, despite the high vapour
pressure of the iodine. In the presence of water or
aqueous solutions, the beads take up liquid and
swell and the iodine is slowly released.

Iodosorb Ointment consists of similar beads
incorporated into a macrogol ointment base. The
iodine content of the beads used to produce the
paste is increased so that, like Iodosorb itself, the
final concentration of iodine in the ointment is
0.9% w/w.

When the beads are placed upon a sloughy or
infected wound, bacteria and cellular debris are
taken up by capillary action and become trapped
in the spaces between the beads. When the
dressing is changed, this debris is washed away.
The iodine which is released as the beads take up
fluid also imparts antibacterial properties to the
dressing.

Indications

Iodosorb beads are recommended for the
treatment of moist, sloughy wounds such as
pressure sores and leg ulcers. Iodosorb Ointment
is also used for the treatment of chronic leg ulcers,
particularly those which are infected or covered
with slough or necrotic tissue or areas that are
difficult to dress with the free-flowing beads.

Contra-indications

As Iodosorb contains iodine, it should not be used
on patients with known or suspected iodine
sensitivity. It is also contra-indicated in
Hashimoto's thyroiditis, and should not be used
on patients with Graves' disease.

Method of Use

A layer of Iodosorb beads or Iodosorb Ointment,
approximately 3 mm thick, is applied to the
wound and covered with a suitable pad or dressing
retention material held in place with tape or a
bandage as appropriate. Removal is best
accomplished by irrigating the wound with sterile
water or normal saline, using a syringe. Once the
wound has been cleansed, a new layer of beads
or ointment is applied while the area is still
moist.

Warnings and Precautions

Iodine is absorbed systemically and therefore
Iodosorb should be used with care on patients
who have a history of thyroid disorders. A single
application should not exceed 50 grams of ointment (5 tubes) or 16 sachets of the beads. Not
more than 150 grams of Iodosorb should be
applied during the course of one week.

Iodosorb should not be applied to pregnant
women or lactating mothers.

Because there is a potential interaction between
iodine and lithium, sulphafurazole and the
sulphonylureas, co-administration is not
recommended.

Iodosorb should not be used on dry wounds.
On lightly exuding wounds there is a danger that
the beads may dry out and form a crust, which
may be difficult to remove.

Iodosorb should not be applied near the eye,
or introduced into sinuses from which removal
may be difficult.

Frequency of Dressing Changes

The frequency of dressing changes will depend
entirely upon the nature of the wound. Initially,
twice daily changes may be required if the beads
become saturated with exudate as indicated by a
loss of colour; but after the first two days, the
interval between changes may be extended until
eventually the dressing is changed about three
times per week.

Shelf Life and Storage Precautions

Iodosorb Ointment should be stored at room
temperature or below.

Presentation

Iodosorb is available in unit dose foil/laminate
sachets, and Iodosorb Ointment in unit dose tubes
each containing 10 grams. Both preparations are
sterilised by irradiation.

Iodosorb sachet

3 g   NSV No. ELU 011
       (PL No. 3863/0001)

Iodosorb Ointment

10 g   NSV No. ELU 031
        (PL No. 3863/0004)

Legal Category

Prescription Only Medicines [POM]

JELONET™

Classification Name

Dressing Paraffin Gauze BP (Normal Loading)

Manufacturers

Smith & Nephew

Product Description

Jelonet consists of a leno-weave fabric of cotton or cotton and viscose, which has been impregnated with white soft paraffin. The dressing is used as a primary wound contact layer and the paraffin is present to reduce the adherence of the product to the surface of a granulating wound.

Two formulations of Paraffin Gauze Dressing are described in the British Pharmacopoeia: they differ in the weight of paraffin present on the gauze. Jelonet, which is an example of the 'normal loading' product, contains not less than 175 grams of paraffin per square metre of cloth. The alternative formulation bears a lower loading of paraffin, in the range 90–130 g/m² (see Paratulle™).

Indications

Jelonet is used as a primary wound contact layer in the treatment of burns, ulcers, skin grafts (both donor and receptor sites), and a variety of traumatic injuries. The material is also used as a transfer medium for skin during grafting.

Contra-indications

Although there are no absolute contra-indications to the use of Jelonet, if the dressing is placed upon a heavily exuding wound its semi-occlusive nature may cause tissue maceration by preventing the free movement of exudate away from the surface of the wound. This is less likely to occur if a dressing bearing the lower loading of paraffin base is used.

Method of Use

Jelonet is applied directly to the surface of the wound and covered with an absorbent pad held in place with tape or a bandage, as appropriate.

Frequency of Dressing Changes

The frequency of dressing changes will depend entirely upon the nature of the wound. If Jelonet is left in position for prolonged periods of time, it can become adherent and cause tissue damage upon removal.

Shelf Life and Storage Precautions

Jelonet should be stored in a cool place.

Presentation

Jelonet is available in two forms: individually wrapped in an aluminium peel pouch, sterilised by irradiation; or packed in bulk in a tin, also sterilised by irradiation.

Individually wrapped

5 cm × 5 cm	NSV No. EKA 009
10 cm × 10 cm*	NSV No. EKA 011
10 cm × 40 cm	NSV No. EKA 013
15 cm × 2 m	NSV No. EKA 015

Bulk

10 cm × 10 cm (10)*	NSV No. EKA 031
10 cm × 10 cm (36)	NSV No. EKA 037
10 cm × 7 m	NSV No. EKA 039

*Available on Drug Tariff.

KALTOSTAT™
KALTOCLUDE™

Classification Name
Kaltostat – Dressing Calcium/Sodium Alginate
Kaltoclude – Dressing Calcium/Sodium Alginate
   Film Backed Adhesive

Manufacturer
BritCair

Product Description

Kaltostat is a fibrous fleece consisting of the mixed sodium and calcium salts of alginic acid in the ratio of 20:80. The dressing is available as a ball for packing cavities, and a flat non-woven pad for application to larger surface wounds. When the dressing is placed on a moist wound surface it absorbs liquid, and the sodium alginate rapidly forms a moist hydrogel. In the presence of exudate or other body fluids containing sodium ions, the calcium alginate is partially converted to the soluble sodium salt, and further gel is formed, which overlays the wound and provides a micro-environment that facilitates wound healing.

Kaltoclude consists of a piece of non-woven alginate fleece bonded on to a semipermeable copolymer film forming an adhesive island dressing. Although the film is permeable to moisture vapour it has the effect of reducing water vapour loss from the surface of the wound and hence prevents the alginate gel formed by interaction with wound exudate from drying out.

Indications

Kaltostat is indicated for use as a primary dressing for split-skin donor sites; for the management of bleeding wounds including cuts, lacerations, and nose bleeds; and for the staunching of bleeding in post-extraction haemorrhage, though this indication is for professional dental use only. The dressing may also be applied to a wide range of exuding lesions including leg ulcers, pressure areas and most other granulating wounds.

Kaltoclude is indicated for the management of superficial low exudate wounds for which the plain alginate fleece would not be suitable.

Contra-indications

Although there are no known contra-indications to the use of Kaltostat or Kaltoclude, neither dressing will be of much value if applied to wounds that are very dry, or covered with hard black necrotic tissue.

Method of Use

Kaltostat is placed onto the surface of the wound and covered with a second sterile dressing pad held in place with surgical tape or a bandage, as appropriate. The selection of the secondary dressing will be governed by the condition of the wound. If large quantities of exudate are anticipated, a simple absorbent dressing pad will be required; but as the wound heals and less exudate is produced, a thinner pad bearing a low adherence plastic film may help to conserve moisture and prevent the wound drying out too quickly. Deeper wounds may be treated using the Kaltostat ball, which should be laid into the cavity but not packed in tightly. It should not be inserted into narrow sinuses or similar wounds from which removal may be difficult. Because the alginate fibre reacts with sodium ions to form a soluble gel, removal of the dressing may be facilitated by first soaking it with sterile normal saline.

Prior to application of Kaltoclude, the skin surrounding the wound should be clean and dry. Kaltoclude is presented on a second transparent plastic film which acts as a carrier for the dressing itself. The carrier bears a blue plastic tab to facilitate removal of the dressing from the backing sheet which is present on the adhesive surface of the film. Once the dressing has been placed in position over the wound, the carrier is removed from the outer surface of the film by means of a second white tab and the film smoothed firmly into position.

Frequency of Dressing Changes

When used as a haemostat, Kaltostat need only be removed when the dry scab is ready to separate from the underlying healthy tissue; but for exuding wounds, such as ulcers and pressure areas, the interval between dressing changes will depend entirely upon the state of the wound. On heavily exuding or sloughy wounds, a daily change may be required at the beginning of treatment, but this may be reduced to alternate days or even less frequently as healing progresses. Wounds that show signs of clinical infection may be dressed with Kaltostat, which should be changed daily; systemic antibiotic therapy should be initiated at the discretion of the medical officer in charge.

When used on clean superfical wounds, Kaltoclude may be left undisturbed until healing is complete unless the accumulation of fluid becomes a problem and makes a change of dressing necessary.

Presentation

Kaltostat and Kaltoclude are presented individually wrapped in a peel pouch, sterilised by gamma irradiation.

Kaltostat pads

5.0 cm × 5.0 cm*	NSV No. ELS 229	
	(PL No. 6079/0002)	
7.5 cm × 12.0 cm	NSV No. ELS 231	
	(PL No. 6079/0002)	
10.0 cm × 20.0 cm	NSV No. ELS 233	
	(PL No. 6079/0002)	
15.0 cm × 25.0 cm	NSV No. ELS 235	
	(PL No. 6079/0002)	

Kaltostat packing

2 g   NSV No. ELS 251
                  (PL No. 6079/0001)

Kaltoclude

10.0 cm × 10.0 cm   NSV No. ELS 331

*Available on Drug Tariff

Legal Category
Pharmacy Only [P]

K-CREPE™

Classification Name
Bandage Light Pressure and Support

Manufacturer
Parema

Product Description

K-Crepe consists of a white knitted fabric containing 86% viscose, 6% nylon and 8% of an elastomeric yarn. A green line runs along its length. The bandage is extensible and highly elastic and may be considered as an alternative to the crêpe bandages in current use, for certain applications. Unlike the crêpes that are made entirely of cotton or cotton and wool, K-Crepe is able to apply and retain a significant level of sub-bandage pressure over a period of days. K-Crepe may be washed if required; when allowed to dry naturally, loosely folded, it will regain much of its original elasticity.

Indications

K-Crepe may be used in the treatment of varicose ulcers, in conjunction with a suitable primary dressing, and for the application of light pressure and support to sprains and strains. However, for this second application, its light weight and high extensibility may make it less suitable than the heavier, less extensible cotton products. As with many other bandages, the pressures that can be achieved and maintained by K-Crepe are limited, but on an average-sized calf, two layers applied in a standard fashion should be able to produce and sustain levels of pressure of the order of 12–15 mmHg; in comparison, products made entirely from cotton would be unlikely to achieve values in excess of 8–10 mmHg under similar conditions. If levels of pressure higher than this are required, or large oedematous legs are to be bandaged, a more powerful product should be selected. Because K-Crepe has the ability to 'follow in', it may be used to maintain compression on limbs as they decrease in circumference as a result of the application of surface pressure.

Contra-indications

K-Crepe should be used with caution on patients who have marked ischaemia or impaired arterial blood supply.

Method of Use

When used to apply support or compression to a leg, the bandage should be held with the bulk roll facing upwards. Working from the inner aspect, a single turn should be made over the top of the foot around the base of the toes to secure the bandage, and a second turn taken up to the base of the heel. After making a figure-of-eight around the ankle, the bandage should be applied up the leg, with each turn overlapping the previous one by 50%, using the line in the centre of the bandage as a guide. Once in place, the bandage may be fastened with clips or tape, as appropriate.

Because of its knitted structure, K-Crepe has a tendency to 'neck', or reduce in width, when under tension. This may have important implications if the 5 or 7 cm width is applied with excessive tension, as there is a possibility that a tourniquet effect might occur. For this reason, the 10 cm size should be considered for routine use, unless particular circumstances dictate otherwise.

Frequency of Dressing Changes

In critical applications where the control of sub-bandage pressure is important, K-Crepe should be reapplied or replaced as frequently as practicable. In other situations, it may be left in place for number of days; although some loss of pressure will undoubtedly occur, this will be less than would have been the case with a product made entirely from cotton.

Warnings and Precautions

K-Crepe should never be applied at full stretch, and care must be taken to ensure that it is not applied so tightly as to restrict blood flow at the knee. The operator should also ensure that a pressure gradient exists beneath the bandage, with the highest levels of pressure at the ankle.

Presentation

K-Crepe is presented individually shrink-wrapped.

5 cm × 4.5 m (stretched)	NSV No. ECA 471
7 cm × 4.5 m (stretched)	NSV No. ECA 473
10 cm × 4.5 m (stretched)	NSV No. ECA 475
15 cm × 4.5 m (stretched)	NSV No. ECA 477

LYOFOAM™
LYOFOAM C ™

Classification Name

Lyofoam – Dressing Polyurethane Foam BP
Lyofoam C – Dressing Polyurethane Foam
  with Activated Charcoal

Manufacturer

Ultra

Product Description

Lyofoam consists of a soft, open cell, hydrophobic, polyurethane foam sheet approximately 8 mm thick. The side of the dressing that is to be placed in contact with the skin has been heat-treated to collapse the cells of the foam, to form a hydrophilic surface. The dressing is freely permeable to gases and water vapour but resists the penetration of aqueous solutions and wound exudate. In use, the dressing absorbs blood or other tissue fluids through the hydrophilic lower surface, and the aqueous component is lost by evaporation through the back of the dressing. Cellular debris and proteinaceous material remain trapped in the small pores in the front of the dressing, which rapidly become occluded if the wound is dirty or producing large volumes of exudate. The dressing maintains a moist warm environment at the surface of the wound, which is conducive to the formation of granulation tissue and epithelialisation. The conditions also favour auto-debridement of the wound, by facilitating rehydration and autolysis of dried necrotic tissue; this process may result in an apparent worsening in the appearance of the wound, initially, as the liquefied slough starts to come away. This is normal and should not give cause for concern, provided there are no clinical signs of infection present.

A special version of Lyofoam is available, which has been cut to fit around tracheostomy tubes and drainage sites.

Lyofoam C consists of a layer of Lyofoam that is heat-bonded around the perimeter to a sheet of plain polyurethane foam. A layer of a non-woven fabric, impregnated with activated carbon granules, is sandwiched between the polyurethane sheets. Lyofoam C serves two functions: it has many of the properties of Lyofoam, maintaining a moist warm environment at the surface of the wound, which is conducive to healing; and it absorbs the noxious odours associated with certain types of wound. The substances that are responsible for the formation of odour appear to be partly retained within the foam itself, but the principal odour-absorbing ability of the dressing is due to the presence of charcoal.

Indications

Lyofoam may be used to dress a variety of exuding wounds, including leg and decubitus ulcers, sutured wounds, burns, and donor sites. Lyofoam C may be indicated if such wounds are malodorous. It is recommended that Lyofoam and Lyofoam C should not be left in position on a shallow drying wound for extended periods, because of the possibility of adherence.

Contra-indications

No absolute contra-indications to the use of Lyofoam or Lyofoam C have been reported, but neither dressing should be applied to wounds that are covered with a dry scab or hard black necrotic tissue, until this has been removed surgically or by some other means.

Method of Use

A suitable size of Lyofoam or Lyofoam C is chosen: the dressing should overlap the edges of the wound by a minimum of 2–3 cm, but in the treatment of leg ulcers and similar exuding wounds, this overlap should be increased to 4–5 cm where possible. The dressing is positioned with the smooth side next to the skin, and held in place with adhesive tape or a bandage, as appropriate.

No secondary dressings are generally required. On areas that are particularly difficult to dress, such as the heels or the sacral region, the dressing may be held in position with a dressing retention sheet, such as Hypafix™ or Mefix™. As sloughy or necrotic wounds are debrided, it is important that they are cleansed thoroughly during dressing changes with sterile normal saline or a solution of a suitable antiseptic agent.

Frequency of Dressing Changes

The frequency with which the dressing should be changed depends entirely upon the nature and condition of the wound. On very dirty sloughy wounds, twice daily changes may be required initially; but as the amount of exudate decreases, the interval between dressing changes may be increased – up to a week, as appropriate.

Presentation

Lyofoam and Lyofoam C are presented individually wrapped in paper peel pouches, sterilised by irradiation.

Lyofoam sheets

7.5 cm × 7.5 cm*	NSV No. ELA 011
10.0 cm × 10.0 cm*	NSV No. ELA 013
17.5 cm × 10.0 cm	NSV No. ELA 015
25.0 cm × 10.0 cm	NSV No. ELA 017
20.0 cm × 15.0 cm	NSV No. ELA 019
30.0 cm × 25.0 cm	NSV No. ELA 021
70.0 cm × 40.0 cm	NSV No. ELA 023

*Available on Drug Tariff

Lyofoam tracheostomy dressing
6.5 cm × 9.0 cm	NSV No. ELA 031

Lyofoam C sheets
10 cm × 10 cm	NSV No. ELV 111
20 cm × 15 cm	NSV No. ELV 115

MEFIX™

Classification Name
Tape Apertured Non-woven Surgical Synthetic Adhesive

Manufacturer
Molnlycke

Product Description

Mefix consists of an apertured, non-woven polyester fabric coated with a layer of an acrylic adhesive, and protected on the roll by a release paper backing. The apertured structure imparts a degree of lateral extensibility and conformability to the product, which has a high tensile strength and must be cut with scissors. Mefix is available in a range of widths and is sometimes referred to as a 'dressing retention sheet'. Because the tape is permeable to water vapour, it is unlikely to cause tissue maceration or be adversely affected by sweating. As both the fabric and the adhesive mass are radio-transparent, Mefix does not have to be removed if the patient is to be X-rayed.

Indications

The high tensile strength and conformability of Mefix make it ideally suited for securing catheters and drainage tubes in position, and for the retention of dressings on joints or awkward body contours. It is particularly useful for retaining dressings on the sacral region in the management of decubitus ulcers. Mefix can also be used to produce island dressings with absorbent pads or hydrogel sheets and probably represents the best method for applying these types of product. As the tape is coated with an acrylic adhesive system, it may generally be used on patients who have exhibited an adverse reaction to adhesives based upon zinc oxide, rubber or resin. The polyester fabric is very 'wear-resistant': once applied, it may be left in position for prolonged periods, if required.

Contra-indications

Mefix should not be applied to patients who are known to be sensitive to acrylic adhesives.

Method of Use

The required length of Mefix is cut from the roll and the backing sheet removed. Care should be taken to ensure that the tape is not applied under tension; if used over a joint, it is recommended that Mefix be orientated so that the direction of maximum extensibility of the fabric coincides with the direction of movement of the limb.

Frequency of Dressing Changes

The frequency of dressing changes will be governed by the condition of the underlying wound.

Warnings and Precautions

Care should be taken to ensure that Mefix is not applied under tension, to prevent shearing forces causing damage to the skin.

Shelf Life and Storage Precautions

In common with all adhesive products, Mefix should be stored in a cool dry place, and not subjected to extremes of temperature or humidity.

Presentation

1.25 cm × 10 m	NSV No. EHR 107
2.5 cm × 10 m	NSV No. EHR 109
5.0 cm × 10 m	NSV No. EHR 111
10.0 cm × 10 m	NSV No. EHR 113
15.0 cm × 10 m	NSV No. EHR 115
20.0 cm × 10 m	NSV No. EHR 117
30.0 cm × 10 m	NSV No. EHR 119

MELOLIN™

Classification Name

Dressing Perforated Film Absorbent BP (Type 1)

Manufacturer

Smith & Nephew

Product Description

Melolin consists of a film of poly(ethylene terephthalate), onto which is bonded an absorbent layer consisting of a mixture of cotton, viscose and polyacrylonitrile fibres, backed with a layer of an apertured non-woven cellulose fabric. The plastic film is present to prevent the dressing adhering to the surface of the wound, and is perforated to allow the passage of exudate from the wound into the body of the pad.

Indications

Melolin may be used on its own to dress dry sutured wounds, superficial cuts and abrasions, and other lightly exuding lesions. It may also be used as the primary wound contact layer for more heavily exuding wounds, if backed by a second absorbent dressing.

Contra-indications

In common with other perforated plastic film dressings, Melolin should be used with caution in the treatment of leg ulcers that produce copious quantities of very viscous exudate, which may be unable to pass through the small holes in the film. Under these circumstances, the exudate may become trapped under the dressing, leading to maceration and inflammation of the surrounding skin.

Method of Use

Melolin has a relatively low absorbent capacity and is therefore intended for use on wounds that do not produce large amounts of exudate. Under these circumstances, a single dressing may simply be secured in position with surgical tape. On more heavily exuding wounds, Melolin may be used as a wound contact layer, beneath a secondary absorbent pad held in position with tape or a bandage.

Frequency of Dressing Changes

The frequency with which the dressing should be changed depends entirely upon the nature and condition of the wound.

Presentation

Melolin is available in two forms: individually wrapped in a paper peel pouch, sterilised by autoclaving; or in bulk, non-sterile.

Individually wrapped

5 cm × 5 cm*	NSV No. EJE 011
10 cm × 10 cm*	NSV No. EJE 013
20 cm × 10 cm*	NSV No. EJE 015

Bulk

5 cm × 5 cm	NSV No. EJE 031
10 cm × 10 cm	NSV No. EJE 033
20 cm × 10 cm	NSV No. EJE 035
20 cm × 30 cm	NSV No. EJE 037
50 cm × 7 m	NSV No. EJE 039

*Available on Drug Tariff.

MICROPORE™

Classification Name

Tape Permeable Non-woven Surgical Synthetic Adhesive BP

Manufacturer

3M

Product Description

Micropore consists of a conformable, non-extensible non-woven fabric manufactured from 100% viscose, coated with a layer of an acrylic adhesive. The tape is easily torn to length. Once applied to the skin, Micropore will withstand limited exposure to water without losing all of its adhesive properties. Because the tape is permeable to both water and water vapour, it will allow the passage of sweat and secretions from the surface of the body to the environment, preventing maceration of the skin.

The tape is radio-transparent, and may be sterilised by ethylene oxide. It is suggested that, if sterile tape is required, strips are removed from the roll and laid over a suitable carrier for introduction into the chamber of the ethylene oxide steriliser. It is important to ensure that any tape so sterilised is adequately aerated before use. Sterilisation of intact rolls of tape is not recommended.

Indications

Micropore may be used for most general purpose applications, but it is most commonly used for dressing retention on non-flexing areas. As the tape is coated with an acrylic adhesive system, it may generally be used on patients who have exhibited an adverse reaction to adhesives based upon zinc oxide, rubber, or resin.

Contra-indications

Although there are no absolute contra-indications to the use of Micropore, it should (like most tapes) be used with caution on patients who have very fragile skin, such as those on long-term steroid therapy.

Warnings and Precautions

It should not be necessary to use skin tackifiers, such as tincture of benzoin, with Micropore. The tape is not extensible, and therefore care should be taken to ensure that it is not applied under tension (which could cause damage to the skin by exerting a shearing force).

Shelf Life and Storage Precautions

In common with all adhesive products, Micropore should be stored in a dry place, and not subjected to extremes of temperature.

Presentation

1.25 cm × 10 m	NSV No. EHU 111
2.5 cm × 10 m	NSV No. EHU 113
5.0 cm × 10 m	NSV No. EHU 115
7.5 cm × 10 m	NSV No. EHU 117
1.2 cm × 5 m*	NSV No. EHU 121
2.5 cm × 5 m*	NSV No. EHU 123
5.0 cm × 5 m*	NSV No. EHU 125
1.25 cm × 9.14 m†	NSV No. EHU 151
2.5 cm × 9.14 m†	NSV No. EHU 153
5.0 cm × 9.14 m†	NSV No. EHU 155

*Available on Drug Tariff
†Pink

OPSITE™
OPSITE CH™
OPSITE I.V. 3000™

Classification Name

Opsite – Dressing Semipermeable Adhesive BP
Opsite CH – Dressing Semipermeable Adhesive Medicated
Opsite I.V. 3000 – Dressing Semipermeable Adhesive

Manufacturer

Smith & Nephew

Product Description

Opsite consists of a thin polyurethane membrane coated with a layer of a vinyl ether adhesive. The dressing, which is permeable to both water vapour and oxygen, is impermeable to micro-organisms; once in position, it provides an effective barrier to external contamination, whilst producing a moist environment at the surface of the wound by reducing water vapour loss from the exposed tissue. Under these conditions in shallow wounds, scab formation is prevented and epidermal regeneration takes place at an enhanced rate, compared with that which occurs in wounds treated with traditional dry dressings. It has been demonstrated that the exudate from human donor sites that accumulates beneath Opsite contains large numbers of neutrophils, high levels of lysozyme, and concentrations of plasma proteins and electrolytes that fall within the normal clinical ranges for blood. In addition, it has been shown that a component of the adhesive system has a pronounced biocidal effect, which imparts anti-bacterial properties to the dressing, and probably accounts for the low incidence of wound infection associated with the use of this material.

Opsite CH differs from Opsite in that the adhesive contains 5% chlorhexidine acetate. Although the manufacturers make no specific claims for this, it is possible that the chlorhexidine may provide some additional protection against infection. It cannot be assumed, however, that sufficient chlorhexidine is available in the dressing to exert any effect upon pre-existing wound or catheter-related infections. A special version of Opsite CH is available as a cannula dressing. One end of the film is reinforced with a second layer of a thicker plastic, through which an elliptical aperture has been made to fit around the injection port of a cannula.

Opsite I.V. 3000 which was developed specifically as a catheter dressing, consists of a hydrophilic polyurethane film coated with an acrylic emulsion adhesive system. The film is much more permeable to water vapour than the original Opsite, approximately 3000 g/m²/24 hours, and is therefore less likely to allow the accumulation of moisture beneath the dressing, reducing the risk of skin maceration and catheter related sepsis. For this reason, it is likely that Opsite I.V. 3000 will eventually replace standard Opsite for this application.

Indications

Opsite may be used in the treatment of scalds, first or second degree burns, donor sites, post-operative wounds, minor injuries (including abrasions and lacerations), and the prevention and treatment of superficial pressure areas. Larger sizes of Opsite are marketed as incise drapes.

Opsite I.V. 3000 and Opsite CH are used for retaining peripheral and central line cannulae, where they allow regular inspection of the site, but prevent contamination. Opsite CH cannula dressing can be used over a cannula with an injection port.

Contra-indications

Although there are no absolute contra-indications to the use of Opsite, it is not recommended that the material be applied over deep cavity wounds, third degree burns, or wounds that show evidence of clinical infection. Opsite CH should not be used on patients who are sensitive to chlorhexidine.

Method of Use

When used as a wound dressing, an appropriate size of Opsite should be chosen, the paper backing removed, and the film lightly smoothed into position. In order to ensure good adhesion, the dressing should be allowed a minimum overlap of 3–4 cm from the margin of the wound onto the surrounding skin. On clean, heavily exuding wounds, such as donor sites, large quantities of fluid sometimes accumulate beneath the film. This should be left undisturbed as far as possible, but if the accumulation becomes excessive, it may be aspirated with a syringe using an aseptic technique. A small patch of Opsite should be applied over the puncture to prevent leakage or contamination.

When Opsite IV 3000 or Opsite CH is used to dress a cannula site, the area should first be thoroughly cleansed with a suitable antiseptic solution and prepared with an alcohol-impregnated swab (to dry and de-fat the skin).

Frequency of Dressing Changes

On clean wounds, such as donor sites and post-operative wounds, Opsite may be left undisturbed for a week or even longer, but in most other situations more frequent changes may be required. Where the dressing is used for the prevention of pressure sores it may be left in position for up to two weeks. When used as a cannula dressing, Opsite I.V. 3000 or Opsite CH may be left in position until the cannula is removed or changed, in accordance with good clinical practice.

Presentation

Opsite, Opsite I.V. 3000 and Opsite CH are presented individually wrapped in peel pouches, sterilised by ethylene oxide.

Opsite sheets

6.0 cm × 8.5 cm†	NSV No. ELW 031
10.0 cm × 10.0 cm	NSV No. ELW 013
10.0 cm × 14.0 cm*	NSV No. ELW 015
25.0 cm × 14.0 cm	NSV No. ELW 019

†Described as an IV dressing

Opsite I.V. 3000

6.0 cm × 8.0 cm	NSV No. ELW 037
6.0 cm × 8.5 cm	NSV No. ELW 039
10.0 cm × 14.0 cm	NSV No. ELW 041

Opsite CH sheets

6.0 cm × 8.0 cm	NSV No. ELW 053
10.0 cm × 14.0 cm	NSV No. ELW 055

Opsite CH cannula dressing
6.0 cm x 8.0 cm   NSV No. ELW 057

*Available on Drug Tariff.

ORTHOFLEX™

Classification Name
Bandage Plaster of Paris Elasticated

Manufacturer
Johnson & Johnson Orthopaedics

Product Description

Orthoflex consists of an elasticated gauze fabric that is coated with a blend of the alpha and beta forms of calcium sulphate hemihydrate (plaster of Paris), together with binders and accelerators. The fabric is held in a slightly pre-tensioned condition by the plaster mass; when the bandage is dipped into water, the tension is released and the elasticity that is inherent in the bandage ensures the formation of a close-fitting cast. Orthoflex can be used on its own or as the first layer in the production of a standard plaster of Paris cast.

The bandage is supplied wrapped around a plastic spool which allows rapid, even wetting of the bandage upon immersion. Once wet, the calcium sulphate hemihydrate is converted to the dihydrate, and the bandage sets to form a hard rigid structure, which is both porous and absorbent. The rate of setting is largely governed by the temperature of the water, but if the bandage is used in accordance with the manufacturer's intructions, an initial set will take place in about two minutes. After about 3−5 minutes, the cast should be fully set − although it may not achieve its maximum strength and become weight-bearing for up to 24−48 hours, depending upon its thickness. The principal disadvantages of Orthoflex lie in its weight, its opacity to X-rays, and its susceptibility to damage by moisture.

Indications

Orthoflex may be used for most orthopaedic applications, and other situations in which rigid immobilisation is required, including the management of fresh or unstable fractures. The enhanced conformability of the material is said to make it particularly suitable for use in mould making, and for holding manipulations and splinting soft tissue repairs.

Method of Use

Orthoflex should be applied over a layer of stockinette and orthopaedic padding. Prior to application, the first 10−15 cm of the bandage should be unrolled to enable the rapid location of the end after dipping. The bandage is held lightly in one hand, and immersed in a suitable container of water at a temperature of around 29°C, at an angle of 45°, for 3−5 seconds. After the bandage is removed from the container, any excess water is gently squeezed out. The bandage is then rolled evenly around the limb, without tension, avoiding the formation of wrinkles. The conformability of the bandage is such that the need for pleats or tucks is reduced. As each successive bandage is applied, it should be constantly moulded and smoothed with wet hands to ensure the formation of a homogeneous cast. Any areas of potential weakness may be strengthened by the addition of five or six layers of bandage, previously formed into a slab.

Warnings and Precautions

When applying a cast, it is important to ensure that all bony prominences are adequately padded, and operators should take care to ensure that no indentations are made in the soft plaster that could lead to the application of local areas of high pressure and the formation of plaster sores. Rough finishes on the edges of the cast should also be avoided. If the bandage is applied to a fresh fracture, sufficient padding should be used to accommodate any swelling of the limb. This is particularly important in view of the close-fitting nature of casts produced with Orthoflex.

Shelf Life and Storage Precautions

The unopened rolls of Orthoflex should be stored in a cool dry atmosphere.

Presentation

Orthoflex is presented as a roll, wrapped around a plastic core, and sealed in a water-resistant pouch.

4 in × 4 yd   NSV No. EAA 151
5 in × 5 yd   NSV No. EAA 153

PARATULLE™

Classification Name
Dressing Paraffin Gauze BP (Light Loading)

Manufacturer
Seton

Product Description

Paratulle consists of a leno-weave fabric of cotton or cotton and viscose, which has been impregnated with yellow soft paraffin. The dressing is used as a primary wound contact layer and the paraffin is present to reduce the adherence of the product to the surface of a granulating wound. Two formulations of Paraffin Gauze Dressing are described in the British Pharmacopoeia: they differ in the weight of paraffin base present on the gauze. Paratulle, which is an example of a 'light loading' product, contains between 90 and 130 grams of paraffin base per square metre of cloth. The alternative formulation bears a higher loading of paraffin, not less than 175 g/m² (see Jelonet™).

Indications

Paratulle is used as a primary wound contact layer in the treatment of burns, ulcers, skin grafts (both donor and receptor sites), and a variey of traumatic injuries.

Contra-indications

Although there are no absolute contra-indications to the use of Paratulle, if the dressing is placed upon a heavily exuding wound its semi-occlusive nature may cause tissue maceration by preventing the free movement of exudate away from the surface of the wound. This is less likely to occur than if a dressing bearing the higher loading of paraffin were to be used.

Method of Use

Paratulle is applied directly to the surface of the wound and covered with an absorbent pad held in place with tape or a bandage, as appropriate.

Frequency of Dressing Changes

The frequency of dressings changes will depend entirely upon the nature of the wound. If Paratulle is left in position for prolonged periods of time, it can become adherent and cause tissue damage upon removal.

Shelf Life and Storage Precautions

Paratulle should be stored in a cool place.

Presentation

Paratulle is presented individually wrapped in a paper/polyethylene peel pouch, sterilised by irradiation.

10 cm × 10 cm*   NSV No. EKA 071
10 cm × 40 cm   NSV No. EKA 077

*Available on Drug Tariff.

SCHERISORB™

Classification Name
Dressing Hydrogel Amorphous

Manufacturer
Smith & Nephew

Product Description

Scherisorb is a colourless to pale yellow transparent aqueous gel, which contains 2% of a modified co-polymer (derived from corn starch), together with propylene glycol as a humectant and preservative. When placed in contact with a wound, the dressing absorbs excess exudate and produces a moist environment at the surface of the wound, without causing tissue maceration.

Indications

Scherisorb may be applied to many different types of wound, including leg and decubitus ulcers. Recent experience has shown that it may also be useful in the management of extravasation injuries, especially in neonates. It is of particular value in the treatment of dry sloughy or necrotic wounds in which it promotes rapid debridement by facilitating rehydration and autolysis of dead tissue. In the management of granulating wounds, Scherisorb prevents desiccation, which facilitates re-epithelialisation and minimises scar formation. Early clinical evidence suggests that the gel can form a useful vehicle for the topical application of antimicrobial agents such as metronidazole. Such preparations may be used, in combination with systemic therapy, in the management of malodorous wounds infected with sensitive anaerobic bacteria.

Contra-indications

Although there are no known contra-indications to the use of Scherisorb as a topical wound dressing, the material is not ideally suited for application to wounds that are exuding very heavily.

Method of Use

Scherisorb should be introduced into the wound to a depth of approximately 5 mm, and covered with a sterile secondary dressing. The selection of the secondary dressing will be governed by the condition of the wound. If significant quantities of exudate are expected, a simple absorbent pad may be used, held in position with tape or a bandage, as appropriate. On lightly exuding wounds, a less permeable secondary dressing may be required, such as a perforated film absorbent dressing (Melolin™ or Telfa™, for example). If the wound is very dry, a more occlusive covering may be used to reduce water vapour loss and prevent the dressing drying out. In the management of extravasations in infants, the dressing may be retained on the wound in a suitably shaped plastic bag, forming a simple glove or boot.

Frequency of Dressing Changes

The interval between dressing changes will depend entirely upon the state of the wound. On heavily exuding or malodorous wounds, daily changes will be required; but on dry wounds, the dressing may be changed on alternate days. It is recommended that the dressing is not left for longer than three days between changes. At the discretion of the medical officer in charge, wounds that show evidence of clinical infection may be dressed with Scherisorb, which should be changed daily. Systemic antibiotic therapy may be commenced, as appropriate.

Warnings and Precautions

Scherisorb contains propylene glycol, which has been reported to be a potential irritant and sensitising agent in a very small number of patients. If a patient should exhibit any signs or symptoms of an adverse reaction to Scherisorb, treatment should be discontinued at once.

Scherisorb may cause a blue discoloration if used in conjunction with topical iodine products.

Each sachet should only be used for a single patient, and any unused gel should be discarded.

Shelf Life and Storage Precautions

Scherisorb should be stored in a cool dry place. The shelf life is three years.

Presentation

Scherisorb is presented individually packed in a laminated aluminium foil sachet, sterilised by autoclaving.

25 g sachet   NSV No. ELG 011
15 g sachet*   NSV No. ELG 013

*Available on Drug Tariff

SCOTCHCAST 2™
SCOTCHCAST PLUS™
SCOTCHFLEX™

Classification Name
Bandage Orthopaedic Resin

Manufacturer
3M

Product Description

Scotchcast 2 consists of a knitted fibreglass substrate impregnated with a polyurethane resin. Scotchcast Plus differs, in that a surface-modifying agent has been added to the resin. This makes the bandage less tacky to handle during application than the majority of synthetic casting materials, and results in a cast with a somewhat smoother surface. The base fabric used in both Scotchcast 2 and Scotchcast Plus is extensible in all directions, which makes the bandage very conformable in use. In Scotchflex, the polyurethane resin is carried on a lightweight knitted fibreglass substrate.

When Scotchcast 2, Scotchcast Plus, or Scotchflex is exposed to moisture vapour or immersed in water, the resin undergoes a polymerisation reaction, which causes the tape to harden and become rigid. A cast made from Scotchcast 2 will set in approximately 3–4 minutes, and be weight-bearing some 20 minutes after setting. Scotchcast Plus and Scotchflex have a slightly longer initial setting time, about 3–5 minutes.

The casts are lightweight, strong, porous, and translucent to X-rays.

Indications

Scotchcast 2 and Scotchcast Plus may be used in most situations where rigid immobilisation is required. These include the formation of standard orthopaedic casts and specialised prosthetic appliances.

Although Scotchflex may be used in most situations where rigid immobilisation is required, casts prepared entirely from this material do not have the same strength and load-bearing capabilities as some of the other fibreglass materials. Additional strength can be imparted by the inclusion of Scotchcast reinforcing strip, a heavy duty, wide-mesh fabric which is used for reinforcing casts.

Contra-indications

In common with all polyurethane casting tapes, Scotchcast 2, Scotchcast Plus, and Scotchflex should be applied with caution on fresh fractures where swelling of the injured limb may be anticipated (which could make rapid removal of the cast necessary).

Method of Use

Scotchcast 2, Scotchcast Plus, and Scotchflex should be applied over a layer of stockinette and orthopaedic padding. Although any suitable product may be used, some workers prefer to use non-absorbent materials based upon synthetic fibres such as polyester, rather than the cotton-based materials usually used in conjunction with plaster of Paris (which will retain moisture, should the final cast become wet).

Prior to application, the bandage should be immersed in water at 21–27°C, and squeezed several times under the surface to ensure complete penetration of water into the body of the bandage. If a slightly slower setting time is required, the bandage should be immersed in water for a couple of seconds only. The tack-reducing agent in Scotchcast Plus is also activated by water, so firm squeezing will enhance the ease of application of the bandage.

The tape should be applied in the form of a spiral, each turn overlapping the previous one by about one-third to one-half of the width of the tape. Three layers of Scotchcast 2 or Scotchcast Plus are usually sufficient in most non-weight-bearing situations, but four or five layers may be required at the heel and toe of a weight-bearing cast. If splints are required, these may be produced from three or four layers of tape. When Scotchflex is used, three or four layers of tape will usually suffice for a non-weight-bearing cast, but more will be required in a weight-bearing situation. Alternatively, a few layers of Scotchcast reinforcing tape may be included in the cast, to provide additional strength.

The cast may be moulded to its final shape during the last 30 seconds of its setting cycle, after which time it may be windowed or trimmed with shears or a standard cast saw. The casts may be repaired or reinforced by the application of additional tape. Although this will adhere successfully to the existing cast, a complete layer should be applied, if possible, to achieve the maximum adhesive bond.

Warnings and Precautions

Prior to setting, the polyurethane resin will adhere firmly to unprotected skin and clothing. Operators should always wear gloves when handling Scotchcast 2, Scotchcast Plus, or Scotchflex, and care should be taken to ensure that the uncured tape does not come into contact with the patient's skin. Once set, the cast is not adversely affected by moisture, but immersion of the cast in water is not recommended, as it may prove very difficult to dry the underlying padding. This in turn may lead to maceration and irritation of the skin.

If the cast is removed with a reciprocating cast saw, the use of dust extraction apparatus is advisable.

Shelf Life and Storage Precautions

The unopened rolls of casting tape should be stored in a cool dry atmosphere below 24°C. Above this temperature, the shelf life will be decreased.

Presentation

Scotchcast 2, Scotchcast Plus, and Scotchflex are all available in the form of a roll, wrapped around a hollow core, and heat-sealed in a poly/foil/poly laminate pouch.

Scotchcast 2

2 in × 4 yd   NSV No. EAF 231

3 in × 4 yd	NSV No. EAF 233
4 in × 4 yd	NSV No. EAF 235
5 in × 4 yd	NSV No. EAF 237

Scotchcast Plus

2 in × 4 yd	NSV No. EAF 331
3 in × 4 yd	NSV No. EAF 333
4 in × 4 yd	NSV No. EAF 335
5 in × 4 yd	NSV No. EAF 337

Scotchflex

2 in × 5 yd	NSV No. EAF 053
3 in × 5 yd	NSV No. EAF 055
4 in × 5 yd	NSV No. EAF 057
5 in × 5 yd	NSV No. EAF 059

SILASTIC™ FOAM

Classification Name

Dressing Silicone Foam Cavity Wound BP

Manufacturer

Dow Corning, distributed by Calmic

Product Description

Silastic Foam dressing is a two-part, room-temperature vulcanising foam, produced from a poly(dimethylsiloxane) base and a stannous octanoate catalyst, which react together to form a soft, pliable, slightly absorbent and non-adherent pale beige foam, which can be used to replace gauze packs or other dressings for certain defined applications. When cured, the final volume of the foam 'stent' is approximately four times that of the original mixture.

Indications

The use of Silastic Foam is indicated in the management of a variety of acute granulating and post-surgical wounds. It has been found to be particularly valuable after surgical excision of a pilonidal sinus, and in the management of other perianal and perineal wounds after surgery for cancer or inflammatory bowel disease. Its successful use has also been reported in the treatment of oro-cutaneous fistulae, hidradenitis suppurativa, sacral and trochanteric decubitus ulcers, and cases of abdominal wall breakdown.

Contra-indications

Silastic Foam should not be introduced into deep narrow wounds that might contain constrictions or hidden pockets or sinuses, as these could result in small pieces of the cured foam becoming detached, remaining undetected in the wound, and leading to problems later on.

Method of Use

Although the dressing is easy to use, it does differ significantly from traditional materials, and requires particular attention to the manufacture of the foam stent. The base and catalyst must be mixed in the ratio of 100:6 – full details of the technique involved are given on the insert that comes with each pack. The exact volumes of the two components used will depend upon the size of the wound, but for convenience, 10 mL of base and 0.6 mL of catalyst are frequently used. These volumes are taken up from the bulk container in appropriately sized syringes, transferred to a suitable mixing vessel, and stirred thoroughly for 15 seconds, before the resulting mixture is poured into the wound. If the foam is to be used after surgical excision, it is usual to pack the wound with a suitable gauze dressing for the first 2–3 days to produce a firm-walled cavity before instituting treatment with Silastic Foam.

Frequency of Dressing Changes

The dressing should be removed at least once a day and the wound cleansed with normal saline. For larger perineal or perianal wounds, the patient may be given a salt bath, where appropriate. The stent should be soaked in a 0.5% aqueous solution of chlorhexidine for 5–10 minutes, and rinsed thoroughly under running water, before being replaced into the wound. Antiseptic solutions containing cetrimide are not recommended. Each dressing may be used for up to a week – or even longer, depending upon circumstances – but as healing progresses, successively smaller stents will need to be produced.

Warnings and Precautions

The catalyst used in the production of Silastic Foam is an irritant, and should not be allowed to come into contact with skin or eyes.

Shelf Life and Storage Precautions

Silastic Foam should be stored in a cool place. The

shelf life is three years from the date of manufacture.

Presentation

20 g kit (for ward use)	NSV No. ELC 111
500 g kit	NSV No. ELC 113

SILASTIC™ GEL SHEETING

Classification Name
Dressing Sheet Silicone Gel

Manufacturer
Dow Corning, distributed by Calmic

Product Description

Silastic Gel Sheeting consists of a transparent sheet of an inert silicone gel, 3–4 mm thick, formed upon an open-mesh nylon net, which provides support and allows the material to be handled normally without disintegrating. The structure of the supporting net is such that the material is extensible in one direction, which imparts a degree of conformability to the product. The gel is impermeable to micro-organisms, and has a moisture vapour permeability of the order of 4.5 g/m^2/hour, which is approximately half that of normal skin. Although the dressing feels 'tacky', it does not leave adhesive residues on the surface of the skin, and will not remain in place without the aid of tape or a bandage.

Indications

Silastic Gel Sheeting may be applied to newly healed skin grafts, or other wounds, as soon as there is epithelial cover. The dressing prevents or reduces scar formation by controlling shrinkage and contracture. Existing hypertrophic scarring also responds to treatment: it has been shown that the affected tissue becomes flatter, relaxed, and less livid. Although Silastic Gel Sheeting has been shown to be of value in the treatment of hypertrophic scars, its precise mode of action is unknown; it is thought that it might be associated with the liberation of low molecular weight silicone fluid and the hydration of the stratum corneum, although this is by no means certain. Unlike previous treatments for hypertrophic scar formation, the product does not require the application of pressure with bandages or specially designed garments. The use of the dressing is also claimed to reduce the need for surgical release, and its early use is thought to prevent scarring from interfering with function. Although the product is primarily intended for application to raised scar tissue, there are some early indications that it may be of use in the treatment of depressed scars (although this remains to be confirmed in larger clinical studies).

Contra-indications

No absolute contra-indications to the use of Silastic Gel Sheeting have been reported, but it is recommended that it should not be applied to tissue until epithelial cover has been established.

Method of Use

Silastic Gel Sheeting is removed from the pack and laid onto the affected area. Depending upon the site, it may be held in position with adhesive tape, a bandage, or a piece of dressing retention sheet (such as Hypafix™ or Mefix™). In areas that are difficult to dress, such as anatomical depressions, the dressing may be stuck in position with Dow Corning medical adhesive. The sheeting can be washed in mild soap solution, rinsed in clean water, and reused. The scar area should be cleansed 12-hourly using clean warm water. Silastic Gel Sheeting may be left in place upon mature scar tissue for 24 hours a day, but in the management of newly healed wounds, the sheeting should be applied initially for about eight hours per day, gradually increasing up to 24 hours over a period of two weeks. If continuous application of the dressing is impractical, it may be applied for 12-hourly periods, to good effect.

Frequency of Dressing Changes

If the the washing instructions are carefully followed, it should be possible to reuse the dressing for 4–7 days on flexion sites and 7–14 days on flat sites, although this will depend upon the nature and position of the scar.

Presentation

Silastic Gel Sheeting is presented individually wrapped in a plastic peel pouch, sterilised by irradiation.

14.5 cm × 12 cm   NSV No. ELY 011

SOFRA-TULLE™

Classification Name
Dressing Framycetin Gauze BP

Manufacturer
Roussel

Product Description

Sofra-Tulle consists of a cotton leno-weave fabric, impregnated with a base composed of white soft paraffin, anhydrous lanolin, and 1.0% w/w framycetin sulphate. Framycetin is an antibiotic of the aminoglycoside group with a wide spectrum of antibacterial activity. Organisms sensitive to framycetin include *Staphylococcus aureus, Escherischia coli, Klebsiella* species, and some strains of *Pseudomonas aeruginosa;* it is not active against yeasts, fungi or viruses. The dressing is used as a primary wound contact layer in the management of infected wounds, combining low adherence with antimicrobial activity.

Indications

Sofra-Tulle may be used in the management of a variety of infected wounds, including minor traumatic injuries, ulcers, burns, and other lesions that are clinically infected by organisms shown to be sensitive to framycetin.

Contra-indications

Sofra-Tulle is contra-indicated in patients who are allergic to lanolin, or who have previously demonstrated a sensitivity to framycetin, neomycin, or any other chemically related product. The dressing should not be used in the treatment of wounds that are free of clinical infection, or infected by organisms that are resistant to the antibiotic.

Method of Use

The wound should be cleansed with a suitable sterile solution, such as normal saline; a single layer of Sofra-Tulle should then be applied and covered with an absorbent pad, held in place with tape or a bandage, as appropriate. When used to dress ulcers, Sofra-Tulle should be shaped to fit the crater and not allowed to extend over the surrounding skin.

Frequency of Dressing Changes

The frequency of dressing changes will depend entirely upon the nature of the wound, but infected wounds that are exuding heavily should be dressed at least once a day.

Warnings and Precautions

Cross-sensitisation to framycetin may occur in patients known to be allergic to chemically related antibiotics (such as neomycin and kanamycin). In normal use, absorption of the antibiotic from Sofra-Tulle is negligible; however, where large areas of the body are being treated, the possibility of ototoxicity caused by prolonged application should be borne in mind.

Shelf Life and Storage Precautions

Sofra-Tulle should be stored in a cool place.

Presentation

Sofra-Tulle is presented individually wrapped in an aluminium peel pouch, manufactured under aseptic conditions.

10 cm × 10 cm*	NSV No. EKB 051 (PL No. 0109/5047R)
10 cm × 30 cm	NSV No. EKB 053 (PL No. 0109/5047R)

*Available on Drug Tariff.

Legal Category

Prescription Only Medicine [POM]

SORBSAN™
SORBSAN PLUS™
SORBSAN SA™

Classification Name
Sorbsan – Dressing Calcium Alginate
Sorbsan Plus – Dressing Calcium Alginate and Viscose
Sorbsan SA – Dressing Calcium Alginate Foam Backed Adhesive

Manufacturer
Steriseal

Product Description

Sorbsan is made from the calcium salt of alginic acid, prepared as a textile fibre, and presented as a rope (for packing cavities), a ribbon (for narrow wounds or sinuses), and a flat non-woven pad (for application to larger open wounds). When in contact with serum, wound exudate, or solutions containing sodium ions, the insoluble calcium alginate is partially converted to the soluble sodium salt, and a hydrophilic gel is produced, which overlays the wound and provides a micro-environment that facilitates wound healing.

Sorbsan Plus consists of a layer of alginate fibre bonded on to an absorbent viscose pad which in turn is backed with a pink viscose/polyester layer to indicate the outer surface of the dressing.

Sorbsan SA consists of a layer of alginate fibre bonded centrally onto a thin sheet of polyurethane foam, which is coated with an acrylic adhesive to form a self-adhesive island dressing. Although the foam is permeable to water vapour, it has the effect of reducing moisture vapour loss from the surface of a lightly exuding wound and thus prevents the dressing from drying out.

Indications

Sorbsan sheets may be applied to a wide range of exuding lesions including leg ulcers, pressure areas, donor sites, and most other granulating wounds but for deeper cavity wounds and sinuses, the rope and ribbon forms are generally more suitable. Sorbsan Plus has the same general indications as the plain Sorbsan sheet but is particularly indicated for heavily exuding lesions. Sorbsan SA should be reserved for lightly exuding wounds which are unsuitable for treatment with a plain alginate sheet.

Contra-indications

Although there are no known contra-indications to the use of Sorbsan, all types will be of little value if applied to wounds that are very dry, or covered with hard black necrotic tissue.

Method of Use

Sorbsan is placed onto the surface of the wound and covered with a sterile dressing pad held in place with surgical tape or a bandage as appropriate. The selection of the secondary dressing will be governed by the condition of the wound. If large quantities of exudate are anticipated, a simple absorbent dressing pad will be required; but as the wound heals and less exudate is produced, a thinner pad bearing a low adherence plastic film may help to conserve moisture and prevent the wound drying out too quickly. Alternatively, in the early stages of treatment Sorbsan Plus may be applied to the wound, held in place with tape or a suitable bandage; secondary dressings are not usually required because of the extra absorbency imparted by the integral absorbent pad. As the wound heals and exudate production diminishes, Sorbsan Plus may be replaced by Sorbsan SA to conserve moisture and prevent the wound from drying out. Deeper cavity wounds or sinuses may be dressed with Sorbsan rope or ribbon, which should be placed gently in position but not packed in too tightly.

Because the alginate fibre reacts with sodium ions to form a soluble gel, the dressing may be removed by irrigation with sterile normal saline, which may be accomplished without causing damage to the wound or pain to the patient.

It has been reported that a small percentage of patients experience a mild 'drawing' or 'burning' sensation immediately after the application of an alginate dressing to a dry wound bed. This sensation, which is usually transient, is thought to be due to the hydrophilic nature of the dressing causing temporary localised drying of the surface of the wound. In most instances, this discomfort may be prevented by moistening the surface of the wound with a small quantity of sterile normal saline immediately prior to the application of the dressing.

Frequency of Dressing Changes

The interval between dressing changes will depend entirely upon the state of the wound and the type of dressing chosen. Sorbsan or Sorbsan Plus applied to heavily exuding or sloughy wounds may need replacing daily at the beginning of treatment but as healing progresses and the amount of exudate decreases, the interval between changes may be extended to two or three days. Clean wounds in the final stages of the healing process should be dressed with Sorbsan SA. A translucent bubble visible through the back of the foam indicates that a change is required although on low exudate wounds the dressing may often be left in place for up to a week.

Wounds that show signs of clinical infection

may be dressed with Sorbsan or Sorbsan Plus, which should be changed daily; systemic antibiotic therapy should be initiated at the discretion of the medical officer in charge.

Presentation

The dressings are presented individually packed in peel pouches, sterilised by ethylene oxide.

Sorbsan

5 cm × 5 cm*	NSV No. ELS 209
10 cm × 10 cm	NSV No. ELS 211
10 cm × 20 cm	NSV No. ELS 215
Packing 30 cm long	NSV No. ELS 213
Ribbon 40 cm long	NSV No. ELS 217

Sorbsan Plus

7.5 cm × 10 cm	NSV No. ELS 271
10 cm × 15 cm	NSV No. ELS 273

Sorbsan SA

9 cm × 11 cm	NSV No. ELS 311

*Available on Drug Tariff

TEGADERM™
TEGADERM PLUS™

Classification Name

Tegaderm – Dressing Semipermeable Adhesive BP

Tegaderm Plus – Dressing Semipermeable Adhesive Medicated

Manufacturer

3M

Product Description

Tegaderm consists of a thin polyurethane membrane coated with a layer of an acrylic adhesive. The dressing, which is permeable to both water vapour and oxygen, is impermeable to micro-organisms; once in position, it provides an effective barrier to external contamination, whilst producing a moist environment at the surface of the wound by reducing water vapour loss from the exposed tissue. Under these conditions in shallow wounds, scab formation is prevented and epidermal regeneration takes place at an enhanced rate, compared with that which occurs in wounds treated with traditional dry dressings. Tegaderm Plus differs from Tegaderm in that the adhesive contains 2% available iodine in the form of an iodophor. In contact with skin, the iodophor slowly releases iodine, which has bactericidal activity and provides protection against infection.

Indications

Tegaderm may be used in the treatment of minor burns, pressure areas, donor sites, post-operative wounds, and a variety of minor injuries (including abrasions and lacerations). It is also used as a protective cover to prevent skin breakdown due to friction or continuous exposure to moisture. Tegaderm and Tegaderm Plus are used to retain peripheral and central IV catheters. The transparent nature of the dressing allows the site to be constantly monitored for signs of infection, leakage or catheter misplacement.

Contra-indications

Although there are no absolute contra-indications to the use of Tegaderm, it is not recommended that the material be applied over deep cavity wounds, third degree burns, or wounds that show evidence of clinical infection. The dressing should not be used to retain in-dwelling arterial catheters. Tegaderm Plus should not be applied to patients who are known or suspected to be sensitive to iodine.

Method of Use

Tegaderm utilises a novel system to facilitate application of the dressing to the surface of the wound. The film is enclosed between two liners: on the adhesive surface is a printed sheet of release paper, and on the outer, non-adhesive surface is a slightly more rigid sheet of thin card. The central portion of the card may be removed, leaving the film suspended on a frame, which facilitates easy precise placement of the dressing and reduces wrinkling. Once in position, the frame is removed and the film is lightly smoothed into position. In order to ensure good adhesion, the dressing should be allowed a minimum overlap of 4–5 cm from the margin of the wound onto the surrounding dry skin. On clean, heavily exuding wounds, such as donor sites, large quantities of fluid sometimes accumulate beneath the film. This should be left undisturbed as far as possible, but if the accumulation becomes excessive, it may be aspirated with a syringe using an aseptic technique. A small patch of Tegaderm should be applied over the puncture to prevent leakage or contamination.

When Tegaderm or Tegaderm Plus is used to dress a cannula site, the area should first be cleansed with alcohol or saline and carefully dried, ensuring that all traces of creams or detergents have been removed.

Frequency of Dressing Changes

In general, Tegaderm should not be left in position for longer than seven days. This is particularly important where the dressing is being used to retain an intravenous catheter.

Provided there is no evidence of infection or any other problem, Tegaderm Plus may be left in position for an extended period, or until the catheter is removed or changed, in accordance with good nursing practice.

Presentation

Tegaderm and Tegaderm Plus are presented individually wrapped in peel pouches, sterilised by gamma irradiation.

Tegaderm

6 cm × 7 cm†	NSV No. ELW 221
6 cm × 7 cm	NSV No. ELW 211
10 cm × 12 cm*	NSV No. ELW 213
10 cm × 25 cm	NSV No. ELW 215
15 cm × 20 cm	NSV No. ELW 217
20 cm × 30 cm	NSV No. ELW 219

†Described as an IV dressing, as the design facilitates placement over intravenous catheter hubs
*Available on Drug Tariff

Tegaderm Plus

6 cm × 8 cm	NSV No. ELW 711
10 cm × 15 cm	NSV No. ELW 713

TELFA™

Classification Name
Dressing Perforated Film Absorbent BP (Type 2)

Manufacturer
Kendall

Product Description

Telfa consists of a thin layer of absorbent cotton fibres, enclosed in a sleeve of poly(ethylene terephthalate) that is perforated in a regular pattern and sealed along two edges. The plastic film is present to prevent the dressing adhering to the surface of the wound, and is perforated to allow the passage of exudate from the wound into the body of the pad.

Indications

Telfa may be used on its own to dress dry sutured wounds, superficial cuts and abrasions, and other lightly exuding wounds. It may also be used as the primary wound contact layer for more heavily exuding wounds, if backed by a second absorbent dressing.

Contra-indications

In common with other perforated plastic film dressings, Telfa should be used with caution in the treatment of leg ulcers that produce copious quantities of very viscous exudate, which may be unable to pass through the small holes in the film. Under these circumstances, the exudate may become trapped under the dressing, leading to maceration and inflammation of the surrounding skin.

Method of Use

Telfa has a low absorbent capacity and is therefore intended for use on wounds that do not produce large amounts of exudate. Under these circumstances, a single dressing may simply be secured in position with surgical tape. On more heavily exuding wounds, Telfa may be used as a wound contact layer, beneath a secondary absorbent pad held in position with tape or a bandage.

Frequency of Dressing Changes

The frequency with which the dressing should be changed depends entirely upon the nature and condition of the wound.

Presentation

Telfa is available in two forms: individually wrapped in paper peel pouches, sterilised by ethylene oxide; or as a dressing with the perforated film on one side only, supplied in bulk, non-sterile.

Individually wrapped

5 cm × 7.5 cm	NSV No. EJE 051
10 cm × 7.5 cm	NSV No. EJE 053

15 cm × 7.5 cm   NSV No. EJE 055
20 cm × 7.5 cm   NSV No. EJE 057

Bulk
20 cm × 7.5 cm   NSV No. EJE 071
25 cm × 20 cm   NSV No. EJE 073

TENSOPRESS™

Classification Name
Bandage Compression

Manufacturer
Smith & Nephew

Product Description

Tensopress consists of a warp-knitted bandage composed of cotton and viscose, incorporating elastomeric threads made from polyurethane. A yellow line runs up the centre of the bandage. The fabric is soft and light, and possesses a degree of lateral extensibility that makes the product very conformable and easy to apply. Tensopress is highly elastic, by virtue of the elastomeric threads, which also give it considerable 'power'. If required, Tensopress may be washed repeatedly without affecting its performance significantly.

Indications

Tensopress is one of the more powerful compression bandages available, and may be used to apply a wide range of sub-bandage pressures. It is primarily intended for the application of controlled levels of pressure in the treatment of venous ulcers and other conditions where compression therapy is required, such as sclerotherapy. Because the bandage has the ability to 'follow in', or maintain compression on limbs as they decrease in circumference, it can be used to reduce existing gross oedema, unlike products made from cotton or lightweight nylon fabrics.

Contra-indications

Because of the power inherent in the bandage, care must be taken to ensure that it is not applied with excessive tension. The pressure that is produced beneath Tensopress will not decrease significantly with time, unlike that beneath a cotton bandage.

All extensible bandages should be used with caution on patients who have marked ischaemia or impaired arterial blood supply, but the incorrect use of Tensopress in these situations could have very serious consequences.

Method of Use

When Tensopress is used to apply support or compression, the leg should be positioned with the knee flexed and the foot at right angles to the leg. With the bulk roll facing upwards, a single turn should be made around the ankle and down over the top of the foot and around the base of the toes. A second turn is then made over the top of the foot and down to cover the heel. After making a further turn around the ankle, the application is completed with a simple spiral up the leg, using the yellow line in the centre of the bandage as a guide for the overlap. Once in place, the bandage may be fastened with clips, tapes, or pins, as appropriate. Care should be taken to ensure that the bandage does not cause a tourniquet effect at the knee, and the operator should ensure that a pressure gradient exists beneath the bandage, with the highest levels of pressure at the ankle.

Frequency of Dressing Changes

Provided the bandage has been correctly applied and does not become displaced, it will continue to apply the desired levels of compression over an extended period. However, it is sometimes recommended that high performance products such as Tensopress should be removed at night and reapplied before the patient gets out of bed in the morning.

Presentation

Tensopress is presented individually boxed.

7.5 cm × 3 m   NSV No. EBA 075
10.0 cm × 3 m   NSV No. EBA 077

TRANSITE™

Classification Name
Dressing Permeable Plastic Film

Manufacturer
Smith & Nephew

Product Description

Transite consists of two layers of thin plastic sheet bonded together to form a transparent film. The dressing is perforated by a series of narrow slits arranged in rows, through which exudate may pass into an absorbent pad placed upon the outer surface of the film. One of the polymers used in the construction of the dressing is hydrophilic, the other is hydrophobic. When placed upon a heavily exuding wound, the hydrophilic component of the film takes up moisture and swells; this causes changes to take place in the geometry of the slits, which effectively open up, facilitating the removal of wound exudate. As the wound heals and the amount of exudate decreases, the hydrophilic layer dries out and the slits revert to their original shape. This process results in the maintenance of a controlled environment at the surface of the wound, which is conducive to wound healing. The smooth continuous surface of the film will not adhere to a granulating wound, and hence will not cause pain or trauma upon removal. Transite itself is not adhesive, but is held in position by means of two self-adhesive handles located on opposite edges of the dressing.

Indications

Transite is recommended for use on heavily exuding wounds, such as donor sites and burns, where marked changes in the rate of exudate formation may be anticipated as healing progresses.

Contra-indications

No absolute contra-indications to the use of Transite have been reported.

Method of Use

An appropriate size of Transite is chosen, and the paper backing removed from one of the handles, which is pressed firmly into position. The backing is then removed from the second handle, and, without applying any tension to the film, the dressing is laid gently over the wound and fastened into place. During the application process, it is important to ensure that the film is not stretched, or the slits will be opened and Transite will be unable to function correctly. A suitable absorbent dressing pad is placed on the back of the film and held in place with tape or a bandage, as appropriate. When the absorbent layer requires changing, this may be done without disturbing the wound contact layer; in theory, this may be left in position until the wound is completely healed.

Frequency of Dressing Changes

The absorbent dressing pad should be changed as often as circumstances dictate, depending upon the condition of the wound; but unless there is a good clinical reason for removing the Transite film, it should be left undisturbed for as long as possible.

Presentation

Transite is presented individually wrapped in a peel pouch, sterilised by ethylene oxide.

10 cm × 10 cm	NSV No. ELW 731
15 cm × 20 cm	NSV No. ELW 733
30 cm × 40 cm	NSV No. ELW 735

TRANSPORE™

Classification Name
Tape Permeable Plastic Surgical Synthetic Adhesive BP

Manufacturer
3M

Product Description

Transpore consists of an extensible, perforated plastic film composed of low density polyethylene, coated with a layer of an acrylic adhesive. The perforations in the tape serve a dual function: they allow the passage of water vapour from the skin (reducing the possibility of maceration and bacterial proliferation), and enable the tape to be torn easily in both directions. Transpore can be worn in the bath or shower, but after exposure to wet conditions it should be patted dry with a towel. The permeability of the dressing is such that its performance is unlikely to be significantly affected by sweating.

The tape is radio-transparent, and may be sterilised by ethylene oxide. It is suggested that, if sterile tape is required, strips are removed from the roll and laid over a suitable carrier for introduction into the chamber of the ethylene oxide steriliser. It is important to ensure that any tape so sterilised is adequately aerated before use.

Sterilisation of intact rolls of tape is not recommended.

Indications

Although Transpore may be used for most general purpose applications, its elasticity and flexibility make it particularly well suited for securing dressings on areas that are subject to movement, and for securing catheters, and anaesthetic and other forms of surgical tubing. As the tape is coated with an acrylic adhesive system, it may generally be used on patients who have exhibited an adverse reaction to adhesives based upon zinc oxide, rubber, or resin.

Contra-indications

Although there are no absolute contra-indications to the use of Transpore, it should (like most tapes) be used with caution on patients who have very fragile skin, such as those on long-term steroid therapy.

Warnings and Special Precautions

It should not be necessary to use skin tackifiers, such as tincture of benzoin, with Transpore. The tape is both extensible and elastic, which makes it well suited for anchoring tubes or dressings to difficult body contours. If applied with excess tension, however, the elastic regain in the tape could lead to the production of a tourniquet effect, or cause damage to the skin by shearing. As with all plastic tapes, Transpore should be applied with the minimum possible tension.

Shelf Life and Storage Precautions

In common with all adhesive products, Transpore should be stored in a dry place, and not subjected to extremes of temperature.

Presentation

1.25 cm × 9.14 m	NSV No. EHA 011
2.50 cm × 9.14 m	NSV No. EHA 013
5.00 cm × 9.14 m	NSV No. EHA 015
7.50 cm × 9.14 m	NSV No. EHA 017

VEINOPLAST™
VEINOPRESS™

Classification Name

Veinopress – Bandage Light Pressure and Support
Veinoplast – Bandage Elastic Synthetic Adhesive

Manufacturer

Molinier, distributed by Steriseal

Product Description

Veinopress consists of a pink-coloured woven fabric, the weft threads of which are made of cotton, and the warp threads of false-twist nylon and elastane (which together impart a high degree of elasticity to the bandage). Veinopress may be washed repeatedly without any adverse effect upon its performance.

Veinoplast is based upon the same fabric, with the addition of a thin layer of an acrylic adhesive.

Indications

Unlike bandages manufactured entirely from cotton and other non-elastomeric fibres, Veinopress and Veinoplast are capable of applying and maintaining significant levels of sub-bandage pressure. Using standard application techniques, either product may be expected to achieve maximum pressures of the order of 35 mmHg at the ankle and 25 mmHg at the calf, assuming a limb of average proportions. The bandages are suitable for the management of venous insufficiency and the control of oedema. They are also used for the application of pressure and support in the treatment of sprains and strains, and varicose veins, and as an aid to rehabilitation following orthopaedic surgery. Veinopress may also be used with advantage, in conjunction with a suitable primary dressing, in the treatment of varicose ulcers.

Contra-indications

Although Veinopress and Veinoplast are suitable for the application of relatively high levels of sub-bandage pressure to normal limbs, they are not ideally suited for the application of such pressures to large limbs that are also grossly oedematous. For these and similar indications, where the highest levels of pressure are required, more powerful products are available. In common with all extensible bandages, Veinopress and Veinoplast should be used with caution on patients who have marked ischaemia or impaired arterial blood supply, and care should be taken to ensure that the bandage is not applied with excessive tension. Veinoplast should also be used with caution on patients who have previously demonstrated a sensitivity reaction to other products bearing acrylic adhesives.

Method of Use

When used to apply support or compression to a leg, the bandage should be held with the bulk roll facing upwards. Working from the inner aspect of the leg, a single turn should be made over the top of the foot around the base of the toes to secure the bandage, and a second turn taken up to the base of the heel. After making a figure-of-eight around the ankle, the bandage should be applied up the leg, with each turn overlapping the previous one by 50%. Once in place, Veinopress may be fastened with clips or tape, as appropriate. Veinoplast does not require further securing. Care should be taken to ensure that the bandage does not cause a tourniquet effect at the knee, and the operator should ensure that a pressure gradient exists beneath the bandage, with the highest levels of pressure at the ankle. If localized areas of higher pressure are required (following sclerotherapy, for example), the bandage may be used in conjunction with foam wedges. In these circumstances, care should be taken to ensure that the pressure applied is not sufficient to cause local tissue damage.

Frequency of Dressing Changes

In very critical applications where the control of sub-bandage pressure is important, the bandage should be replaced (or, for Veinopress, reapplied) as frequently as practicable; in most other situations, the bandage may be left undisturbed for a number of days. Some decrease in sub-bandage pressure is inevitable, but this will be less with Veinoplast than with Veinopress. Veinopress, in turn, produces sub-bandage pressures that persist for longer than those under traditional crêpe-type products.

Presentation

Veinopress and Veinoplast are individually boxed.

Veinopress

8 cm × 3 m (unstretched)	NSV No. ECA 451
10 cm × 3 m (unstretched)	NSV No. ECA 453

Veinoplast

8 cm × 3 m (unstretched)	NSV No. ECJ 051
10 cm × 3 m (unstretched)	NSV No. ECJ 053

VIGILON™

Classification Name
Dressing Hydrogel Sheet

Manufacturer
Bard, distributed by Seton

Product Description

Vigilon is a hydrogel sheet, consisting of cross-linked polyethylene oxide, and containing 96% water, supported upon a net of low density polyethylene, which provides strength. The gel, which is capable of absorbing approximately its own weight of wound exudate, is permeable to water vapour and oxygen, but impermeable to water and bacteria. The dressing provides a moist environment upon the surface of the wound in which healing can take place; provided it is not allowed to dry out, it will not adhere to the underlying tissue upon removal.

Indications

Vigilon may be used in the treatment of a variety of wounds in which there has been limited epidermal damage, such as dermabrasions, minor burns, and superficial pressure areas. The dressing is cool and soothing to the touch and is said to reduce local pain and discomfort in some types of injury.

Contra-indications

Vigilon should not be used on wounds that are exuding heavily, or as a covering for cavities or sinuses.

Method of Use

When Vigilon is removed from the pack, it is covered on both surfaces with a sheet of poly-ethylene film. One sheet of film is removed before use, and the gel placed directly in contact with the wound. The second sheet (on the outer surface of the dressing) may be left in position to conserve moisture, if the wound is relatively dry; on a wound that produces significant quantities of exudate, the second sheet should be removed to facilitate the passage of water vapour through the gel, and prevent tissue maceration due to excessive fluid build-up. Once applied, the dressing is usually covered with an absorbent pad held in place with tape or a bandage, as appropriate. For lightly exuding wounds on areas that are difficult to dress with Vigilon, such as the sacral region, a dressing retention sheet (such as Hypafix™ or Mefix™) may be used to form an island dressing. On dry wounds, there is sometimes a possibility that the dressing will dry out. If this occurs, Vigilon may be readily rehydrated with sterile water or normal saline prior to removal.

Frequency of Dressing Changes

The frequency of dressing changes will depend entirely upon the nature and condition of the wound. On clean, lightly exuding wounds, the dressing may be left undisturbed for 3–4 days, or sometimes longer; but on more heavily exuding wounds, daily changes may be required.

Warnings and Precautions

Vigilon should not be applied to wounds that have been found to contain *Pseudomonas aeruginosa*, or that show evidence of clinical infection.

Shelf Life and Storage Precautions

Vigilon should be stored in a cool place.

Presentation

Vigilon is presented in a plastic pouch, sterilised by ethylene oxide, inside a non-sterile aluminium peel pouch.

4 in × 4 in   NSV No. ELE 051
6 in × 3 in   NSV No. ELE 053

Surgical Dressings Classification and Cross-reference Indexes

The classification reproduced below attempts to bring together products that are similar in performance, or used for similar indications, and forms the basis of section E of the nationally agreed National Supplies Vocabulary (NSV) used in the National Health Service. In this system, a simple primary classification is followed by a more detailed breakdown of all the products that come under the major heading. Although the full NSV records data on all dressings (including generic products such as cotton wool and gauzes) together with information on the sizes of the products concerned, much of this has been omitted from these cross-reference lists for the sake of clarity and simplicity.

The classification is followed by a cross-reference index that lists products by classification code, effectively grouping together products that are similar in function or use. Additional indexes list the dressings by generic name (generally that of the British Pharmacopoeia) and by proprietary or trade name. An index of the products of each manufacturer is followed by a list of manufacturers' addresses and telephone numbers.

By using these cross-reference indexes, it is possible for a purchasing department to identify the nature or function of an unfamiliar dressing, and to check whether an alternative material may already be available in stock. For example, if Fixomull Stretch is requested, it will be found by reference to the proprietary name index that this is known as 'Tape Apertured Non-woven Surgical Synthetic Adhesive'. In the generic listing, four other products have this same description, one of which may already be available in stock and therefore be offered as an alternative.

Classification of Dressings

BANDAGES

Orthopaedic casting materials — EA –

Bandages plaster of Paris	EAA
Bandages plaster of Paris resin reinforced	EAB
Bandages synthetic resin (moisture cured)	EAF
Bandages synthetic resin (heat cured)	EAJ
Bandages polyurethane foam based	EAK

Compression bandages — EB –

One-way stretch	EBA
Two-way stretch	EBB

Bandages for providing light pressure and support — EC –

Plain fabric based	ECA
Foam based	ECB
Cohesive	ECD
Self-adhesive (rubber-based adhesive)	ECG
Self-adhesive (synthetic adhesive)	ECJ
Self-adhesive (diachylon adhesive)	ECK

Extensible bandages used for dressing retention — ED –

Cotton conforming	EDA
Conforming stretch	EDB
Conforming stretch (cohesive)	EDG

Non-extensible retention/support bandages — EE –

Roll	EEA
Shaped/preformed (woven)	EED
Shaped/preformed (non-woven)	EEG
Suspensory	EEJ

Paste bandages — EF –

Bandages with zinc and/or other medicaments	EFA

TUBULAR BANDAGES/STOCKINETTES — EG –

Light pressure and support

Bandages tubular elastic plain	EGA

Bandages tubular elastic shaped	EGB
Garments produced from tubular elastic bandages	EGC

Support and protection

Bandages tubular elastic with foam pad	EGG

Retention and protection

Stockinettes	EGJ
Stockinette lightweight	EGP

Retention only

Bandages tubular net	EGT
Garments produced from tubular net bandages	EGU

SURGICAL TAPES   EH –

Plastic film backing

Permeable plastic synthetic adhesive	EHA
Semipermeable plastic synthetic adhesive	EHB
Occlusive plastic synthetic adhesive	EHC
Permeable plastic rubber-based adhesive	EHF
Semipermeable plastic rubber-based adhesive	EHG
Occlusive plastic rubber-based adhesive	EHH

Woven fabric backing

Permeable woven synthetic adhesive	EHK
Occlusive woven synthetic adhesive	EHL
Permeable woven rubber-based adhesive	EHO
Occlusive woven rubber-based adhesive	EHP
Elastic woven rubber-based adhesive	EHQ

Non-woven fabric backing

Apertured non-woven synthetic adhesive	EHR
Permeable non-woven synthetic adhesive	EHU

Foam based

Permeable foam backed synthetic adhesive	EHX

ADHESIVE DRESSINGS   EI –

Dressings with integral absorbent pad

Plastic backed synthetic adhesive	EIA
Plastic backed synthetic adhesive electromagnetically detectable	EIB

Plastic backed rubber-based adhesive	EIC
Plastic backed rubber-based adhesive electromagnetically detectable	EID
Woven fabric backed synthetic adhesive	EIG
Woven fabric backed rubber-based adhesive	EIH
Non-woven fabric backed synthetic adhesive	EIJ

Dressing strips with integral absorbent pad

Plastic backed synthetic adhesive	EIL
Plastic backed rubber-based adhesive	EIM
Fabric backed synthetic adhesive	EIO
Fabric backed rubber-based adhesive	EIP
Non-woven fabric backed synthetic adhesive	EIQ

Wound closures

Non-woven/fabric based plain	EIR
Non-woven/fabric based medicated	EIS
Plastic based plain	EIT
Plastic based medicated	EIU

Adhesive plasters

Self-adhesive	EIX

WOUND MANAGEMENT PRODUCTS

Wound dressing pads   EJ –

Absorbent high exudate	EJA
Absorbent low exudate	EJB
Absorbent low adherence face low exudate	EJE
Absorbent low adherence face high exudate	EJF
Wound dressing pads with integral bandage (standard dressings)	EJI
Dressings absorbent drain/intravenous	EJK

Wound contact materials low adherence   EK –

Dressings 'tulle gras' type fabric unmedicated	EKA
Dressings 'tulle gras' type fabric medicated	EKB
Dressings knitted fabric	EKG

Absorbent/interactive wound management products   EL –

Dressings foam preformed	ELA
Dressings foam formed *in situ*	ELC
Dressings hydrogel sheet	ELE
Dressings hydrogel sheet medicated	ELF

Dressings hydrogel amorphous	ELG	Cotton applicators	ENV
Dressings hydrogel amorphous medicated	ELH	Foam	ENW
Dressings hydrogel formed *in situ*	ELI		
Dressings hydrogel formed *in situ* medicated	ELJ	*Maternity/sanitary products*	EO–
Dressings hydrocolloid sheet	ELM	Maternity/sanitary pads plain	EOA
Dressings hydrocolloid sheet medicated	ELN	Maternity/sanitary pads looped	EOB
Dressings hydrocolloid amorphous	ELO	Maternity/sanitary pads with adhesive strip	EOC
Dressings hydrocolloid amorphous medicated	ELP	Tampons	EOF
Dressings absorbable haemostatic	ELS		
Polysaccharide beads/granules	ELT		
Polysaccharide beads/granules medicated	ELU		
Dressings containing activated charcoal	ELV	**PROTECTIVES**	
Dressings film	ELW		
Biological products	ELX	*Orthopaedic wadding*	EP–
Miscellaneous	ELY	Cellulose based autoclavable	EPA
		Cellulose based non-autoclavable	EPB
		Synthetic fibre based autoclavable	EPE
SURGICAL ABSORBENTS		Synthetic fibre based non-autoclavable	EPF
		Foam based	EPH
Surgical absorbents X-ray-detectable	EM–		
		Eye pads	EQ–
Ribbon gauze	EMA	Plain	EQA
Ribbon gauze coloured	EMB	Adhesive	EQB
Gauze/fabric rolls	EME	Eye pads with integral bandage	EQC
Gauze/fabric throat packs coloured	EMG		
Gauze/fabric swabs	EMI	*Chiropodial/surgical protectives*	ER–
Gauze/fabric swabs coloured	EMJ	Felts plain compressed	ERA
Gauze/fabric swabs stitched	EMM	Felts plain semi-compressed	ERB
Gauze/fabric swabs stitched with tapes	EMQ	Felts plain soft	ERC
Pledgets	EMU	Felts adhesive compressed	ERF
Neuropatties woven	EMV	Felts adhesive semi-compressed	ERG
Neuropatties non-woven	EMW	Felts adhesive soft	ERH
		Foam padding plain	ERJ
Surgical/clinical absorbents		Foam padding adhesive	ERK
non-X-ray-detectable	EN–	Tubular foam bandages	ERN
		Miscellaneous chiropodial protectives	ERP
Ribbon gauze	ENA		
Gauze/fabric rolls	ENE		
Swabs gauze/fabric woven	ENI		
Swabs gauze/fabric woven filmated	ENJ	**ORTHOPAEDIC PRODUCTS**	ES–
Swabs non-woven fabric	ENK		
Swabs non-woven fabric filmated	ENL	Traction kits rubber-based adhesive	ESA
Gauze and cellulose wadding	ENM	Traction kits synthetic adhesive	ESB
Gauze and cotton tissue	ENN	Traction kits non-adhesive	ESC
Nursing/breast pads	ENO	Extension plasters zinc oxide adhesive	ESE
Dental napkins/rolls/throat packs	ENP	Extension plasters synthetic adhesive	ESF
Cellulose wadding	ENQ	Bandages skin traction foam	ESJ
Lint	ENR	Miscellaneous orthopaedic appliances	ESM
Cotton/fibre rolls	ENT		
Cotton balls	ENU		

Index of Classifications, General Product Descriptions, and Proprietary/Trade Names

CLASSIFICATION	GENERAL PRODUCT DESCRIPTION	PROPRIETARY/TRADE NAME
EAA	Orthopaedic Casting Material Plaster Based	Cellona Elastic Cellona SR Gypsona Gypsona S Orthoflex Plastrona
EAB	Orthopaedic Casting Material Plaster Based Resin Reinforced Orthopaedic Casting Material Resin Based	Cellamin Crystona
EAF	Orthopaedic Casting Material Polyurethane Based	Cellacast Delta-Cast Delta-Cast Plus Delta–Lite Conformable Delta–LiteS Dynacast Dynacast Extra Scotchcast 2 Scotchcast Plus Scotchflex Zim-flex
EAK	Orthopaedic Casting Material Polyurethane Foam Based	Neofract
EBA	Compression Bandages	Bilastic Forte Bilastic Medium Bilastic Normal Biscard Blue Line Webbing Elastoweb Granuflex Hydrocolloid Bandage Lastobind Lastodur Rowden Foote Bandage Setopress Tensopress Varico
ECA	Light Pressure and Support Bandages	Comprilan Covic Crevic Elastocrepe Elastovic Elset Elset S Stump Bandage

CLASSIFICATION	GENERAL PRODUCT DESCRIPTION	PROPRIETARY/TRADE NAME
		Elvic
		Grip
		Idealast
		J Plus
		K-Crepe
		Lenkelast
		Leukocrepe
		Rayvic
		Sanicrepe
		Tensolastic
		Varicrepe
		Veinopress
ECB	Light Pressure and Support Bandages Foam	Lyoband
ECD	Light Pressure and Support Bandages Cohesive	Coban
		Cohepress
		Gazofix
		Idealhaft
		Secure Forte
ECG	Light Pressure and Support Bandages coated with Rubber Based Adhesive	Elastoplast Elastic Adhesive Bandage
		Flexoplast Plain Spread
		Flexoplast Ventilated
		Leukoband
		Zopla-Band EAB Standard
ECJ	Light Pressure and Support Bandages coated with Synthetic Adhesive	Acrylastic
		Hapla-Band
		Lite-Flex
		Poroplast
		Veinoplast
ECK	Light Pressure and Support Bandages coated with Diachylon Adhesive	Lestreflex Plain
		Lestreflex Ventilated
EDA	Dressing Retention Bandages Cotton	Crinx
		Kling
EDB	Dressing Retention Bandages Elasticated	Creplux
		Gauzelast
		Gauzex
		J Fast
		K-Band
		Lastotel
		Mollelast
		Nephlex
		Nylex
		Peha-Crep
		Slinky
		Stayform
		Tensofix Forte
		Transelast

CLASSIFICATION	GENERAL PRODUCT DESCRIPTION	PROPRIETARY/TRADE NAME
EDG	Dressing Retention Bandages Cohesive	Peha-Haft Secure Tensoplus Lite
EFA	Medicated Paste Bandages	Calaband Coltapaste Ichthopaste Icthaband Quinaband Tarband Viscopaste PB7 Zincaband
EGA	Tubular Support Bandages	Lastogrip Rediform Stulpa Tensogrip Tricodur Tubigrip

EGC	Garments for Pressure and Support	Tubigrip Hip Spica
		Tubigrip Lumbar Abdominal
		   Support Bandage
		Tubigrip Post-mastectomy
		   Bandage

EGG	Tubular Support Bandages Foam Padded	Tubipad
EGJ	Tubular Stockinettes	TG-Tubular Bandage Tubegauz Tubinette Tubiton
EGP	Tubular Stockinette Lightweight Elasticated	Tubifast
EGT	Tubular Net Bandages	Macrofix Netelast Netgrip Setonet Stulpa-fix Surgifix
EHA	Surgical Tapes Plastic Backed with Synthetic Adhesive	Leukofix Omnipor Transpore

EHB	Surgical Tapes Plastic Backed
	   Semipermeable with Synthetic Adhesive
		Airstrip Electromagnetically
		   Detectable Strapping

EHC	Surgical Tapes Plastic Backed Occlusive with Synthetic Adhesive	Blenderm Leukoflex Omniflex

CLASSIFICATION	GENERAL PRODUCT DESCRIPTION	PROPRIETARY/TRADE NAME
EHF	Surgical Tapes Plastic Backed Permeable with Rubber-based Adhesive	Dermiclear
EHH	Surgical Tapes Plastic Backed Occlusive with Rubber-based Adhesive	Setonplast Sleek
EHK	Surgical Tapes Woven Fabric Backed with Synthetic Adhesive	Dermicel Durapore Hapla-Tape Leukosilk Omnisilk
EHO	Surgical Tapes Woven Fabric Backed Permeable with Rubber-based Adhesive	Leukoplast
EHP	Surgical Tapes Woven Fabric Backed Occlusive with Rubber-based Adhesive	Hartmannplast Hospital Tape Leukoplast (Waterproof) Leukotape Omniplast Paragon Tensotape Zopla Rigid Strapping Chiropodial Thin Zopla Rigid Strapping Standard
EHQ	Surgical Tapes Woven Fabric Backed Elasticated with Rubber-based Adhesive	Elastoplast Plaster
EHR	Surgical Tapes Non-woven Fabric Backed Apertured	Chirofix Curafix Fixomull Stretch Hypafix Medipore Dressing Cover Mefix
EHU	Surgical Tapes Non-woven Fabric Backed	Albupore Dermilite Leukopor Micropore Omnivlies Pharmaclusive Tenderskin
EHX	Surgical Tapes Foam Backed	Microfoam
EIA	Adhesive Dressings Plastic Backed	Airstrip Airstrip Post-operative Dressing Band Aid Steripad Post-operative Dressing

CLASSIFICATION	GENERAL PRODUCT DESCRIPTION	PROPRIETARY/TRADE NAME
EIB	Adhesive Dressings Plastic Backed Electromagnetically Detectable	Airstrip Electromagnetically Detectable Eyetec
EIH	Adhesive Dressings Woven Fabric Backed with Rubber-based Adhesive	Coverlet Elastoplast Island Dressings
EIJ	Adhesive Dressings Non-woven Fabric Backed with Synthetic Adhesive	Curapor Post-operative Dressing Cutiplast Steril Hansapor Steril Plus Mepore Micropore Dressing Primapore
EIL	Dressing Strip Plastic Backed with Synthetic Adhesive	Airstrip Strip
EIO	Dressing Strip Fabric Backed with Synthetic Adhesive	Band Aid Fabric Dressing Strip
EIP	Dressing Strip Fabric Backed with Rubber-based Adhesive	Elastoplast Dressing Strip
EIQ	Dressing Strip Non-woven Fabric Backed with Synthetic Adhesive	Curapor Dressing Strip Hansamed Dressing Strip Mepore Roll
EIR	Wound Closure Strips Fabric Based	Cicagraf Neatseal Steri-Strip Suture Strip Suture Strip Plus
EIT	Wound Closure Strips Plastic Based	Steri-Strip Primaclear
EJA	Absorbent Dressings	ABD Dressing Pad ABD Plus Dressing Pad Cestra Dressing Pad Cutisorb Mesorb Steraid Dressing Pad Surgipad Multisorb
EJE	Absorbent Dressings with Low Adherence Face (Low Exudate)	Absderma Alutex Cuticell ETE Melolin Melolite

CLASSIFICATION	GENERAL PRODUCT DESCRIPTION	PROPRIETARY/TRADE NAME
		Metalline Release II Sk-Intact Telfa
EJF	Absorbent Dressings with Low Adherence Face (High Exudate)	Intrasite Cavity Wound Dressing Perfron
EJK	Drain or Tracheostomy Dressings	Lyofoam Tracheostomy Dressing Metalline Drainage Dressing Metalline Tracheostomy Dressing Sof-Wick
EKA	Primary Wound Contact Materials Impregnated with Ointment Basis	Branolind Grassolind Jelonet Lomatuell Paranet Paratulle Unitulle Vaseline Petrolatum Gauze
EKB	Primary Wound Contact Materials Impregnated with Ointment Basis Medicated	Bactigras Branolind L Clorhexitulle Fucidin Intertulle Inadine M and M Tulle Scarlet Red Dressing Serotulle Sofra-Tulle Xeroflow Xeroform
EKG	Primary Wound Contact Materials Plain	N-A Dressing Tricotex
ELA	Foam Dressings	Allevyn Coraderm (temporarily discontinued) Lyofoam Silastic Foam Sheeting Synthaderm (temporarily discontinued)
ELC	Foam Dressings formed *in situ*	Silastic Foam
ELE	Hydrogel Dressing Sheets	Geliperm Sheet

CLASSIFICATION	GENERAL PRODUCT DESCRIPTION	PROPRIETARY/TRADE NAME
		Geliperm Sheet (Dry) Spenco 2nd Skin Vigilon
ELG	Amorphous Hydrogels	Bard Absorption Dressing Geliperm Granulated Gel Scherisorb
ELH	Hydrogel Dressing with Metronidazole	Metrotop
ELM	Hydrocolloid Sheet Dressings	Biofilm Comfeel Comfeel Pressure Relieving Dressing Dermiflex Granuflex Granuflex E Granuflex Extra Thin Intrasite Tegasorb
ELO	Hydrocolloid Pastes Powders or Granules	Biofilm Powder Comfeel Paste Comfeel Powder Granuflex Granules Granuflex Paste
ELS	Alginate Dressings	Kaltostat Sorbsan Stop Hemo Tegagel Ultraplast
	Alginate Island Dressings	Sorbsan SA Kaltoclude
	Alginate Dressing with Absorbent Pad	Sorbsan Plus
	Absorbable Haemostats	Oxycell Spongostan Spongostan Anal Surgicel
ELT	Polysaccharide Bead Dressings Plain	Debrisan Debrisan Absorbent Pad Debrisan Paste
ELU	Polysaccharide Bead Dressings Medicated	Iodosorb Iodosorb Ointment
ELV	Dressings Containing Activated Charcoal	Actisorb Plus

CLASSIFICATION	GENERAL PRODUCT DESCRIPTION	PROPRIETARY/TRADE NAME
		Carbonet
		Carbosorb
		Kaltocarb
		Lyofoam C
ELW	Transparent Film Dressings	Bioclusive
		Cutifilm
		Dermafilm
		Dermoclude
		Ensure-it
		Granuflex Transparent
		Omiderm
		Opraflex
		Opsite
		Opsite I.V. 3000
		Opsite CH Cannula Dressing
		Tegaderm
		Transite
	Transparent Film Dressings Composite	Tegaderm Pouch Dressing
		Transigen
	Transparent Film Dressings Medicated	Tegaderm Plus
		Opsite CH
ELX	Biological Materials	Corethium 1
		Corethium 2
		E-Z Derm
		Zenoderm
ELY	Aerosol Dressings	Hansaplast Spray
		Nobecutane
		Opsite Spray
	Net Nylon Non-adhesive	Pharmanet
—	Silicone Gel Sheets	Silastic Gel Sheeting
		Spenco Silicone Gelsheets
ENJ	Filmated Gauze Swabs	Cotfil
ENK	Non-woven Gauze Swabs	Cutisoft
		Mesoft
		Mesoft Sponge
		Multisorb Plus
		Nu Gauze
		Topper
ENL	Filmated Non-woven Gauze Swabs	Regal
ENP	Dental Absorbents	Dentanaps

CLASSIFICATION	GENERAL PRODUCT DESCRIPTION	PROPRIETARY/TRADE NAME
		Oratex Dental Napkins
		Oratex Dental Rolls
		Oratex Throat Pack Material
		Oratex Sterile Coiled Dental Wadding
ENR	Medicated Absorbent Lint	Boric Lint
ENV	Cotton Applicators	Cotton Bud
ENW	Foam Applicators	Lyoswab
EOF	Tampons	Lil-Lets Tampon
		Tampax Tampon
EPA	Undercast Padding Cellulose Fibre Based	Orthoban
		Soffban Natural
		Velband
		Webril
EPE	Undercast Padding Synthetic Fibre Based	Cellona Undercast Padding
		Delta-Rol
		Soffban
		Soxtexe
		Web Wrap
EPH	Undercast Padding Foam Based	Cellona Pretape
		Delta-Tape
		Tensoban
EQB	Eye Pads	Coverlet Eye Occlusor
		Elastoplast Eye Occlusion Patch
		Opticlude
ERJ	Foam Padding Plain	Dalzofoam Plain
		Hindafome Plain
		Nuprene Plain
		Silcofoam Plain
		Swanfoam Plain
ERK	Foam Padding Adhesive	Dalzofoam Adhesive
		Hapla Nuprene
		Hapla Swanfoam
		Nuprene DS
		Reston Foam
		Reston Foam
		Zopla Foam-O-Felt
		Zopla Hindafome
		Zopla Silcofoam CB
		Zopla Silcofoam DS
		Zopla Sponge Rubber
		Zopla Swanfoam

CLASSIFICATION	GENERAL PRODUCT DESCRIPTION	PROPRIETARY/TRADE NAME
ERN	Tubular Foam Bandages	Foamband Tubifoam
ERP	Miscellaneous Chiropodial Protectives	Hapla Fleecy Web Hapla Moleskin Hapla Stockinette Standard Hapla Stockinette Thin Zopla Fleecy Web Zopla Moleskin Zopla Stockinette
ESA	Traction Kits Rubber-based Adhesive	Elastoplast Skin Traction Kit
ESB	Traction Kits Synthetic Adhesive	Elastoplast Skin Traction Kit Synthetic Adhesive Tractac
ESC	Traction Kits Non-adhesive	Elastoplast Traction Kit Notac Specialist Foam Traction Kit
ESE	Extension Plaster Rubber-based Adhesive	Elastoplast Extension Plaster Zopla Extension Strapping
ESJ	Skin Traction Bandages Foam Based	Ventfoam
ESM	Miscellaneous Orthopaedic Products	Arthro-Pad Collafoam Collar'n'cuff Tensoflex

Index of Generic Names, Proprietary/Trade Names, and Classifications

GENERIC NAME	PROPRIETARY/ TRADE NAME	CLASSI- FICATION
Bandage Elastic Web BP (with Footloop)	Varico	EBA
Bandage Elasticated Tubular	Stulpa	EGA
	Tricodur	EGA
Bandage Elasticated Tubular BP	Lastogrip	EGA
	Rediform	EGA
	Tensogrip	EGA
	Tubigrip	EGA
Bandage Elasticated Tubular Foam Padded	Tubipad	EGG
Bandage Light Pressure and Support	Comprilan	ECA
	Covic	ECA
	Elastovic	ECA
	Elset	ECA
	Elset S Stump Bandage	ECA
	Elvic	ECA
	Idealast	ECA
	J Plus	ECA
	K-Crepe	ECA
	Lenkelast	ECA
	Rayvic	ECA
	Tensolastic	ECA
	Varicrepe	ECA
	Veinopress	ECA
Bandage Light Pressure and Support Cohesive	Coban	ECD
	Cohepress	ECD
	Gazofix	ECD
	Idealhaft	ECD
	Secure Forte	ECD
Bandage Light Pressure and Support Foam	Lyoband	ECB
Bandage Lumbar Abdominal Support	Tubigrip Lumbar Abdominal Support	EGC
Bandage Orthopaedic Alumino-silicate Resin	Crystona	EAB
Bandage Orthopaedic Foam	Cellona Pretape	EPH
	Delta-Tape	EPH
	Tensoban	EPH
Bandage Orthopaedic Polyurethane Foam Based	Neofract	EAK
Bandage Orthopaedic Resin	Cellacast	EAF
	Delta-Cast	EAF
	Delta-Cast Plus	EAF
	Delta-Lite Conformable	EAF
	Delta-Lite S	EAF
	Dynacast	EAF
	Dynacast Extra	EAF
	Scotchcast 2	EAF
	Scotchcast Plus	EAF
	Scotchflex	EAF
	Zim-flex	EAF
Bandage Orthopaedic Wadding (Cellulose Fibre)	Orthoban	EPA
	Soffban Natural	EPA
	Velband	EPA
	Webril	EPA
Bandage Orthopaedic Wadding (Synthetic Fibre)	Cellona Undercast Padding	EPE

GENERIC NAME	PROPRIETARY/ TRADE NAME	CLASSI- FICATION
	Delta-Rol	EPE
	Soffban	EPE
	Soxtexe	EPE
	Web Wrap	EPE
Bandage Plaster of Paris	Cellona SR	EAA
	Gypsona S	EAA
	Plastrona	EAA
Bandage Plaster of Paris BP	Gypsona	EAA
Bandage Plaster of Paris Elasticated	Cellona Elastic	EAA
	Orthoflex	EAA
Bandage Plaster of Paris Resin Reinforced	Cellamin	EAB
Bandage Polyamide and Cellulose Contour BP	Slinky	EDB
	Stayform	EDB
Bandage Post-mastectomy	Tubigrip Post-mastectomy Bandage	EGC
Bandage Skin Traction Foam	Ventfoam	ESJ
Bandage Titanium Dioxide Adhesive	Poroplast	ECJ
Bandage Tubular Elastic Net	Macrofix	EGT
	Netelast	EGT
	Netgrip	EGT
	Setonet	EGT
	Stulpa-fix	EGT
	Surgifix	EGT
Bandage Tubular Foam	Foamband	ERN
	Tubifoam	ERN
Bandage Zinc Paste BP	Viscopaste PB7	EFA
	Zincaband	EFA
Bandage Zinc Paste Calamine and Clioquinol BP	Quinaband	EFA
Bandage Zinc Paste and Calamine Drug Tariff	Calaband	EFA
Bandage Zinc Paste and Coal Tar BP	Coltapaste	EFA
	Tarband	EFA
Bandage Zinc Paste and Ichthammol BP	Ichthopaste	EFA
	Icthaband	EFA
Collar Cervical	Collafoam	ESM
Dressing Absorbent Cavity Wound	Intrasite Cavity Wound Dressing	EJF
Dressing Absorbent Fenestrated	Sof-Wick	EJK
Dressing Absorbent Low Adherence Face	Absderma	EJE
	Alutex	EJE
	Cuticell	EJE
	ETE	EJE
	Melolite	EJE
	Metalline	EJE
	Release II	EJE
	Sk-Intact	EJE
Dressing Absorbent Silicone Foam	Silastic Foam Sheeting	ELA
Dressing Absorbent with Activated Charcoal Cloth	Carbonet	ELV
	Carbosorb	ELV
Dressing Activated Charcoal Cloth with Silver	Actisorb Plus	ELV
Dressing Calcium Alginate	Sorbsan	ELS
	Stop Hemo	ELS
	Tegagel	ELS

GENERIC NAME	PROPRIETARY/ TRADE NAME	CLASSI- FICATION
Dressing Calcium Alginate Foam Backed Adhesive	Sorbsan SA	ELS
Dressing Calcium Alginate and Viscose	Sorbsan Plus	ELS
Dressing Calcium/Sodium Alginate	Kaltostat	ELS
Dressing Calcium/Sodium Alginate Film Backed Adhesive	Kaltoclude	ELS
Dressing Calcium/Sodium Alginate with Activated Charcoal	Kaltocarb	ELV
Dressing Cannula Semipermeable Adhesive Medicated	Opsite CH Cannula Dressing	ELW
Dressing Chlorhexidine Gauze BP	Bactigras	EKB
	Clorhexitulle	EKB
	Serotulle	EKB
Dressing Cod Liver Oil and Honey Gauze	M and M Tulle	EKB
Dressing Collagen Absorbable	Corethium 2	ELX
Dressing Collagen Temporary	Corethium 1	ELX
Dressing Collagen with Silver Cross-linked	E-Z Derm	ELX
Dressing Cover Apertured Non-woven Adhesive	Medipore Dressing Cover	EHR
Dressing Cover Semipermeable Non-woven Synthetic Adhesive	Pharmaclusive	EHU
Dressing Drainage Absorbent Low Adherence Face	Metalline Drainage Dressing	EJK
Dressing Elastic Adhesive	Coverlet	EIH
Dressing Elastic Adhesive BP	Elastoplast Island Dressing	EIH
Dressing Elastic Adhesive BP (Strip)	Elastoplast Dressing Strip	EIP
Dressing Film Aerosol	Hansaplast Spray	ELY
	Nobecutane	ELY
	Opsite Spray	ELY
Dressing Framycetin Gauze BP	Sofra-Tulle	EKB
Dressing Hydrocolloid Granules	Granuflex Granules	ELO
Dressing Hydrocolloid Impermeable	Dermiflex	ELM
Dressing Hydrocolloid Paste	Comfeel Paste	ELO
	Granuflex Paste	ELO
Dressing Hydrocolloid Permeable	Biofilm	ELM
Dressing Hydrocolloid Powder	Biofilm Powder	ELO
	Comfeel Powder	ELO
Dressing Hydrocolloid Semipermeable	Comfeel	ELM
	Granuflex	ELM
	Intrasite	ELM
	Tegasorb	ELM
Dressing Hydrocolloid Semipermeable Extra Absorbent	Granuflex E	ELM
Dressing Hydrocolloid Semipermeable Pressure Relieving	Comfeel Pressure Relieving Dressing	ELM
Dressing Hydrocolloid Semipermeable Thin	Granuflex Extra Thin	ELM
Dressing Hydrocolloid Semipermeable Transparent	Granuflex Transparent	ELW
Dressing Hydrogel Amorphous	Bard Absorption Dressing	ELG
	Scherisorb	ELG
Dressing Hydrogel Amorphous with Metronidazole	Metrotop	ELH
Dressing Hydrogel Granulated	Geliperm Granulated Gel	ELG
Dressing Hydrogel Sheet	Geliperm Sheet	ELE
	Spenco 2nd Skin	ELE
	Vigilon	ELE
Dressing Hydrogel Sheet Dry	Geliperm Sheet (Dry)	ELE

GENERIC NAME	PROPRIETARY/ TRADE NAME	CLASSI- FICATION
Dressing Island Electromagnetically Detectable Impermeable Adhesive Dressing	Eyetec	EIB
Dressing Island Electromagnetically Detectable Semipermeable Adhesive	Airstrip Electromagnetically Detectable	EIB
Dressing Island Non-woven Fabric Adhesive	Curapor Post-operative Dressing	EIJ
	Cutiplast Steril	EIJ
	Hansapor Steril Plus	EIJ
	Mepore	EIJ
	Micropore Dressing	EIJ
	Primapore	EIJ
Dressing Island Permeable Plastic Adhesive	Steripad Post-operative Dressing	EIA
Dressing Knitted Viscose Primary BP	N-A Dressing	EKG
	Tricotex	EKG
Dressing Pad Absorbent	ABD Dressing Pad	EJA
	ABD Plus Dressing Pad	EJA
	Cestra Dressing Pad	EJA
	Cutisorb	EJA
	Mesorb	EJA
	Multisorb	EJA
	Steraid Dressing Pad	EJA
	Surgipad	EJA
Dressing Pad Absorbent Low Adherence Face	Perfron	EJF
Dressing Paraffin Gauze	Grassolind	EKA
	Lomatuell	EKA
Dressing Paraffin Gauze (Fine Weave)	Vaseline Petrolatum Gauze	EKA
Dressing Paraffin Gauze BP (Light Loading)	Paratulle	EKA
	Unitulle	EKA
Dressing Paraffin Gauze BP (Normal Loading)	Jelonet	EKA
	Paranet	EKA
Dressing Paraffin Gauze Compound	Branolind	EKA
Dressing Paraffin Gauze Compound with Stadacain	Branolind L	EKB
Dressing Perforated Film Absorbent BP (Type 1)	Melolin	EJE
Dressing Perforated Film Absorbent BP (Type 2)	Telfa	EJE
Dressing Permeable Plastic Adhesive	Band Aid	EIA
Dressing Permeable Plastic Film	Transite	ELW
Dressing Polysaccharide Bead	Debrisan	ELT
Dressing Polysaccharide Bead Medicated	Iodosorb	ELU
Dressing Polysaccharide Bead Paste	Debrisan Paste	ELT
Dressing Polysaccharide Bead Paste Medicated	Iodosorb Ointment	ELU
Dressing Polysaccharide Bead Paste Pad	Debrisan Absorbent Pad	ELT
Dressing Polyurethane Film Hydrophilic	Omiderm	ELW
Dressing Polyurethane Foam BP	Lyofoam	ELA
Dressing Polyurethane Foam Hydrophilic	Allevyn	ELA
Dressing Polyurethane Foam Primary BP	Coraderm (temporarily discontinued)	ELA
	Synthaderm (temporarily discontinued)	ELA
Dressing Polyurethane Foam with Activated Charcoal	Lyofoam C	ELV
Dressing Povidone-Iodine/Polyethylene Glycol	Inadine	EKB
Dressing Scarlet Red Gauze	Scarlet Red Dressing	EKB
Dressing Semipermeable Adhesive	Dermafilm	ELW
	Dermoclude	ELW

GENERIC NAME	PROPRIETARY/ TRADE NAME	CLASSI- FICATION
	Ensure-it	ELW
	Opraflex	ELW
	Opsite I.V. 3000	ELW
Dressing Semipermeable Adhesive BP	Bioclusive	ELW
	Cutifilm	ELW
	Opsite	ELW
	Tegaderm	ELW
Dressing Semipermeable Adhesive Composite	Tegaderm Pouch Dressing	ELW
	Transigen	ELW
Dressing Semipermeable Adhesive Medicated	Opsite CH	ELW
	Tegaderm Plus	ELW
Dressing Semipermeable Waterproof Plastic Wound BP	Airstrip	EIA
	Airstrip Post-operative Dressing	EIA
Dressing Sheet Silicone Gel	Silastic Gel Sheeting	ELY
	Spenco Silicone Gelsheets	ELY
Dressing Silicone Foam Cavity Wound BP	Silastic Foam	ELC
Dressing Sodium Alginate	Ultraplast	ELS
Dressing Sodium Fusidate Gauze BP	Fucidin Intertulle	EKB
Dressing Strip Fabric Adhesive	Band Aid Fabric Dressing Strip	EIO
Dressing Strip Non-woven Fabric	Curapor Dressing Strip	EIQ
Dressing Strip Non-woven Fabric Backed	Hansamed Dressing Strip	EIQ
	Mepore Roll	EIQ
Dressing Strip Semipermeable Plastic	Airstrip Strip	EIL
Dressing Tracheostomy Low Adherence Face	Metalline Tracheostomy Dressing	EJK
Dressing Tracheostomy Polyurethane Foam	Lyofoam Tracheostomy Dressing	EJK
Dressing Tribromophenate and Oil Emulsion Gauze	Xeroflow	EKB
Dressing Tribromophenate and Paraffin Gauze	Xeroform	EKB
Fleecy Web Synthetic Adhesive	Hapla Fleecy Web	ERP
Fleecy Web Zinc Oxide Adhesive	Zopla Fleecy Web	ERP
Foam Backed with Swansdown	Swanfoam Plain	ERJ
Foam Padding Latex	Hindafome Plain	ERJ
Foam Padding Latex Zinc Oxide Adhesive	Zopla Hindafome	ERK
Foam Polyurethane Plain	Dalzofoam Plain	ERJ
	Nuprene Plain	ERJ
	Silcofoam Plain	ERJ
Foam Polyurethane Synthetic Adhesive	Hapla Nuprene	ERK
Foam Polyurethane Zinc Oxide Adhesive	Dalzofoam Adhesive	ERK
	Nuprene DS	ERK
Foam Synthetic Adhesive Backed with Swansdown	Hapla Swanfoam	ERK
Foam Zinc Oxide Adhesive Backed with Swansdown	Zopla Swanfoam	ERK
Foam/Felt Combination Zinc Oxide Adhesive	Zopla Foam-O-Felt	ERK
Hip Spica (Bandage Elasticated Tubular)	Tubigrip Hip Spica	EGC
Implant Porcine Dermis	Zenoderm	ELX
Lint Boric Acid BPC	Boric Lint	ENR

GENERIC NAME	PROPRIETARY/ TRADE NAME	CLASSI- FICATION
Moleskin Synthetic Adhesive	Hapla Moleskin	ERP
Moleskin Zinc Oxide Adhesive	Zopla Moleskin	ERP
Napkin Dental Absorbent Gauze	Oratex Dental Napkin	ENP
Napkin Dental Non-woven Fabric	Dentanaps	ENP
Net Nylon Non-adhesive	Pharmanet	ELY
Oxidised Cellulose BP	Oxycell	ELS
	Surgicel	ELS
Pack Throat Absorbent Cotton with Non-woven Fabric Cover	Oratex Throat Pack Material	ENP
Pad Eye Self-adhesive	Coverlet Eye Occlusor	EQB
	Elastoplast Eye Occlusion Patch	EQB
	Opticlude	EQB
Plaster Extension BP	Elastoplast Extension Plaster	ESE
	Zopla Extension Strapping	ESE
Polyurethane Foam Cloth Backed Zinc Oxide Adhesive	Zopla Silcofoam CB	ERK
Polyurethane Foam Synthetic Adhesive	Reston Foam	ERK
Polyurethane Foam Zinc Oxide Adhesive	Zopla Silcofoam DS	ERK
Roll Dental Absorbent	Oratex Dental Roll	ENP
Sling Foam Padded	Collar'n'cuff	ESM
Sponge Absorbable Gelatin	Spongostan	ELS
Sponge Absorbable Gelatin (Anal)	Spongostan Anal	ELS
Sponge Non-woven Fabric	Mesoft Sponge	ENK
Sponge Rubber Zinc Oxide Adhesive	Zopla Sponge Rubber	ERK
Stockinette Cotton BP	Tubegauz	EGJ
Stockinette Cotton and Viscose BP	Tubiton	EGJ
Stockinette Elasticated Lightweight	Tubifast	EGP
Stockinette Paraffined	TG-Tubular Bandage	EGJ
Stockinette Synthetic Adhesive	Hapla Stockinette Standard	ERP
Stockinette Thin Synthetic Adhesive	Hapla Stockinette Thin	ERP
Stockinette Viscose BP	Tubinette	EGJ
Stockinette Zinc Oxide Adhesive	Zopla Stockinette	ERP
Support Ankle Elasticated	Tensoflex	ESM
Support Joint Elasticated Foam Padded	Arthro-Pad	ESM
Swab Absorbent Foam Preparation	Lyoswab	ENW
Swab Gauze Filmated	Cotfil	ENJ
Swab Muslin Electromagnetically Detectable	Super Chex X-Ray-Detectable Muslin Swab	EMM
Swab Non-woven Fabric	Cutisoft	ENK
	Mesoft	ENK
	Multisorb Plus	ENK
	Nu Gauze	ENK
	Topper	ENK
Swab Non-woven Fabric Filmated	Regal	ENL

GENERIC NAME	PROPRIETARY/ TRADE NAME	CLASSI- FICATION
Tampon (Non-applicator)	Lil-Lets Tampon	EOF
Tampon with Applicator	Tampax Tampon	EOF
Tape Apertured Non-woven Surgical Synthetic Adhesive	Chirofix	EHR
	Curafix	EHR
	Fixomull Stretch	EHR
	Hypafix	EHR
	Mefix	EHR
Tape Elastic Surgical Adhesive BP	Elastoplast Plaster	EHQ
Tape Electromagnetically Detectable Semipermeable Surgical Synthetic Adhesive	Airstrip Electromagnetically Detectable Strapping	EHB
Tape Impermeable Plastic Surgical Adhesive BP	Setonplast	EHH
	Sleek	EHH
Tape Impermeable Plastic Surgical Synthetic Adhesive	Omniflex	EHC
Tape Impermeable Plastic Surgical Synthetic Adhesive BP	Blenderm	EHC
	Leukoflex	EHC
Tape Permeable Foam Surgical Synthetic Adhesive	Microfoam	EHX
Tape Permeable Non-woven Surgical Synthetic Adhesive	Omnivlies	EHU
Tape Permeable Non-woven Surgical Synthetic Adhesive BP	Albupore	EHU
	Dermilite	EHU
	Leukopor	EHU
	Micropore	EHU
	Tenderskin	EHU
Tape Permeable Plastic Surgical Adhesive BP	Dermiclear	EHF
Tape Permeable Plastic Surgical Synthetic Adhesive	Omnipor	EHA
Tape Permeable Plastic Surgical Synthetic Adhesive BP	Leukofix	EHA
	Transpore	EHA
Tape Permeable Woven Surgical Synthetic Adhesive	Omnisilk	EHK
Tape Permeable Woven Surgical Synthetic Adhesive BP	Dermicel	EHK
	Durapore	EHK
	Leukosilk	EHK
Tape Permeable Woven Thin Surgical Synthetic Adhesive	Hapla-Tape	EHK
Tape Zinc Oxide Porous Surgical Adhesive	Leukoplast	EHO
Tape Zinc Oxide Surgical Adhesive	Hospital Tape	EHP
	Leukotape	EHP
	Omniplast	EHP
	Tensotape	EHP
	Zopla Rigid Strapping Standard	EHP
Tape Zinc Oxide Surgical Adhesive BP	Paragon	EHP
Tape Zinc Oxide Thin Surgical Adhesive	Zopla Rigid Strapping Chiropodial Thin	EHP
Tape Zinc Oxide Waterproof Fabric Surgical Adhesive	Hartmannplast	EHP
	Leukoplast (Waterproof)	EHP

GENERIC NAME	PROPRIETARY/ TRADE NAME	CLASSI- FICATION
Traction Kit Non-adhesive	Elastoplast Traction Kit	ESC
	Notac	ESC
	Specialist Foam Traction Kit	ESC
Traction Kit Rubber Adhesive	Elastoplast Skin Traction Kit	ESA
Traction Kit Synthetic Adhesive	Elastoplast Skin Traction Kit Synthetic Adhesive	ESB
	Tractac	ESB
Wadding Dental in Coils Sterile	Oratex Sterile Coiled Dental Wadding	ENP
Wound Closure Fabric	Neatseal	EIR
Wound Closure Strip	Cicagraf	EIR
	Steri-Strip	EIR
	Suture Strip	EIR
	Suture Strip Plus	EIR
Wound Closure Strip Transparent	Steri-Strip Primaclear	EIT

Index of Proprietary/Trade Names, Generic Names, Manufacturers, and Classification

PROPRIETARY/TRADE NAME	GENERIC NAME	MANU-FACTURER	CLASSI-FICATION
ABD Dressing Pad	Dressing Pad Absorbent	Ken	EJA
ABD Plus Dressing Pad	Dressing Pad Absorbent	Ken	EJA
Absderma	Dressing Absorbent Low Adherence Face	LIC	EJE
Acrylastic	Bandage Elastic Synthetic Adhesive	BDF	ECJ
Actisorb Plus	Dressing Activated Charcoal Cloth with Silver	JJ	ELV
Airstrip	Dressing Semipermeable Waterproof Plastic Wound BP	SN	EIA
Airstrip Electromagnetically Detectable	Dressing Island Electromagnetically Detectable Semipermeable Adhesive	SN	EIB
Airstrip Electromagnetically Detectable Strapping	Tape Electromagnetically Detectable Semipermeable Surgical Synthetic Adhesive	SN	EHB
Airstrip Post-operative Dressing	Dressing Semipermeable Waterproof Plastic Wound BP	SN	EIA
Airstrip Strip	Dressing Strip Semipermeable Plastic	SN	EIL
Albupore	Tape Permeable Non-woven Surgical Adhesive Synthetic BP	SN	EHU
Allevyn	Dressing Polyurethane Foam Hydrophilic	SN	ELA
Alutex	Dressing Absorbent Low Adherence Face	Ort	EJE
Arthro-Pad	Support Joint Elasticated Foam Padded	Set	ESM
Bactigras	Dressing Chlorhexidine Gauze BP	SN	EKB
Band Aid	Dressing Permeable Plastic Adhesive	JJ	EIA
Band Aid Fabric Dressing Strip	Dressing Strip Fabric Adhesive	JJ	EIO
Bard Absorption Dressing	Dressing Hydrogel Amorphous	Set	ELG
Bilastic Forte	Bandage Compression	Mol	EBA
Bilastic Medium	Bandage Compression	Ste	EBA
Bilastic Normal	Bandage Compression	Ste	EBA
Bioclusive	Dressing Semipermeable Adhesive BP	JJ	ELW
Biofilm	Dressing Hydrocolloid Permeable	Cli	ELM
Biofilm Powder	Dressing Hydrocolloid Powder	Cli	ELO
Biscard	Bandage Elastic Web BP	Mar	EBA
Blenderm	Tape Impermeable Plastic Surgical Synthetic Adhesive BP	3M	EHC
Blue Line Webbing	Bandage Elastic Web BP	Set	EBA
Boric Lint	Lint Boric Acid BPC	LN	ENR
Branolind	Dressing Paraffin Gauze Compound	Har	EKA
Branolind L	Dressing Paraffin Gauze Compound with Stadacain	Har	EKB
Calaband	Bandage Zinc Paste and Calamine Drug Tariff	Set	EFA

PROPRIETARY/TRADE NAME	GENERIC NAME	MANU-FACTURER	CLASSI-FICATION
Carbonet	Dressing Absorbent with Activated Charcoal Cloth	SN	ELV
Carbosorb	Dressing Absorbent with Activated Charcoal Cloth	Set	ELV
Cellacast	Bandage Orthopaedic Resin	Loh	EAF
Cellamin	Bandage Plaster of Paris Resin Reinforced	Loh	EAB
Cellona Elastic	Bandage Plaster of Paris Elasticated	Loh	EAA
Cellona Pretape	Bandage Orthopaedic Foam	Loh	EPH
Cellona SR	Bandage Plaster of Paris	Loh	EAA
Cellona Undercast Padding	Bandage Orthopaedic Wadding (Synthetic Fibre)	Loh	EPE
Cestra Dressing Pad	Dressing Pad Absorbent	Rob	EJA
Chirofix	Tape Apertured Non-woven Surgical Synthetic Adhesive	HL	EHR
Cicagraf	Wound Closure Strip	SN	EIR
Clorhexitulle	Dressing Chlorhexidine Gauze BP	Rou	EKB
Coban	Bandage Light Pressure and Support Cohesive	3M	ECD
Cohepress	Bandage Light Pressure and Support Cohesive	Ste	ECD
Collafoam	Collar Cervical	Set	ESM
Collar'n'cuff	Sling Foam Padded	Set	ESM
Coltapaste	Bandage Zinc Paste and Coal Tar BP	SN	EFA
Comfeel	Dressing Hydrocolloid Semipermeable	Col	ELM
Comfeel Paste	Dressing Hydrocolloid Paste	Col	ELO
Comfeel Powder	Dressing Hydrocolloid Powder	Col	ELO
Comfeel Pressure Relieving Dressing	Dressing Hydrocolloid Semipermeable Pressure Relieving	Col	ELM
Comprilan	Bandage Light Pressure and Support	BDF	ECA
Coraderm (temporarily discontinued)	Dressing Polyurethane Foam Primary BP		ELA
Corethium 1	Dressing Collagen Temporary	JJ	ELX
Corethium 2	Dressing Collagen Absorbable	JJ	ELX
Cotfil	Swab Gauze Filmated	VC	ENJ
Cotton Bud	Applicator Absorbent Cotton	JJ	ENV
Coverlet	Dressing Elastic Adhesive	BDF	EIH
Coverlet Eye Occlusor	Pad Eye Self-adhesive	BDF	EQB
Covic	Bandage Light Pressure and Support	Gro	ECA
Creplux	Bandage Conforming Stretch	Mol	EDB
Crevic	Bandage Cotton Crêpe BP	Gro	ECA
Crinx	Bandage Cotton Conforming BP (Type A)	SN	EDA
Crystona	Bandage Orthopaedic Alumino-silicate Resin	SN	EAB
Curafix	Tape Apertured Non-woven Surgical Synthetic Adhesive	Loh	EHR
Curapor Dressing Strip	Dressing Strip Non-woven Fabric	Loh	EIQ
Curapor Post-operative Dressing	Dressing Island Non-woven Fabric Adhesive	Loh	EIJ
Cuticell	Dressing Absorbent Low Adherence Face	BDF	EJE
Cutifilm	Dressing Semipermeable Adhesive BP	BDF	ELW

PROPRIETARY/TRADE NAME	GENERIC NAME	MANU-FACTURER	CLASSI-FICATION
Cutiplast Steril	Dressing Island Non-woven Fabric Adhesive	BDF	EIJ
Cutisoft	Swab Non-woven Fabric	BDF	ENK
Cutisorb	Dressing Pad Absorbent	BDF	EJA
Dalzofoam Adhesive	Foam Polyurethane Zinc Oxide Adhesive	Set	ERK
Dalzofoam Plain	Foam Polyurethane Plain	Set	ERJ
Debrisan	Dressing Polysaccharide Bead	Pha	ELT
Debrisan Absorbent Pad	Dressing Polysaccharide Bead Paste Pad	Pha	ELT
Debrisan Paste	Dressing Polysaccharide Bead Paste	Pha	ELT
Delta-Cast	Bandage Orthopaedic Resin	JJO	EAF
Delta-Cast Plus	Bandage Orthopaedic Resin	JJO	EAF
Delta-Lite Conformable	Bandage Orthopaedic Resin	JJO	EAF
Delta-Lite S	Bandage Orthopaedic Resin	JJO	EAF
Delta-Rol	Bandage Orthopaedic Wadding (Synthetic Fibre)	JJO	EPE
Delta-Tape	Bandage Orthopaedic Foam	JJO	EPH
Dentanaps	Napkin Dental Non-woven Fabric	VC	ENP
Dermafilm	Dressing Semipermeable Adhesive	Vyg	ELW
Dermicel	Tape Permeable Woven Surgical Synthetic Adhesive BP	JJ	EHK
Dermiclear	Tape Permeable Plastic Surgical Adhesive BP	JJ	EHF
Dermiflex	Dressing Hydrocolloid Impermeable	JJ	ELM
Dermilite	Tape Permeable Non-woven Surgical Synthetic Adhesive BP	JJ	EHU
Dermoclude	Dressing Semipermeable Adhesive	Bri	ELW
Durapore	Tape Permeable Woven Surgical Synthetic Adhesive BP	3M	EHK
Dynacast	Bandage Orthopaedic Resin	SN	EAF
Dynacast Extra	Bandage Orthopaedic Resin	SN	EAF
E-Z Derm	Dressing Collagen with Silver Cross-linked	Bio	ELX
Elastocrepe	Bandage Cotton Crêpe BP	SN	ECA
Elastoplast Dressing Strip	Dressing Elastic Adhesive BP (Strip)	SN	EIP
Elastoplast Elastic Adhesive Bandage	Bandage Elastic Adhesive BP (Porous)	SN	ECG
Elastoplast Extension Plaster	Plaster Extension BP	SN	ESE
Elastoplast Eye Occlusion Patch	Pad Eye Self-adhesive	SN	EQB
Elastoplast Island Dressing	Dressing Elastic Adhesive BP	SN	EIH
Elastoplast Plaster	Tape Elastic Surgical Adhesive BP	SN	EHQ
Elastoplast Skin Traction Kit	Traction Kit Rubber Adhesive	SN	ESA
Elastoplast Skin Traction Kit Synthetic Adhesive	Traction Kit Synthetic Adhesive	SN	ESB
Elastoplast Traction Kit	Traction Kit Non-adhesive	SN	ESC
Elastovic	Bandage Light Pressure and Support	Gro	ECA
Elastoweb	Bandage Elastic Heavy Cotton and Rubber BP	SN	EBA
Elset	Bandage Light Pressure and Support	Set	ECA
Elset S Stump Bandage	Bandage Light Pressure and Support	Set	ECA

PROPRIETARY/TRADE NAME	GENERIC NAME	MANU-FACTURER	CLASSI-FICATION
Elvic	Bandage Light Pressure and Support	Gro	ECA
Ensure-it	Dressing Semipermeable Adhesive	Bec	ELW
ETE	Dressing Absorbent Low Adherence Face	Mln	EJE
Eyetec	Dressing Island Electromagnetically Detectable Impermeable Adhesive	Rob	EIB
Fixomull Stretch	Tape Apertured Non-woven Surgical Synthetic Adhesive	BDF	EHR
Flexoplast Plain Spread	Bandage Elastic Adhesive BP (Plain Spread)	Rob	ECG
Flexoplast Ventilated	Bandage Elastic Adhesive BP (Ventilated)	Rob	ECG
Foamband	Bandage Tubular Foam	Foa	ERN
Fucidin Intertulle	Dressing Sodium Fusidate Gauze BP	Leo	EKB
Gauzelast	Bandage Conforming Stretch	BDF	EDB
Gauzex	Bandage Conforming Stretch	Mol	EDB
Gazofix	Bandage Light Pressure and Support Cohesive	BDF	ECD
Geliperm Granulated Gel	Dressing Hydrogel Granulated	Gei	ELG
Geliperm Sheet	Dressing Hydrogel Sheet	Gei	ELE
Geliperm Sheet (Dry)	Dressing Hydrogel Sheet Dry	Gei	ELE
Granuflex	Dressing Hydrocolloid Semipermeable	Con	ELM
Granuflex E	Dressing Hydrocolloid Semipermeable Extra Absorbent	Con	ELM
Granuflex Extra Thin	Dressing Hydrocolloid Semipermeable Thin	Con	ELM
Granuflex Granules	Dressing Hydrocolloid Granules	Con	ELO
Granuflex Hydrocolloid Bandage	Bandage Compression	Con	EBA
Granuflex Paste	Dressing Hydrocolloid Paste	Con	ELO
Granuflex Transparent	Dressing Hydrocolloid Semipermeable Transparent	Con	ELW
Grassolind	Dressing Paraffin Gauze	Har	EKA
Grip	Bandage Cotton Stretch BP	Oxf	ECA
Gypsona	Bandage Plaster of Paris BP	SN	EAA
Gypsona S	Bandage Plaster of Paris	SN	EAA
Hansamed Dressing Strip	Dressing Strip Non-woven Fabric Backed	BDF	EIQ
Hansaplast Spray	Dressing Film Aerosol	BDF	ELY
Hansapor Steril Plus	Dressing Island Non-woven Fabric Adhesive	BDF	EIJ
Hapla Fleecy Web	Fleecy Web Synthetic Adhesive	HL	ERP
Hapla Moleskin	Moleskin Synthetic Adhesive	HL	ERP
Hapla Nuprene	Foam Polyurethane Synthetic Adhesive	HL	ERK
Hapla Stockinette Standard	Stockinette Synthetic Adhesive	HL	ERP
Hapla Stockinette Thin	Stockinette Thin Synthetic Adhesive	HL	ERP
Hapla Swanfoam	Foam Synthetic Adhesive Backed with Swansdown	HL	ERK
Hapla-Band	Bandage Elastic Thin Synthetic Adhesive	HL	ECJ
Hapla-Tape	Tape Permeable Woven Thin Surgical Synthetic Adhesive	HL	EHK
Hartmannplast	Tape Zinc Oxide Waterproof Fabric Surgical Adhesive	Har	EHP
Hindafome Plain	Foam Padding Latex	HL	ERJ
Hospital Tape	Tape Zinc Oxide Surgical Adhesive	JJ	EHP

PROPRIETARY/TRADE NAME	GENERIC NAME	MANU-FACTURER	CLASSI-FICATION
Hypafix	Tape Apertured Non-woven Surgical Synthetic Adhesive	SN	EHR
Ichthopaste	Bandage Zinc Paste and Ichthammol BP	SN	EFA
Icthaband	Bandage Zinc Paste and Ichthammol BP	Set	EFA
Idealast	Bandage Light Pressure and Support	Har	ECA
Idealhaft	Bandage Light Pressure and Support Cohesive	Har	ECD
Inadine	Dressing Povidone-Iodine/Polyethylene Glycol	JJ	EKB
Intrasite	Dressing Hydrocolloid Semipermeable	SN	ELM
Intrasite Cavity Wound Dressing	Dressing Absorbent Cavity Wound	SN	EJF
Iodosorb	Dressing Polysaccharide Bead Medicated	Per	ELU
Iodosorb Ointment	Dressing Polysaccharide Bead Paste Medicated	Per	ELU
J Fast	Bandage Conforming Stretch	JJ	EDB
J Plus	Bandage Light Pressure and Support	JJ	ECA
Jelonet	Dressing Paraffin Gauze BP (Normal Loading)	SN	EKA
K-Band	Bandage Conforming Stretch	Par	EDB
K-Crepe	Bandage Light Pressure and Support	Par	ECA
Kaltocarb	Dressing Calcium/Sodium Alginate with Activated Charcoal	Bri	ELV
Kaltoclude	Dressing Calcium/Sodium Alginate Film Backed Adhesive	Bri	ELS
Kaltostat	Dressing Calcium/Sodium Alginate	Bri	ELS
Kling	Bandage Cotton Conforming BP (Type B)	JJ	EDA
Lastobind	Bandage Compression	Har	EBA
Lastodur	Bandage Compression	Har	EBA
Lastogrip	Bandage Elasticated Tubular BP	Har	EGA
Lastotel	Bandage Conforming Stretch	Har	EDB
Lenkelast	Bandage Light Pressure and Support	Har	ECA
Lestreflex Plain	Bandage Diachylon Adhesive BPC 1973 (Plain)	Set	ECK
Lestreflex Ventilated	Bandage Diachylon Adhesive BPC 1973 (Ventilated)	Set	ECK
Leukoband	Bandage Elastic Adhesive	BDF	ECG
Leukocrepe	Bandage Cotton Stretch BP	BDF	ECA
Leukofix	Tape Permeable Plastic Surgical Synthetic Adhesive BP	BDF	EHA
Leukoflex	Tape Impermeable Plastic Surgical Synthetic Adhesive BP	BDF	EHC
Leukoplast	Tape Zinc Oxide Porous Surgical Adhesive	BDF	EHO
Leukoplast (Waterproof)	Tape Zinc Oxide Waterproof Fabric Surgical Adhesive	BDF	EHP

PROPRIETARY/TRADE NAME	GENERIC NAME	MANU-FACTURER	CLASSI-FICATION
Leukopor	Tape Permeable Non-woven Surgical Synthetic Adhesive BP	BDF	EHU
Leukosilk	Tape Permeable Woven Surgical Synthetic Adhesive BP	BDF	EHK
Leukotape	Tape Zinc Oxide Surgical Adhesive	BDF	EHP
Lil-Lets Tampon	Tampon (Non-applicator)	SN	EOF
Lite-Flex	Bandage Elastic Synthetic Adhesive	JJ	ECJ
Lomatuell	Dressing Paraffin Gauze	Loh	EKA
Lyoband	Bandage Light Pressure and Support Foam	Ult	ECB
Lyofoam	Dressing Polyurethane Foam BP	Ult	ELA
Lyofoam C	Dressing Polyurethane Foam with Activated Charcoal	Ult	ELV
Lyofoam Tracheostomy Dressing	Dressing Tracheostomy Polyurethane Foam	Ult	EJK
Lyoswab	Swab Absorbent Foam Preparation	Ult	ENW
M and M Tulle	Dressing Cod Liver Oil and Honey Gauze	Mal	EKB
Macrofix	Bandage Tubular Elastic Net	HMS	EGT
Medipore Dressing Cover	Dressing Cover Apertured Non-woven Adhesive	3M	EHR
Mefix	Tape Apertured Non-woven Surgical Synthetic Adhesive	Mln	EHR
Melolin	Dressing Perforated Film Absorbent BP (Type 1)	SN	EJE
Melolite	Dressing Absorbent Low Adherence Face	SN	EJE
Mepore	Dressing Island Non-woven Fabric Adhesive	Mln	EIJ
Mepore Roll	Dressing Strip Non-woven Fabric Backed	Mln	EIQ
Mesoft	Swab Non-woven Fabric	Mln	ENK
Mesoft Sponge	Sponge Non-woven Fabric	Mln	ENK
Mesorb	Dressing Pad Absorbent	Mln	EJA
Metalline	Dressing Absorbent Low Adherence Face	Loh	EJE
Metalline Drainage Dressing	Dressing Drainage Absorbent Low Adherence Face	Loh	EJK
Metalline Tracheostomy Dressing	Dressing Tracheostomy Low Adherence Face	Loh	EJK
Metrotop	Dressing Hydrogel Amorphous with Metronidazole	Til	ELH
Microfoam	Tape Permeable Foam Surgical Synthetic Adhesive	3M	EHX
Micropore	Tape Permeable Non-woven Surgical Synthetic Adhesive BP	3M	EHU
Micropore Dressing	Dressing Island Non-woven Fabric Adhesive	3M	EIJ
Mollelast	Bandage Conforming Stretch	Loh	EDB
Multisorb	Dressing Pad Absorbent	SN	EJA
Multisorb Plus	Swab Non-woven Fabric	SN	ENK
N-A Dressing	Dressing Knitted Viscose Primary BP	JJ	EKG
Neatseal	Wound Closure Fabric	Rob	EIR
Neofract	Bandage Orthopaedic Polyurethane Foam Based	JJO	EAK

PROPRIETARY/TRADE NAME	GENERIC NAME	MANU-FACTURER	CLASSI-FICATION
Nephlex	Bandage Conforming Stretch	SN	EDB
Netelast	Bandage Tubular Elastic Net	Rou	EGT
Netgrip	Bandage Tubular Elastic Net	BDF	EGT
Nobecutane	Dressing Film Aerosol	Ast	ELY
Notac	Traction Kit Non-adhesive	Set	ESC
Nu Gauze	Swab Non-woven Fabric	JJ	ENK
Nuprene DS	Foam Polyurethane Zinc Oxide Adhesive	HL	ERK
Nuprene Plain	Foam Polyurethane Plain	HL	ERJ
Nylex	Bandage Conforming Stretch	Mol	EDB
Omiderm	Dressing Polyurethane Film Hydrophilic	Per	ELW
Omniflex	Tape Impermeable Plastic Surgical Synthetic Adhesive	Har	EHC
Omniplast	Tape Zinc Oxide Surgical Adhesive	Har	EHP
Omnipor	Tape Permeable Plastic Surgical Synthetic Adhesive	Har	EHA
Omnisilk	Tape Permeable Woven Surgical Synthetic Adhesive	Har	EHK
Omnivlies	Tape Permeable Non-woven Surgical Synthetic Adhesive	Har	EHU
Opraflex	Dressing Semipermeable Adhesive	Loh	ELW
Opsite	Dressing Semipermeable Adhesive BP	SN	ELW
Opsite CH	Dressing Semipermeable Adhesive Medicated	SN	ELW
Opsite CH Cannula Dressing	Dressing Cannula Semipermeable Adhesive Medicated	SN	ELW
Opsite I.V. 3000	Dressing Semipermeable Adhesive	SN	ELW
Opsite Spray	Dressing Film Aerosol	SN	ELY
Opticlude	Pad Eye Self-adhesive	3M	EQB
Oratex Dental Napkin	Napkin Dental Absorbent Gauze	VC	ENP
Oratex Dental Roll	Roll Dental Absorbent	VC	ENP
Oratex Sterile Coiled Dental Wadding	Wadding Dental in Coils Sterile	VC	ENP
Oratex Throat Pack Material	Pack Throat Absorbent Cotton with Non-woven Fabric Cover	VC	ENP
Orthoban	Bandage Orthopaedic Wadding (Cellulose Fibre)	Cow	EPA
Orthoflex	Bandage Plaster of Paris Elasticated	JJO	EAA
Oxycell	Oxidised Cellulose BP	AHS	ELS
Paragon	Tape Zinc Oxide Surgical Adhesive BP	SN	EHP
Paranet	Dressing Paraffin Gauze BP (Normal Loading)	VC	EKA
Paratulle	Dressing Paraffin Gauze BP (Light Loading)	Set	EKA
Peha-Crep	Bandage Conforming Stretch	Har	EDB
Peha-Haft	Bandage Conforming Stretch Cohesive	Har	EDG
Perfron	Dressing Pad Absorbent Low Adherence Face	JJ	EJF
Pharmaclusive	Dressing Cover Semipermeable Non-woven Synthetic Adhesive	Pha	EHU
Pharmanet	Net Nylon Non-adhesive	Pha	ELY

PROPRIETARY/TRADE NAME	GENERIC NAME	MANU-FACTURER	CLASSI-FICATION
Plastrona	Bandage Plaster of Paris	Har	EAA
Poroplast	Bandage Titanium Dioxide Adhesive	Sch	ECJ
Primapore	Dressing Island Non-woven Fabric Adhesive	SN	EIJ
Quinaband	Bandage Zinc Paste Calamine and Clioquinol BP	Set	EFA
Rayvic	Bandage Light Pressure and Support	Gro	ECA
Rediform	Bandage Elasticated Tubular BP	Sal	EGA
Regal	Swab Non-woven Fabric Filmated	JJ	ENL
Release II	Dressing Absorbent Low Adherence Face	JJ	EJE
Reston Foam	Polyurethane Foam Synthetic Adhesive	3M	ERK
Rowden Foote Bandage	Bandage Compression	HMS	EBA
Sanicrepe	Bandage Cotton Stretch BP	CG	ECA
Scarlet Red Dressing	Dressing Scarlet Red Gauze	She	EKB
Scherisorb	Dressing Hydrogel Amorphous	SN	ELG
Scotchcast 2	Bandage Orthopaedic Resin	3M	EAF
Scotchcast Plus	Bandage Orthopaedic Resin	3M	EAF
Scotchflex	Bandage Orthopaedic Resin	3M	EAF
Secure	Bandage Conforming Stretch Cohesive	JJ	EDG
Secure Forte	Bandage Light Pressure and Support Cohesive	JJ	ECD
Serotulle	Dressing Chlorhexidine Gauze BP	Set	EKB
Setonet	Bandage Tubular Elastic Net	Set	EGT
Setonplast	Tape Impermeable Plastic Surgical Adhesive BP	Set	EHH
Setopress	Bandage Compression	Set	EBA
Silastic Foam	Dressing Silicone Foam Cavity Wound BP	Cal	ELC
Silastic Foam Sheeting	Dressing Absorbent Silicone Foam	Cal	ELA
Silastic Gel Sheeting	Dressing Sheet Silicone Gel	Cal	ELY
Silcofoam Plain	Foam Polyurethane Plain	HL	ERJ
Sk-Intact	Dressing Absorbent Low Adherence Face	Rob	EJE
Sleek	Tape Impermeable Plastic Surgical Adhesive BP	SN	EHH
Slinky	Bandage Polyamide and Cellulose Contour BP	CG	EDB
Sof-Wick	Dressing Absorbent Fenestrated	JJ	EJK
Soffban	Bandage Orthopaedic Wadding (Synthetic Fibre)	SN	EPE
Soffban Natural	Bandage Orthopaedic Wadding (Cellulose Fibre)	SN	EPA
Sofra-Tulle	Dressing Framycetin Gauze BP	Rou	EKB
Sorbsan	Dressing Calcium Alginate	Ste	ELS
Sorbsan Plus	Dressing Calcium Alginate and Viscose	Ste	ELS
Sorbsan SA	Dressing Calcium Alginate Foam Backed Adhesive	Ste	ELS
Soxtexe	Bandage Orthopaedic Wadding (Synthetic Fibre)	CG	EPE
Specialist Foam Traction Kit	Traction Kit Non-adhesive	JJO	ESC
Spenco 2nd Skin	Dressing Hydrogel Sheet	Spe	ELE
Spenco Silicone Gelsheets	Dressing Sheet Silicone Gel	Spe	ELY

PROPRIETARY/TRADE NAME	GENERIC NAME	MANU-FACTURER	CLASSI-FICATION
Spongostan	Sponge Absorbable Gelatin	TMP	ELS
Spongostan Anal	Sponge Absorbable Gelatin (Anal)	TMP	ELS
Stayform	Bandage Polyamide and Cellulose Contour BP	Rob	EDB
Steraid Dressing Pad	Dressing Pad Absorbent	RB	EJA
Steri-Strip	Wound Closure Strip	3M	EIR
Steri-Strip Primaclear	Wound Closure Strip Transparent	3M	EIT
Steripad Post-operative Dressing	Dressing Island Permeable Plastic Adhesive	JJ	EIA
Stop Hemo	Dressing Calcium Alginate	Win	ELS
Stulpa	Bandage Elasticated Tubular	Har	EGA
Stulpa-fix	Bandage Tubular Elastic Net	Har	EGT
Super Chex X-Ray-Detectable Muslin Swab	Swab Muslin Electromagnetically Detectable	VC	EMM
Surgicel	Oxidised Cellulose BP	JJ	ELS
Surgifix	Bandage Tubular Elastic Net	HMS	EGT
Surgipad	Dressing Pad Absorbent	JJ	EJA
Suture Strip	Wound Closure Strip	Bio	EIR
Suture Strip Plus	Wound Closure Strip	Bio	EIR
Swanfoam Plain	Foam Backed with Swansdown	HL	ERJ
Synthaderm (temporarily discontinued)	Dressing Polyurethane Foam Primary BP		ELA
TG-Tubular Bandage	Stockinette Paraffined	Loh	EGJ
Tampax Tampon	Tampon with Applicator	Tam	EOF
Tarband	Bandage Zinc Paste and Coal Tar BP	Set	EFA
Tegaderm	Dressing Semipermeable Adhesive BP	3M	ELW
Tegaderm Plus	Dressing Semipermeable Adhesive Medicated	3M	ELW
Tegaderm Pouch Dressing	Dressing Semipermeable Adhesive Composite	3M	ELW
Tegagel	Dressing Calcium Alginate	3M	ELS
Tegasorb	Dressing Hydrocolloid Semipermeable	3M	ELM
Telfa	Dressing Perforated Film Absorbent BP (Type 2)	Ken	EJE
Tenderskin	Tape Permeable Non-woven Surgical Synthetic Adhesive BP	Ken	EHU
Tensoban	Bandage Orthopaedic Foam	SN	EPH
Tensofix Forte	Bandage Conforming Stretch	SN	EDB
Tensoflex	Support Ankle Elasticated	SN	ESM
Tensogrip	Bandage Elasticated Tubular BP	SN	EGA
Tensolastic	Bandage Light Pressure and Support	SN	ECA
Tensoplus Lite	Bandage Conforming Stretch Cohesive	SN	EDG
Tensopress	Bandage Compression	SN	EBA
Tensotape	Tape Zinc Oxide Surgical Adhesive	SN	EHP
Topper	Swab Non-woven Fabric	JJ	ENK
Tractac	Traction Kit Synthetic Adhesive	JJO	ESB
Transelast	Bandage Conforming Stretch	Loh	EDB
Transigen	Dressing Semipermeable Adhesive Composite	SN	ELW
Transite	Dressing Permeable Plastic Film	SN	ELW
Transpore	Tape Permeable Plastic Surgical Synthetic Adhesive BP	3M	EHA

PROPRIETARY/TRADE NAME	GENERIC NAME	MANU-FACTURER	CLASSI-FICATION
Tricodur	Bandage Elasticated Tubular	BDF	EGA
Tricotex	Dressing Knitted Viscose Primary BP	SN	EKG
Tubegauz	Stockinette Cotton BP	Set	EGJ
Tubifast	Stockinette Elasticated Lightweight	Set	EGP
Tubifoam	Bandage Tubular Foam	Set	ERN
Tubigrip	Bandage Elasticated Tubular BP	Set	EGA
Tubigrip Hip Spica	Hip Spica (Bandage Elasticated Tubular)	Set	EGC
Tubigrip Lumbar Abdominal Support Bandage	Bandage Lumbar Abdominal Support	Set	EGC
Tubigrip Post-mastectomy Bandage	Bandage Post-mastectomy	Set	EGC
Tubinette	Stockinette Viscose BP	Set	EGJ
Tubipad	Bandage Elasticated Tubular Foam Padded	Set	EGG
Tubiton	Stockinette Cotton and Viscose BP	Set	EGJ
Ultraplast	Dressing Sodium Alginate	WC	ELS
Unitulle	Dressing Paraffin Gauze BP (Light Loading)	Rou	EKA
Varico	Bandage Elastic Web BP (with Footloop)	Set	EBA
Varicrepe	Bandage Light Pressure and Support	CG	ECA
Vaseline Petrolatum Gauze	Dressing Paraffin Gauze (Fine Weave)	She	EKA
Veinoplast	Bandage Elastic Synthetic Adhesive	Ste	ECJ
Veinopress	Bandage Light Pressure and Support	Ste	ECA
Velband	Bandage Orthopaedic Wadding (Cellulose Fibre)	JJO	EPA
Ventfoam	Bandage Skin Traction Foam	Sch	ESJ
Vigilon	Dressing Hydrogel Sheet	Set	ELE
Viscopaste PB7	Bandage Zinc Paste BP	SN	EFA
Web Wrap	Bandage Orthopaedic Wadding (Synthetic Fibre)	3M	EPE
Webril	Bandage Orthopaedic Wadding (Cellulose Fibre)	Ken	EPA
Xeroflow	Dressing Tribromophenate and Oil Emulsion Gauze	She	EKB
Xeroform	Dressing Tribromophenate and Paraffin Gauze	She	EKB
Zenoderm	Implant Porcine Dermis	Eth	ELX
Zim-flex	Bandage Orthopaedic Resin	Zim	EAF
Zincaband	Bandage Zinc Paste BP	Set	EFA
Zopla Extension Strapping	Plaster Extension BP	HL	ESE
Zopla Fleecy Web	Fleecy Web Zinc Oxide Adhesive	HL	ERP
Zopla Foam-O-Felt	Foam/Felt Combination Zinc Oxide Adhesive	HL	ERK
Zopla Hindafome	Foam Padding Latex Zinc Oxide Adhesive	HL	ERK
Zopla Moleskin	Moleskin Zinc Oxide Adhesive	HL	ERP
Zopla Rigid Strapping Chiropodial Thin	Tape Zinc Oxide Thin Surgical Adhesive	HL	EHP

PROPRIETARY/TRADE NAME	GENERIC NAME	MANU-FACTURER	CLASSI-FICATION
Zopla Rigid Strapping Standard	Tape Zinc Oxide Surgical Adhesive	HL	EHP
Zopla Silcofoam CB	Polyurethane Foam Cloth Backed Zinc Oxide Adhesive	HL	ERK
Zopla Silcofoam DS	Polyurethane Foam Zinc Oxide Adhesive	HL	ERK
Zopla Sponge Rubber	Sponge Rubber Zinc Oxide Adhesive	HL	ERK
Zopla Stockinette	Stockinette Zinc Oxide Adhesive	HL	ERP
Zopla Swanfoam	Foam Zinc Oxide Adhesive Backed with Swansdown	HL	ERK
Zopla-Band EAB Standard	Bandage Elastic Adhesive BP (Plain Spread)	HL	ECG

Index of Manufacturers, Proprietary/Trade Names

MANU-FACTURER	PROPRIETARY/TRADE NAME	MANU-FACTURER	PROPRIETARY/TRADE NAME
	Hapla Swanfoam		Dressing Strip
	Hapla-Band		Bioclusive
	Hapla-Tape		Corethium 1
	Hindafome Plain		Corethium 2
	Nuprene DS		Cotton Bud
	Nuprene Plain		Dermicel
	Silcofoam Plain		Dermiclear
	Swanfoam Plain		Dermiflex
	Zopla Extension Strapping		Dermilite
	Zopla Fleecy Web		Hospital Tape
	Zopla Foam-O-Felt		Inadine
	Zopla Hindafome		J Fast
	Zopla Moleskin		J Plus
	Zopla Rigid Strapping Chiropodial Thin		Kling
			Lite-Flex
	Zopla Rigid Strapping Standard		N-A Dressing
			Nu Gauze
	Zopla Silcofoam CB		Perfron
	Zopla Silcofoam DS		Regal
	Zopla Sponge Rubber		Release II
	Zopla Stockinette		Secure
	Zopla Swanfoam		Secure Forte
	Zopla-Band EAB Standard		Sof-Wick
HMS	Macrofix		Steripad Post-operative Dressing
	Rowden Foote Bandage		
	Surgifix		Surgicel
Har	Branolind		Surgipad
	Branolind L		Topper
	Grassolind	JJO	Delta-Cast
	Hartmannplast		Delta-Cast Plus
	Idealast		Delta-Lite Conformable
	Idealhaft		Delta-Lite S
	Lastobind		Delta-Rol
	Lastodur		Delta-Tape
	Lastogrip		Neofract
	Lastotel		Orthoflex
	Lenkelast		Specialist Foam Traction Kit
	Omniflex		Tractac
	Omniplast		Velband
	Omnipor	Ken	ABD Dressing Pad
	Omnisilk		ABD Plus Dressing Pad
	Omnivlies		Telfa
	Peha-Crep		Tenderskin
	Peha-Haft		Webril
	Plastrona	LIC	Absderma
	Stulpa	LN	Boric Lint
	Stulpa-fix	Leo	Fucidin Intertulle
JJ	Actisorb Plus	Loh	Cellacast
	Band Aid		Cellamin
	Band Aid Fabric		Cellona Elastic

MANU-FACTURER	PROPRIETARY/TRADE NAME	MANU-FACTURER	PROPRIETARY/TRADE NAME
	Primapore		Tubigrip Lumbar Abdominal Support Bandage
	Scherisorb		Tubigrip Post-mastectomy Bandage
	Sleek		
	Soffban		Tubinette
	Soffban Natural		Tubipad
	Tensoban		Tubiton
	Tensofix Forte		Varico
	Tensoflex		Vigilon
	Tensogrip		Zincaband
	Tensolastic	She	Scarlet Red Dressing
	Tensoplus Lite		Vaseline Petrolatum Gauze
	Tensopress		Xeroflow
	Tensotape		Xeroform
	Transigen	Spe	Spenco 2nd Skin
	Transite		Spenco Silicone Gelsheets
	Tricotex	Ste	Bilastic Medium
	Viscopaste PB7		Bilastic Normal
Sal	Rediform		Cohepress
Sch	Poroplast		Sorbsan
	Ventfoam		Sorbsan Plus
Set	Arthro-Pad		Sorbsan SA
	Bard Absorption Dressing		Veinoplast
	Blue Line Webbing		Veinopress
	Calaband	TMP	Spongostan
	Carbosorb		Spongostan Anal
	Collafoam	Tam	Tampax Tampon
	Collar'n'cuff	Til	Metrotop
	Dalzofoam Adhesive	Ult	Lyoband
	Dalzofoam Plain		Lyofoam
	Elset		Lyofoam C
	Elset S Stump Bandage		Lyofoam Tracheostomy Dressing
	Icthaband		
	Lestreflex Plain		Lyoswab
	Lestreflex Ventilated	VC	Cotfil
	Notac		Dentanaps
	Paratulle		Oratex Dental Napkin
	Quinaband		Oratex Dental Roll
	Serotulle		Oratex Sterile Coiled Dental Wadding
	Setonet		
	Setonplast		Oratex Throat Pack Material
	Setopress		Paranet
	Tarband		Super Chex X-Ray-Detectable Muslin Swab
	Tubegauz		
	Tubifast	Vyg	Dermafilm
	Tubifoam	WC	Ultraplast
	Tubigrip	Win	Stop Hemo
	Tubigrip Hip Spica	Zim	Zim-flex

Manufacturers' Names and Addresses

AHS   Associated Hospital Supply,
Sherwood Rd, Aston Fields,
Bromsgrove,
Worcs B60 3DR
Bromsgrove (0527) 76776

Ast   Astra Pharmaceuticals Ltd,
Home Park Estate,
Kings Langley,
Herts WD4 8DH
Kings Langley (09277) 66191

RB   Robert Bailey & Son PLC,
Dysart St, Great Moor,
Stockport,
Cheshire SK7 7PF
061-483 1133

Brd   C.R. Bard International Ltd,
Pennywell Industrial Estate,
Sunderland SR4 9EW
091-534 3131

BDF   B.D.F. Medical Ltd,
Yeomans Drive, Blakelands,
Milton Keynes,
Bucks MK14 5LS
Milton Keynes (0908) 617171

Bec   Becton Dickinson UK Ltd,
Between Towns Rd,
Cowley,
Oxford OX4 3LY
Oxford (0865) 777722

Bio   Bioplasty Ltd,
Unit 8, The Microcentre,
Gillette Way,
Reading,
Berks RG2 0LR
Reading (0734) 755180

Bri   BritCair Laboratories Ltd,
Progress House,
Albert Rd,
Aldershot,
Hants GU11 1SZ
Aldershot (0252) 333314

Cal   Calmic Medical Division,
The Wellcome Foundation Ltd,
Crewe Hall, Crewe,
Cheshire CW1 1UB
Crewe (0270) 583151

Cli   CliniMed Ltd,
Cavell House, Knaves Beech Way,
Loudwater, High Wycombe,
Bucks HP10 9QY
Bourne End (0628) 850100

Col   Coloplast Ltd,
Peterborough Business Park,
Peterborough PE2 0FX
Peterborough (0733) 239898

Con   ConvaTec Ltd,
Squibb House,
141-149 Staines Rd,
Hounslow,
Middx TW3 3JA
081-572 7422

Cow   Jacob Cowan & Sons Ltd,
Ellers Mill, Dalston,
Carlisle CA5 7QJ
Carlisle (0228) 710205

CG   Cuxson, Gerrard & Co.(IMS) Ltd,
Oldbury, Warley,
West Midlands B69 3BB
021-552 1355

Eth   Ethicon Ltd,
PO Box 408, Bankhead Avenue,
Edinburgh EH11 4HE
031-453 6011

Foa   Foamband Products Ltd,
Tregoniggie Industrial Estate,
Falmouth, Cornwall TR11 4SN
Falmouth (0326) 72897

Gei   Geistlich Sons Ltd,
Newton Bank, Long Lane,
Chester CH2 3QZ
Chester (0244) 47534

Gro   Grout & Co.,
Boundary Rd, Southtown,
Great Yarmouth,
Norfolk NR31 0LW
Great Yarmouth (0493) 2446

Har   Paul Hartmann Ltd,
Unit F, Royale Pennine
Trading Estate, Royale Rd,
Rochdale, Lancs OL11 3EX
Rochdale (0706) 59393

HL
Hinders-Leslies Ltd,
Green Pond Rd,
London E17 6EN
081-523 0116

HMS
Hospital Management & Supplies Ltd,
Selinus Lane,
Dagenham RM8 1QD
081-593 7511

JJ
Johnson & Johnson Patient Care Ltd,
Coronation Rd, Ascot,
Berks SL5 9EY
Ascot (0990) 872626

JJO
Johnson & Johnson Orthopaedics Ltd,
Stem Lane, New Milton,
Hants BH25 5NN
New Milton (0425) 620888

Ken
The Kendall Company (UK) Ltd,
Telford Rd, Houndmills Industrial
Estate, Basingstoke,
Hants RG21 2XZ
Basingstoke (0256) 473212

LN
Lees-Newsome Ltd,
Ashley St, Oldham,
Lancs OL9 6LT
061-6521321

Leo
Leo Laboratories Ltd,
Longwick Rd, Princes
Risborough, Aylesbury,
Bucks HP17 9RR
Princes Risborough (08444) 7333

LIC
LIC Hygien
S-171 83,
Svetsarvagen 20,
Solna, Sweden

Loh
Lohmann UK Ltd,
Credsec House, Oxford Rd,
Stone, Aylesbury,
Bucks HP17 8PL
Aylesbury (0296) 747272

3M
3M Health Care,
3M House, 1 Morley St,
Loughborough,
Leics LE11 1EP
Loughborough (0509) 611611

Mal
Malam Laboratories,
37 Oakwood Rise,
Heaton, Bolton,
Lancs BL1 5EE
Bolton (0204) 41285

Mar
J.G. Marlow & Sons,
Pelham Street Mills,
Derby
Derby (0332) 44148

Mol
Molinier Industries,
Rue des Siccards,
BP4-42340 Veauche,
France
010-33-77947501

Mln
Molnlycke Ltd,
Southfields Rd, Dunstable,
Beds LU6 3EJ
Dunstable (0582) 600211

Oxf
Oxford Mill Co. Ltd,
Taylor Street West,
Accrington,
Lancs BB5 1RA
Accrington (0254) 35644

Par
Parema Ltd,
Sullington Rd,
Shepshed, Nr. Loughborough,
Leics LE12 9JJ
Loughborough (0509) 502051

Per
Perstorp Pharma Ltd,
Wound-Care Division,
Studio 1, Intec 2, Wade Rd,
Basingstoke, Hants RG24 0NE
Basingstoke (0256) 477868

Pha
Pharmacia Ltd,
Pharmacia House,
Midsummer Boulevard,
Milton Keynes MK9 3HP
Milton Keynes (0908) 661101

Rob
Robinson Healthcare,
Hipper House, Chesterfield,
Derbyshire S40 1YF
Chesterfield (0246) 220022

Rou
Roussel Laboratories Ltd,
Broadwater Park, North Orbital Rd,
Uxbridge, Middx UB9 5HP
Uxbridge (0895) 834343

Sal
Salt & Son Ltd,
Saltair House, Lord St,
Nechells, Birmingham B7 4DS
021-359 5123

Sch
Scholl (UK)
182-204 St. John St,
London EC1P 1DH
071-253 2030

Set	Seton Products Ltd, Tubiton House, Medlock St, Oldham, Lancs OL1 3HS 061-652 2222
She	Sherwood Medical Industries, County Oak Way, Crawley, West Sussex RH11 7YQ Crawley (0293) 34501
SN	Smith & Nephew Medical Ltd, PO Box 81, 101 Hessle Rd, Hull HU3 2BN Hull (0482) 25181
Spe	Spenco Medical (UK) Ltd, Burrell Road, Haywards Heath, West Sussex RH16 1TW Wivelsfield Green (0444) 415171
Ste	Steriseal Ltd, Thornhill Rd, Redditch, Worcs B98 9NL Redditch (0527) 64222
Tam	Tambrands Ltd, Dunsbury Way, Lee Park, Havant, Hants PO9 5DG Havant (0705) 474141
Til	Tillots Laboratories Valley Road Industrial Estate, Porters Wood, St. Albans, Herts AL3 6PD St. Albans (0727) 50561
TMP	Tridas Medical Products Ltd, 276 High St, Langley, Berks SL3 8HD Slough (0753) 686969
Ult	Ultra Laboratories Ltd, Trinity Trading Estate, Tribune Drive, Sittingbourne, Kent ME10 2PG Sittingbourne (0795) 70953
VC	Vernon-Carus Ltd, Penwortham Mills, Preston, Lancs PR1 9SN Preston (0772) 744493
Vyg	Vygon UK Ltd, Bridge Rd, Cirencester, Glos GL7 1PT Cirencester (0285) 67051
WC	Wallace, Cameron & Co. Ltd, 303 Drakemire Drive, Glasgow G45 9SU 041-634 6881
Win	Windsor Pharmaceuticals Ltd, Ellesfield Ave, Bracknell, Berks RG12 4YS Bracknell (0344) 484448
Zim	Zimmer, Patient Care Systems, Dunbeath Road, Elgin Industrial Estate, Swindon, Wilts SN2 6EA Swindon (0793) 481441

Index

Dressings not in this Index may be found in the classified Indexes, pp 156—92

Dressings not in this Index may be found in the classified Indexes, pp 156-92

Dressings not in this Index may be found in the classified Indexes, pp 156–92

Dressings not in this Index may be found in the classified Indexes, pp 156–92

Dressings not in this Index may be found in the classified Indexes, pp 156-92

Dressings not in this Index may be found in the classified Indexes, pp 156–92

Dressings not in this Index may be found in the classified Indexes, pp 156–92